The Management of Malignant Disease Series

General Editor: Professor Michael J. Peckham

This book is dedicated
to the memory of Gordon Hamilton Fairley

'There is a way of winning by losing, a way of victory
in defeat which we are going to discover.'

Van der Post, L. (1954)
A Bar of Shadow
The Hogarth Press, London

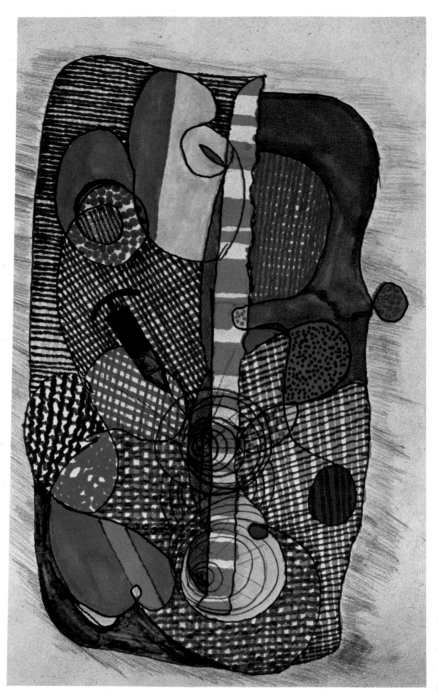

Frontispiece. Picture of his pain, by Mr H.Y.

The Management of Terminal Malignant Disease

Second edition

Edited by Dame Cicely Saunders

DBE, MA, MD, FRCP, Hon DSc(Yale), FRCN
Medical Director, St Christopher's Hospice, London

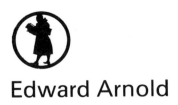

Edward Arnold

© Edward Arnold (Publishers) Ltd 1984

First published in Great Britain 1984 under the title *The Management of Terminal Disease*
by Edward Arnold (Publishers) Ltd,
41 Bedford Square, London WC1B 3DQ
Second edition, 1984

Edward Arnold (Australia) Pty Ltd,
80 Waverley Road, Caulfield East,
Victoria 3145, Australia

Edward Arnold,
300 North Charles Street, Baltimore,
Maryland 21201, U.S.A.

British Library Cataloguing in Publication Data

The Management of terminal malignant disease.—2nd ed.—(The Management of
malignant disease Series; 1)
    1. Cancer patients   2. Terminal care
    3. Cancer—Psychological aspects
    4. Cancer—Social aspects
    I. Saunders, *Dame* Cicely   II. Series
    362.1′96994   RC262
    ISBN 0-7131-4456-4

Whilst the advice and information in this book are believed to be true and accurate at
the date of going to press, neither the authors nor the publisher can accept any legal
responsibility or liability for any errors or omissions that may be made.

Text set in 10/11 Baskerville and printed in Great Britain by
Butler & Tanner Ltd, Frome and London

Contributors

Mary J. Baines, MB, BChir
Physician, St Christopher's Hospice, London

Thelma D. Bates, MB, ChB, FRCR
Consultant Radiotherapist and Oncologist, St Thomas' Hospital, London

Robert Baxter, FFARCS
Consultant Anaesthetist, Pain Relief Unit, Greenwich District Hospital,
London

K. C. Calman, MD, PhD, MRCP, FRCS, FRSE
Professor of Clinical Oncology, University of Glasgow

R. L. Carter, MA, DM, DSc, FRCPath
Reader in Pathology and Consultant Pathologist, Institute of Cancer
Research and Royal Marsden Hospital, Haddow Laboratories, Sutton, Surrey

Harriet Copperman, RGN, NDN Cert, SCM
Nursing Director, North London Hospice Home Care Service

M. J. F. Courtenay, MB, BChir, FRCGP
General Practitioner, Battersea, SW11; Senior Research Fellow, Department
of General Practice, St Thomas's Hospital Medical School, London

G. R. Dunstan, MA, HonDD, FSA
Emeritus Professor of Moral and Social Theology in the University of
London; Honorary Research Fellow in the University of Exeter; Priest in the
Church of England

Gillian Ford, CB, MRCP, FFCM
Deputy Chief Medical Officer, Department of Health and Social Security

Janet Goodall, FRCPE, DCH, DObstRCOG
Consultant Paediatrician, North Staffordshire Hospital Centre, Stoke on
Trent

B. Joan Haram, MRCS, LRCP, FRCPath
Formerly Consultant Pathologist, Elizabeth Garrett Anderson Hospital,
London

Louis Heyse-Moore, DObstRCOG, DCH, MRCGP, MRCP
Medical Director, Trinity Hospice, London

Ian McC. Kennedy, LLB, LLM
Professor of Medical Law and Ethics, King's College, London

Winifred Morris, SRN, ONC, NDN
Senior Nurse, Care of the Terminally Ill, North Tees Hospital, Stockton-on-
Tees

C. Murray Parkes, MD, FRCPsych, DPM
Senior Lecturer, Department of Psychiatry, The London Hospital Medical
College, London

Dame Cicely M. Saunders, DBE, MA, MD, FRCP, Hon DSc(Yale)
Medical Director, St Christopher's Hospice, London

Robert G. Twycross, MA, DM, FRCP
Consultant Physician, Sir Michael Sobell House, The Churchill Hospital,
Oxford

Thérèse Vanier, FRCP
Consultant, St Christopher's Hospice, London

J. Welsh, MRCP, BSc
Director of Medical Services; Honorary Consultant in Clinical Oncology
Hunters Hill Home, Glasgow

T. S. West, OBE, MB, BS
Deputy Medical Director, St Christopher's Hospice, London

Michael R. Williams, BM, BCh, FRCS
Lately Consultant Surgeon, Kent and Canterbury Hospital, Canterbury

Foreword

The first edition of this book was the first in a series of books entitled **The Management of Malignant Disease.** The management of terminal disease is arguably one of the most important topics to be considered—and perhaps one of the most difficult to discuss adequately between a single pair of covers. Dame Cicely brings to the subject unrivalled experience, authority and breadth of vision, and she and her collaborators have produced a book which fills a considerable need. This book reflects the approach adopted at St Christopher's Hospice, London, and it sets out the theory and, above all, the practice which has made St Christopher's justifiably famous but which has been shown to be eminently transferable into other settings. Some of the material is controversial, and no effort has been made to iron out what are sometimes quite marked differences in opinion. In many instances, such differences reflect our underlying ignorance of the complex physical, mental and emotional components which make up the terminal stages of malignant disease. These areas of ignorance, and the directions in which this subject are likely to move in the future, are discussed; but the emphasis throughout lies firmly on practical management. As such, the book is directed to a large medical and non-medical audience who can hardly fail to gain new insights into the practice of this most exacting branch of clinical oncology.

The General Editor

Preface

The first edition of this book was commissioned by Professor Gordon Hamilton Fairley and the first plans were completed at the time of his tragic death. Its dedication is a symbol of the hope that he, with his gifts of sympathetic and original scientific imagination, would approve its many facets.

First, an acknowledgement of my various contributors. Dr Richard Carter is a pathologist with particular interest in advanced malignant disease. This interest was expanded as a result of working for eight years as a week-end clinical assistant at St Joseph's Hospice, Hackney. Professor Calman had already been involved in this area of oncology when he became the secretary of the Terminal Care Study Group, to which most of the authors belong. Dr Colin Murray Parkes has been concerned with the needs of the bereaved for more than twenty-five years and was involved with the planning of St Christopher's Hospice from 1965. Since its opening in 1967, he has spent one or two days weekly among its staff and patients and has directed its psychosocial studies. After ten years' experience in general practice, Dr Mary Baines joined the clinical team of St Christopher's Hospice shortly after the opening. She has developed the daily work of the wards and has also studied the underlying causes of the physical distress which brings over 600 patients a year to the Hospice. She helped to pioneer its domiciliary service, the first such team to carry out hospice home care. Dr Robert Twycross first made contact with me at St Joseph's Hospice while he was still a medical student, and it was a common, continuing interest which drew him to St Christopher's Hospice in 1971. He was invited to undertake comparative studies of diamorphine and morphine as Clinical Research Fellow, supported by the Department of Health and Social Security and the Sir Halley Stewart Trust. This was a development of work on the use of narcotics in terminal care, first observed at St Luke's Hospital, London, and later developed at St Joseph's Hospice in the 1950s and 1960s.

Dr Baxter first came on rounds at St Christopher's with Dr James, then consultant to the Pain Clinic at King's College Hospital, and has maintained his links with hospice practice ever since. In years past, Mr Michael Williams and I met on Mr N.R. Barrett's firm at St Thomas' Hospital, as houseman and medical social worker. In due course, Michael Williams became a Consultant Surgeon at Canterbury and, in his capacity as Surgical Tutor, organized two symposia on Pain and the Care of the Dying, in which I and other members of the staff of St Christopher's Hospice took part. It was Mr Barrett who first directed me from nursing and medical social work to medicine: 'It's the doctors who desert the dying ... go and read medicine ...'. He aroused a similar interest in his houseman. Dr Thelma Bates always visited any of her patients who had been transferred to the Hospice. When the need for a closer look at the common ground between cytotoxic chemotherapy and terminal care first brought Dr Thérèse Vanier to join our team part time, it soon became obvious that there should be a consultant in radiotherapy combined with chemotherapy. Dr Bates has been a regular consultant at the Hospice since 1974, and pioneered the first 'Support Team' in the UK.

Dr Thomas West has extended our involvement with the families of our patients ever since he returned to this country after twelve years in the more closely knit society of Northern Nigeria, and has stimulated the development of our ward meetings and teamwork. Dr Michael Courtenay, general practitioner and Course Organizer of the St Thomas' Hospital Vocational Training Scheme for General Practice (Vice-President of the Society for Psychosomatic Research), was asked to comment on the work described from his position, outside the special centre, and on its relevance to general hospital and family practice. Two nurses have described the applications of the general principles first developed in an in-patient hospice setting. Mrs W.A. Morris, having long had this interest as a ward sister, came to St Christopher's wards on a brief visit and pioneered the post of Nursing Officer in what was termed 'special care' in a district general hospital. Miss Harriet Copperman, first as Nursing Director in the St Joseph's Hospice Home Care Team and later with the Royal Free Hospital Support Team, has long experience with patients and families in their own homes.

Professor Gordon Dunstan is one of three past and present Hospice Council members who have contributed. His insistence on studying ethics, not in philosophical abstraction but among practitioners, brought him as a learner into the medical field.

Dr Joan Haram has worked as a volunteer member of the team since the beginning. Her meticulous and untiring work as recorder has established a unique set of records and retrievable information.

Dr Gillian Ford's chapter is her personal view. For many years before terminal care became one of her concerns at the Department of Health and Social Security, she had also been one of St Christopher's volunteer doctors, spending a weekend a month as doctor on duty.

Mr Ian Kennedy has written elsewhere on this subject, and we have had the pleasure of correspondence and visits with him over the past few years.

Finally, Dr Janet Goodall, a consultant paediatrician who has written and spoken frequently about the problems of children and their families, and who has shared her insights with our Terminal Care Study Group, has contributed to this new edition.

Mention is made in the text of other workers in this field: those on whose experience St Christopher's has drawn, and others who have entered the field since the Hospice opened. One patient has contributed directly and innumerable patients and their families and ward staff, indirectly. To them all, our honour and gratitude.

I am deeply indebted to all the contributors for their hard work and patience, to Mrs Christine Kearney for endless toil with the typewriter, the word processor and the editor, and to Edward Arnold (Publishers) Ltd and the interest and tolerance of Mr Paul Price and Miss Barbara Koster.

London, 1984   CS

Contents

1

Appropriate treatment, appropriate death

Cicely Saunders

'And a certain woman ... had suffered many things of many physicians, and had spent all that she had, and was nothing bettered, but rather grew worse.'
   St Mark's Gospel 5 : 25, 26

'There is a general understanding that terminal care refers to the management of patients in whom the advent of death is felt to be certain and not too far off and for whom medical effort has turned away from therapy and become concentrated on the relief of symptoms and the support of both patient and family.'
   (Holford, 1973)

That nothing can be done to arrest the spread of a tumour does not mean that there is nothing to be done at all, and it is imperative that we recognize the moment when the 'therapy' of 'active treatment' is becoming irrelevant to the needs of a particular patient and an alternative form of 'therapy' is indicated. One important support to everyone concerned will be adequate treatment of the physical distress of dying. The control of symptoms is becoming increasingly sophisticated, and the question 'What is the relative value of the various available methods of treatment in this particular patient?'(Cade, 1963) is as pertinent and positive now as at any stage of a patient's illness. Some recent advances make such decisions increasingly difficult. Terminal care is a facet of oncology, concerned with the control of symptoms instead of with the control of the tumour. There should be an overlap between these areas of the total discipline and it is important that the doctors concerned should be aware of all the possibilities and judge together what is appropriate for each patient.

Movement as indicated in Fig. 1.1 may be mainly in the direction of the

Palliative

Active   Terminal

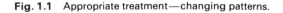

Fig. 1.1   Appropriate treatment—changing patterns.

heavy arrows, but it should be emphasized that this still calls for 'treatment' which is not a soft option, but activity aimed at new, appropriate objectives. No patients should become locked irretrievably in what is (or may become) for them the wrong part of the discipline. The aims of the different areas are not mutually exclusive, and effective control of symptoms may accompany or revive the prospect of further treatment aimed at active palliation or even cure.

As Mount has pointed out, such treatment, operating at times in a setting of crisis intervention, has rewards comparable to those of surgery; calling for the fine titration of drug regimens against troublesome symptoms has some of the satisfactions of medicine, and dealing with the anxious, the depressed and the bereaved is related to those of psychiatry (Mount 1980).

We tend to consider only the doctor's decisions in this field, and patients and families are frequently informed after these decisions have been made and are not really involved in them. Some patients certainly appear to take no interest in the changes being made in their treatment; others demand of their doctors that 'everything possible should be tried', without question as to likely side-effects or chances of benefit. Some offer, with a certain bravado, to have any new treatment 'tried out' on them. Others immediately despair when they suspect cancer and do not present until obliged to do so by advanced, totally incurable, disease.

Yet there are surely many who could and should be involved more often. A woman may, for example, decide to forego further surgery or a course of radio-therapy which would keep her away from home while her children are taking important examinations; another will not tolerate changes in her appearance. Should they not be included in the team making the decisions? People who come to us for treatment sometimes do not realize how much control they have given us; do they always intend to abrogate so much responsibility?

Another definition?

In spite of growing evidence that 'treatment for dying' has become an accepted part of medicine, the terminal stage can still be defined as beginning at the moment when the clinician says, 'There is nothing more to be done,' and then starts to withdraw from his patient. Patients are well aware when this happens and, on their admission to a unit such as St Christopher's Hospice, they reveal this with sad clarity. A few have been so desperate that they have tried to take their own lives. Here lies much of the strength of the appeal for the legislation of euthanasia, and if 'reformed medical care' does not reach all in need of it, 'the evidence of suffering will gradually make it more plausible' (Fletcher, 1982).

We believe that euthanasia would be a negative answer to a problem that can be solved by positive action, for 'To imply that nothing helpful can be done is inexcusable and seldom if ever true' (Smithers, 1960). Nor do we always realize how much we can do simply by coming to see the patient even though we have nothing to offer in the (by now) irrelevant context of radical treatment. We fail to understand what patients with terminal disease ask of us. They are commonly too realistic to expect that we can take away the whole hard thing that is happening to them; instead they ask for concern and care for their distress and symptoms. Above all, they ask for our awareness of them as people, with their own unique personality, past and relationships. At no time in the total care of the cancer patient is this of greater importance.

Hinton (1963) described the high incidence of physical and mental distress among patients dying in the wards of a teaching hospital. Although that was twenty years ago, there is still much that we need to learn and to teach before the proper standards of relief reach every patient. We should aim for the relief that enables a patient not only to die peacefully, but also to live until he dies, as himself and not as what has been termed an 'uncomplaining residue' (Weisman and Hackett, 1962). The patient can hardly be involved in any decisions while he is either swamped by distress or smothered with treatment. We need to be concerned with the quality of living, hard though it is to judge this for another person. At the same time, while we are aware of the possibility of regression even at this stage (and may well share this slender hope with our patient), we have to see that this part of our care, even though it ends with the patient's death, is both positive and important in its own right.

Successful symptomatic treatment should enable a patient to be so relieved of physical distress that he is freed to concentrate on other matters and maintain his sense of personal worth (Vanderpool, 1978). If we are to overcome the feelings of failure which tend to pervade the atmosphere surrounding the dying, we need to be aware of the proper criterion of success in this situation. This is not to be seen primarily in our activities, but rather in what the patient and his family can achieve in the face of progressive physical deterioration. This may be the most important part of his life, and the crises it brings may impel to creative resolution. The spirit often becomes stronger and more mature as the body weakens and superficialities are stripped away.

The management of terminal disease includes everything which will help the patient to find his own way of dying, his own death. Weisman has called this process 'safe conduct' and has developed the concept of an 'appropriate death'. He defines it as 'an absence of suffering, preservation of important relationships, an interval for anticipatory grief, relief of remaining conflicts, belief in timeliness, exercise of feasible options and activities, and consistency with physical limitations, all within the scope of one's ego ideal' (Weisman, in Feifel, 1977). The preservation of important relationships probably requires a certain sharing of truth and may mean that both the patient and the one he is leaving will grieve—alone and together—in anticipation of their parting. I have seen many times that such anticipation can facilitate the resolution of conflicts although the initial stages of realization may bring much anguish. Our own experience is frequently of a positive outcome, especially when open communication between family members can be fostered. Such final resolutions, together with a feeling of completeness and fulfillment, can make this the 'timely' moment to die, even for someone whose age or responsibilities would seem to make this improbable. We may have different ideas concerning the meaning of life and death, but we can all try to help a patient to attain some kind of harmony with what he sees as truth and rightness. Our own continual experience and the challenges to our beliefs and their rethinking in our daily experience may help to encourage such progress in our patients. Words are rarely needed, and may hinder this essentially individual process.

Such preparation for death is possible for those without a sense of existence beyond this world as well as for individuals who believe in some form of immortality and a God into whose hands they may commend their spirits. All humanity shares apprehension of the unknown—most of all the unknown of death. Religion in itself does not necessarily make dying easier, certainly not if it is merely seen as a somewhat magical way of avoiding trouble. Religion is not a way of manipulating the world, but rather a way of responding to it. It is widely held that true faith is rarely met today, but our experience is that many people and their families show quiet confidence and simple faith in unseen Love. We recognize the creative endurance of those who believe that their suffering has been given meaning by something or someone beyond themselves. The beliefs do not allow one to avoid the pains of weakness and parting, but can greatly assuage their bitterness.

Whatever our own beliefs, we should never impose them on another person, least of all any individual who is dependent upon us. But anyone who is trying to live in response to the demands his own life makes upon him, whether he sees this in any kind of religious terms or not, can create a climate in which another may find the strength to reach out trustfully and say 'Yes' to life and to death.

Appropriate truth?

Truth is not merely a matter of words, and we are likely to find the particular truth which is fitted to our patient's need only in some kind of relationship with him. This question is discussed in Chapters 4 and 11, but it bears so directly upon the decisions discussed above, on the whole management of a terminal illness and on all the relationships involved, and is so constantly the theme of a student's questions, that it seems appropriate to consider here some of the arguments in the continuing debate which surrounds the question of 'telling'.

It is still common form to tell a patient little or nothing about his condition but to put the family fully into the picture. What do we do to our patient and to his relationships with his family and friends when we create this kind of barrier of unshared truth between them? A man describing his illness to me said: 'I couldn't think what had happened to my marriage. What had I done that I should suddenly feel so separated from my wife, why was she obviously so sad and anxious?' When his disease recurred, he extracted the truth from the doctors at his treating hospital. I subsequently asked him, 'Back at the beginning, would you rather that your wife had been told less or that you should have been told more?' The patient answered, 'The first—but at least we should have been together.' He had responsibilities, too.

We hesitate to tell the full truth to a patient who is living appropriately, believing his illness, though perhaps serious, is not fatal, and here it may well be kinder to withhold its full implications from the family as well. We can suggest that it would be wise not to undertake new and heavy commitments at this stage without implying that the patient is already mortally ill. There are times when we can honestly say that we do not know precisely how the disease is progressing, and take a more optimistic viewpoint. However, when the patient's confidence in recovery is being undermined by the processes of illness and the impairment of communication with those nearest to him, then the unknown is often more fearful than the most dreaded reality, and it is likely that the time has come for a more frank discussion. This should not be forced nor will it necessarily give the full truth of the situation, as the doctor sees it, delivered at one blow; rather, it shows the clinician's readiness to follow the patient's questions and observe any verbal or non-verbal clues he may give. This is one of the aspects of terminal care which each doctor discovers from his own experience if he is prepared to listen, without any prepared answer or technique, and to respond to each person in a way he feels to be right at the time. Those who see a patient once in consultation may be able to do this helpfully, but we should not assault another person with a truth which he is not yet ready to handle, least of all when we cannot offer continuing support. The doctor who allows or encourages open interchange should normally be the one who can also promise that he will never abandon the patient and who gives the assurance that he will control any physical distress and will discuss and exploit any improvement. He also needs to say that he will share this knowledge with the family and suggest that they can now discuss it together. Some families resist this strongly and try hard to 'protect' the patient. They may sometimes be right, but they are not always the best judges, being much oppressed by their own anxiety, and every effort must be made to support them as well. It is hardly surprising that if a family is asked whether a patient should be informed at the first moment of their shock at being told of a fatal prognosis, their immediate reaction will be that the truth should be kept from him. Nor, later on, that the pain the knowledge is causing them should make them wish to protect the patient from enduring it also. But we meet many patients who have suffered alone with the very truth from which all around them were persuading themselves they were protected. It is possible (as Dr West describes in Chapter 11) to help such a family move from an entrenched position of denial and share at least some of the last part of their life together. Joint discussions are often helpful and the patient may at times be the strongest member of the group.

Doctors may mistrust such openness, but if they speak with care, beginning with somewhat open-ended or even ambiguous remarks, they will learn to judge how much to say at any one time. This demands all we can give of our time and our sensitivity, but opportunities will come for those who have confidence in their patients' courage and common sense—qualities which do not disappear along with good health.

It is seldom appropriate to present full information without testing out the patient's expectations in some way, but I remember giving an unequivocal answer to a man. It would have been an insult to his courage and determination to have done anything else. He asked, 'Was it hard for you to tell me that?' When I replied 'Yes—it was', he said 'Thank you. It is hard to be told but it is hard to tell too,' and repeated 'Thank you'. We have to watch what people do with the truths we give them, and I had no cause to regret this directness. I believe his answer also tells us that if it is *not* hard to tell, then we should hesitate before doing so, for it is a serious commitment from one person to another. Some patients deliberately avoid asking questions or receiving information, and others are reported as reacting adversely to such news. Such silence must be respected, but at times one is tempted to ask, 'But *how* did you tell him?' or 'What did you let him tell you?' These questions are not always justified—there are times when we have all made great efforts to help and still judged incorrectly. It is a comfort to know that many people who do not wish to be led into facing reality are capable of 'forgetting' an entire conversation of this kind. The human mind has an invaluable capacity to repress an unpleasant truth.

Several investigators have shown that many more people are aware of their diagnosis and prognosis that those around them realize. Hinton (1963) carried out a controlled study of a group of dying patients in the wards of a London teaching hospital. He showed that 50 per cent of his 102 dying patients already had a shrewd idea of the severity of their illness when he first interviewed them, and that 'Awareness of dying grew so that three out of every four spoke of this possibility or certainty'. These patients had not been 'told' and the ward staff were often unaware that they had this knowledge. A later paper, 'Talking with people about to die', summarized the comments of 60 patients receiving care for terminal cancer made to Hinton about their discussions with doctors and nurses. Of these, 40 had some awareness of dying and none disapproved of open discussion. Of the 21 reporting little or no truthful conversation with the staff, 9 were critical but the other 12 were not dissatisfied, including some who were aware of their prognosis (Hinton, 1974). However, Hinton later reported that patients were least depressed and anxious at a hospice and preferred the more frank communication available there (Hinton, 1979).

Witzel reported interviews with 110 patients shortly before their deaths and found them resigned, with little or no fear; most were aware that they were dying but expressed no desire for details about their illness. He compared them with a control group with serious but not fatal illness. The second group wanted information about their condition and feared death, though few thought they would actually die (Witzel, 1975).

On the other hand, McIntosh reported on a year's study in a cancer ward where 'the corner-stone of the doctors' philosophy on telling was the belief that the great majority of the patients should not be told'. He found that the over-whelming majority of the patients knew or suspected they had a malignancy, but that 70 per cent of them did not want any confirmation of their prognosis. He did not consider that these patients anticipated that they would adjust better to their illness if they were told (McIntosh, 1977). Brewin (1977) de-scribed in detail ways of communication throughout a prolonged illness, and Graeme wrote of 'the broad road of daily encouragement and support' which lies between 'stark realities on the one hand and the silent evasion of hearty bonhomie on the other' (Graeme, 1975), and found many patients did not want confirmation until the end was near.

The appeal for quantitative studies to add to the 'anecdotal approach' has given us valuable information but not the infallible guidelines which some may have hoped for. We still have to attempt to meet with each individual patient as one person with another and try to assess what his needs may be at that particular moment, being aware that these needs may change throughout the progress of the illness.

Weiseman (1972) has discussed this carefully in his book *On Dying and Denying*, pointing out that patients are quick to sense to whom it is safe to talk. The more secure a patient feels, the more likely he is to ask questions or to feel his way tentatively towards talking freely.

The real presence of another person is a place of security. I recall remarking to two psychiatrists that when patients are in a climate of safety they will come to realize what is happening in their own way and not be afraid. One said:

'How can you speak of a climate of safety when death is the most unsafe thing that can happen?' To which the other replied: 'I think you are using the wrong word. I think it should be "security". A child separated from his mother may be quite safe—but he feels very insecure. A child in his mother's arms during an air raid may be very unsafe indeed—but he feels quite secure.' We have to try to give our patients that feeling of security in which they can begin, when they are ready, to face unsafety. This may not necessarily be the knowledge of their approaching death. It may be apprehensions concerning investigations or treatment, changes in the situation, hospital admission, or the acceptance of increasing weakness. *Security does what deception or denial cannot do.* It may protect a patient from knowledge of the real issues entirely, but it can also help to lighten much of the burden of that knowledge when it comes, for, above all, it relieves that isolation which accentuates all suffering.

Although bad news given starkly can have devastating results, knowledge of a fatal prognosis does not in itself inevitably lead to apathy or despair. There is clinical evidence of such knowledge 'galvanizing a will to live' which was not apparent before. 'Untapped potentials for responsible and effective behaviour as well as less depression and blame for others became evident. Honest and sensitive talk ... tends to attenuate feelings of guilt and inadequacy not only in the patient but also in professional personnel and family as well' (Feifel, 1977). Truth and hope are not mutually exclusive, and the informed patient is frequently better able to fight for his life because he knows the real battlefield. Surely most of us wish to take some responsibility for our dying as well as for our living?

Inept words cannot be unsaid, but they can be softened or forgotten—such is man's capacity for denial. We will learn to do better if we examine our own mistakes and continue to visit the patient and help him as best we can within his own frame of reference. Only occasionally does one have to withdraw completely. We should remember that our sins of commission—too much told and too soon, or a rash answer given to another doctor's patient without previous discussion—will be visited on our heads many times; our sins of omission—our neglect of the isolated, frightened patient who can gain no real reassurance—are not usually apparent and we rarely receive the blame we deserve for them.

Many of us have seen the kind of hope that springs out of realization, from facing and tackling a situation, however bleak that situation may be. Much sorrow would be avoided if we realized that a large element of the defensiveness which surrounds a patient is unnecessary and self-defeating. Most dying patients are aware that time is running out, whether or not the staff looking after them are willing to acknowledge it or the family can face talking about it (Weisman, 1972). They do not commonly blame the family who have tried to spare them pain by deception, and often move into closer and healing relationships once truth is shared (Stedeford, 1981a, 1981b).

Yet, having said all this, we must remember that love does not always need words to convey its meanings, and that a family may share these problems and say their farewells in silence. Doctors or nurses, too, can give their support without direct discussion. Talk of symptoms, which may be used as a way out of involvement with such problems, can also be a way of meeting a patient with reassurance on a much deeper level.

West points out in Chapter 11 that the time of admission may provide a crucial opportunity to bring reality into a family separated by deception. Contrary to much belief, although some patients choose to come because they know what to expect from past family experiences, many people do not associate St Christopher's Hospice solely with death. Its mixed group of patients— the wing for elderly residents, its discharges and the home care and out-patient service— enable those who come for admission to identify with one of these groups. Some who did not realize how ill they were will move gradually towards truth, often asking questions or making oblique comments to students or junior members of staff (whom they think are unlikely to be in a position to give answers) until they are ready to approach the doctor or senior nurse.

Recording a patient's comments helps the ward team to share their knowledge of the patient's feelings; it also sharpens their perceptions. If we believe that it is possible to allow open communication, it does not mean that this will necessarily take place. Words are often unnecessary; communication takes place in other ways. It does mean that all conversations are more relaxed and arise spontaneously out of a personal interchange. Most patients finally realize what is happening even if they prefer not to talk about it. A situation where this was not allowed to happen was described sadly to me by a patient. Mrs S., aged 40, in hospital for a radical mastectomy, found herself in bed next to someone her own age who was dying with metastatic breast cancer. This patient had increasing pain and paralysis and spent much of her time watching the clock, waiting for her next injection. As Mrs S. described it, 'Everybody knew she was dying—and took a step back. She was encouraged to pin all her hopes on a visit from the consultant and in some new treatment that he might suggest—at length he arrived, but his visit came too late, she was already unconscious.' Mrs S. wrote to me, 'Her last three weeks were spent anticipating that visit—to my mind they would have been better spent on more important things than false hopes. I'm convinced that she would have preferred the truth and that the people who were nursing her had passed the buck.' Mrs S. said to a group of students, 'I think "hope" is almost a dirty word to me now.' In discussion she added, 'I can face dying, I can face pain, but what I can't face is being treated as less than a person.'

Erasing fears

The various fears associated with advanced cancer in the public mind include fear of pain, of pain-relieving drugs which they believe will both swamp personality and inevitably lose their effect, of dependence and isolation, and of 'being kept alive by technology' without having any choice in the matter. In this book we are concerned to erase these fears and to present general principles of analysis, assessment and treatment which can be interpreted in any setting and for each individual patient. This has been a largely unexplored field—'an aspect of oncology whose scientific foundations are only just beginning to be laid' (Symington and Carter, 1976). There is still much to be learned of the natural history of advanced disease and the pathological processes at work; the basis for specific symptoms is often imperfectly understood and treatment is haphazard or at best empirical. Myths concerning the use of analgesics, especially the narcotics, still deny relief to many patients. Neither patient nor family receives the emotional and social help which concerned professionals of many disciplines (and volunteers) could offer them. The contributions which radio-therapy, chemotherapy and surgery can make in the care of unremitting disease are not always considered. Often, patients say that they wish to die in their own homes, and many families feel disappointed and guilty when lack of adequate support makes this impossible.

We have tried to draw together on our practical experience and records to present a guide to clinical practice in this field and to look at the mental and social needs of patients with terminal disease. As well as aiming at the highest medical standards, we must consider the philosophy, ethics and theology of our practice. If we are to have the strength to 'watch' with a patient and family in distress and anguish, we have to look to our own beliefs and our own supports. The phrase 'watch with me' comes from the story of Jesus facing death in the Garden of Gethsemane (St Matthew's Gospel, 26 : 38) and sums up the deepest need of any person facing death or desolation. It did not mean 'take away', it could not have meant 'understand or explain'—its simple and costly demand was to 'stay there'. We can offer this as we work for the 'good death' which is a major factor in the continuing life of the surviving family; it is also the incentive and reward of good terminal care.

'I've heard illness out
Until it has nothing to say to me,
And I thank God I have the last word.'
   (Fry, 1954)

References

Brewin, T.B. (1977). The cancer patient: communication and morale. *British Medical Journal* **2,** 1623.

Cade, S. (1963). Cancer: the patient's viewpoint and the clinician's problems. *Proceedings of the Royal Society of Medicine* **56,** 1.

Feifel, H. (Ed.) (1977). Death in contemporary America. In *New Meanings of Death*, p. 7. McGraw-Hill, New York and Maidenhead.

Fletcher, J.C. (1982). Is euthanasia ever justifiable? In *Controversies in Oncology*, p. 297. Ed. by P.H. Wiernik. John Wiley, New York.

Fry, C. (1954). *The Dark is Light Enough*. Oxford University Press, London.

Graeme, P. (1961). The terminal care of the cancer patient. 1. The doctor. *St Mary's Hospital Gazette* **67,** 118.

Hinton, J. (1963). Mental and physical distress in the dying. *Quarterly Journal of Medicine* **32,** 1.

Hinton, J. (1974). Talking with people about to die. *British Medical Journal* **2,** 25.

Hinton, J. (1979). Comparison of places and policies for terminal care. *Lancet* **1,** 29.

Holford, J.M. (1973). *Terminal Care. Care of the Dying*. Proceedings of a National Symposium held on 29 November, 1972. HMSO, London.

McIntosh, J. (1977). *Communication and Awareness in a Cancer Ward*. Croom Helm, London; Prodist, New York.

Mount, B.M. (1980). Editorial: Hospice care. *Journal of the Royal Society of Medicine* **73,** 471.

Smithers, D.W. (1960). *A Clinical Prospect of the Cancer Problem*. Livingstone, Edinburgh.

Stedeford, A. (1981a). Couples facing death I—Psychosocial aspects. *British Medical Journal* **283,** 1033.

Stedeford, A. (1981b). Couples facing death II—Unsatisfactory communication. *British Medical Journal* **283,** 1098.

Symington, T. and Carter, R.L. (Eds.) (1976). Editorial note. In *Scientific Foundations of Oncology*, p. 673. Heinemann Medical, London.

Vanderpool, H.Y. (1978). The ethics of terminal care. *Journal of the American Medical Association* **239**, 850.

Weiseman, A.D. (1972). *On Dying and Denying. A Psychiatric Study of Terminality*, p. 93. Behavioral Publications, New York.

Weiseman, A.D. and Hackett, T.P. (1962). The dying patient. *Forest Hospital Publications* **1**, 742.

Witzel, L. (1975). Behaviour of the dying patient. *British Medical Journal* **2**, 81.

Addenda

I: Editor's comment on frontispiece

Few diseases possess the capacity that cancer has to shut a patient off almost completely from those around him. 'It seemed so strange; no-one seemed to want to look at me,' said a patient on admission. When to this emotional isolation physical distress is added such as constant nausea, intractable dyspnoea or pain, a patient may be held a prisoner in a kind of solitary confinement. If to someone trapped in this situation we offer no more than the injection of a narcotic, can we marvel if he becomes drug dependent or asks us for the quick release of death? This does not exaggerate the situation. Here, one patient illustrates vividly the feelings of a multitude.

The painting reproduced as the Frontispiece to this book was commissioned from Mr H.Y. when he was an in-patient at St Christophers's Hospice. He had an inoperable squamous cell carcinoma of the bronchus, and summarized histories of his two admissions are given below. Painting was his hobby and, as his condition improved, his bed-table became covered with sketches. We suggested that he might try to illustrate his memory of the pain of his thoracotomy and of a painful acute retention which developed shortly after his admission. The urethritis which had precipitated this was treated successfully; he received one dose of narcotic before he was catheterized and the infection treated with antibiotics. Pain was never a problem for the rest of that admission.

Mr H.Y. depicts his pain surrounding him totally as he lies stretched out on his bed. He described the whorled figures to me as the 'knotted muscles' of tension. He is cut off from the world by it.

This was an acute pain which was treated specifically; but the painting could also represent the feelings of many patients with chronic pain for which no specific treatment is available. Too many of them have to endure it or to wait until pain is present before they can expect to be given any relief. 'In our hospital the patients have to earn their morphine' a student reported to us on a hospice ward round.

Summary of Mr H.Y.'s First Admission to St Christopher's Hospice

Aged 51 M   Admitted 25/11/70
                             Discharged 27/2/71

Admitted from home, as an emergency at request of general practitioner.

Carcinoma of left bronchus, since July 1970
Bronchoscopy, September 1970
Thoracotomy, November 1970.

Pain Has had some pain across thoracic spine and in the scar, but this not his main complaint.

History July 1970: cough and slight haemoptysis; reported to GP. X-ray then no appreciable disease (NAD). September 1970: repeat x-ray, then bronchoscopy and biopsy showed squamous cell carcinoma of left bronchus. November 1970: thoracotomy; growth found to be inoperable. Sent home after 2 weeks. Appetite poor, vomiting sometimes, dysphagia, marked loss of weight. Sleeps badly; tries to cough but has no strength. Unable to sit up unaided. Very constipated: frequency of micturition. Increasing weakness of both legs. Breathlessness the main problem. Knows that he has a tumour but not the prognosis. Baptist.

On Examination (OE) Very weak; anaemic; marked signs of breathlessness. Pulse 90. Collapse and consolidation of left chest. Polyneuritis both hands and feet. Paraethesia, loss of feeling and weakness. Very ill and frightened.

Drugs

25/11–27/2	Prednisone	O	5–10 mg t.d.s.
25/11–27/2	Promazine hydrochloride (Sparine)	O	25 mg t.d.s.
27/11–27/2	Liver extract (Minamino Compound)		10 ml t.d.s.
8/12	Diamorphine hydrochloride	O	5 mg s.o.s.
21/12–24/12	Nitrofurantoin (Furadantin)	O	100 mg q.d.s.
12/2–27/2	Nitrofurantoin (Furadantin)	O	100 mg q.d.s.
24/12–27/2	Imipramine hydrochloride (Tofranil)	O	25 mg t.d.s.
11/1–3/2	Co-trimoxazole (Septrin)	O	Tabs 2–1 b.d.
3/2–13/2	Sulphomyxin sodium (Thiosporin)	i.m.	500 000 units 6-hourly

Also courses of Chloramphenicol, cloxacillin, nalidixic acid (Negram), dextropropoxyphene (Distalgesic) from time to time; methagualone hydrochloride (Mandrax) then nitrazepam (Mogadon) at night; chlorpromazine hydrochloride (Largactil) 50 mg at night.

Progress The acute chest infection was fairly rapidly controlled, patient's appetite improved and he felt better. The polyneuritis slowly resolved and he became ambulant. On 8/12 he developed painful retention requiring catheterization. The urinary infection was resistant but finally improved on Thiosporin. Pain went but frequency remained. Developed a large fluctuant swelling over thoracotomy scar on 1/2/71. This discharged copiously. Patient improved greatly in his general condition, was pain-free, went home for several week-ends and was discharged home on 27/2/71. Will be admitted again if necessary.

Footnote When Mr H.Y. became acutely ill a few days after his discharge home following his thoracotomy, his family doctor had not received any notification from the hospital. His doctor believed he needed urgent treatment but the hospital had extra beds up and were not able to readmit him.

b.d. = twice a day; i.m. = intramuscular injection; O = oral; g.d.s. = four times a day; s.o.s. = if circumstances require; t.d.s. = three times a day.

Summary of Mr H.Y.'s Second Admission to St Christopher's Hospice

Aged 51   M

Readmitted 3/6/71
Died 14/8/71

Readmitted from the Out-patient Clinic. *See previous summary.*

Carcinoma of left bronchus

Further history   Patient had been discharged home on 27/2/71, since when he had been visited several times and had attended the OP Clinic. He managed very well at first but had repeated chest infections with purulent sputum, treated with antibiotics. Frequency of micturition was troublesome and, on 3/6, patient was complaining of severe pain and was able to pass very little urine each time. For 2 days he had been very sleepy and his mind had been wandering.

Drugs

3/6–12/8	Prednisone	O	10 mg t.d.s.
3/6–16/6	Promazine hydrochloride (Sparine)	O	25 mt t.d.s.
11/6–19/6	Co-trimoxazole (Septrin)	O	Tabs 2 b.d.
9/7–13/7	Co-trimoxazole (Septrin)	O	Tabs 2 b.d.
20/7–7/8	Co-trimoxazole (Septrin)	O	10 ml b.d.
16/6–5/7	Diamorphine hydrochloride	O	2.5–5 mg 4-hourly q.d.s. b.d. at night
5/8–14/8	Diamorphine hydrochloride (Benylin)	O/l	2.5–5 mg 4-hourly
16/6–5/7	Prochlorperazine (Stemetil)	O	5 mg 4-hourly q.d.s., b.d. o.d.
3/8–11/8	Prochlorperazine (Stemetil)	O/l	5/6.25–12.5 mg 4-hourly p.r.n.
19/6–10/7	Ampicillin	O	250 mg q.d.s.
23/6–24/7	Diphenhydramine hydrochloride (Benylin)	O	5–10 ml 4-hourly t.d.s.
13/7–20/7	Colistin sulphate (Colomycin)	/I	1 000 000 units t.d.s.
4/8–13/8	Cyclizine	O/l	50/50 mg b.d.

Chlorpromazine bydrochloride (Largactil) 25 mg at night; nitrazepam (Mogadon) 2 tablets at night; methadone linctus 5–10 ml at night p.r.n. hyoscine i.m. 0.4 mg 3 times, 13/8. 14/8.

Progress   Catheter passed soon after admission; urine drained well. Remained drowsy and quiet. Cough troublesome and sputum blood-stained. Occasional pain and ab-dominal distension when catheter became blocked. Bladder wash-outs and catheter changed as needed. Pain controlled by small doses of mist. Diamorphine, gradually reduced from 4-hourly to *nocte* only by 5/7. Became brighter and was pushing himself along in his wheelchair and later walking with a Zimmer walking aid. Took Communion on the ward on 21/7. Not so well by the end of the month, again becoming more drowsy and having episodes of vomiting and nausea. Small doses of regular analgesic restarted. Gradually became weaker, with more frequent vomiting. Remained weak, confused from time to time, but mostly peaceful. Bouts of severe coughing and restlessness at times, which responded to medication. Lapsed into unconsciousness on 13/8, remained very peaceful and died at 00.35 hours on 14/8/71.

Footnote   His wife wrote after his death about the extra eight months of his life that the whole family had enjoyed. They still keep in touch with the hospice.

b.d. = twice a day;   i.m. = intramuscular injection;   O = oral;   O/i = oral/injection; I = injection; o.d. = once a day; p.r.n. = as the occasion arises; q.d.s. = four times a day; t.d.s. = three times a day.

II: Facts and figures

B. Joan Haram

The clinical studies team includes two part-time self-styled 'Recorders', both of them retired doctors, whose work it is to compose a summary of each patient's case notes, if possible from the onset of symptoms until discharge or death. Each summary is stuck to a Cope Chat punch card, (Paramount card by Copeland Chatterson Co. Ltd), which is then fitted to a master card, round the periphery of which, about 250 items of information are listed. The card is punched opposite the appropriate items and the resulting information extracted and analysed for statistics and research. A copy is retained in the notes, another copy is sent to the hospital or doctor previously attended by the patient.

The basic format of the summary has remained unchanged, but additional details have been incorporated as the work of the hospice expanded. Data include the history of illness, diagnosis, previous treatment, present symptoms, mobility, insight, home circumstances, reason for admission and whether the patient has been admitted from hospital or home. If the patient has been under the care of the domiciliary service of the hospice, this is reported. Pain, being of special significance, is mentioned under a separate heading. All this material is culled from various sources such as doctors' letters, nurses' notes and hospital reports. Examination by the doctor admitting the patient follows. Drugs prescribed are listed, with dates of starting and stopping each drug, increased dosages give, and when possible any change from oral to parenteral administration. The progress of the illness is described and, if the patient remains at St Christopher's for any length of time, particular events are noted. These would include visits home, further active treatment, insight during stay, and unexpected developments. If death occurs, the terminal symptoms and mode of dying are recorded.

Since July 1967 when the hospice opened, until the end of 1982, the number of summaries completed was 9102. The annual figure rose from 321 in 1968 to reach a peak of 785 in 1981. This increase has been due in part to the growing number of patients being discharged from St Christopher's to be cared for by the domiciliary service. Many are re-admitted, sometimes more than once, thus needing additional summaries to record their subsequent history. Over the years there has been a steady increase in the number and variety of drugs prescribed, and sorting drug sheets may be very time consuming. Most of the summaries take about 40–60 minutes to compile, but exceptionally they may need several hours of diligent work. They continue to provide a simple basis for monitoring and modifying clinical results, and numerous studies using their basic data have been carried out.

January 1984.

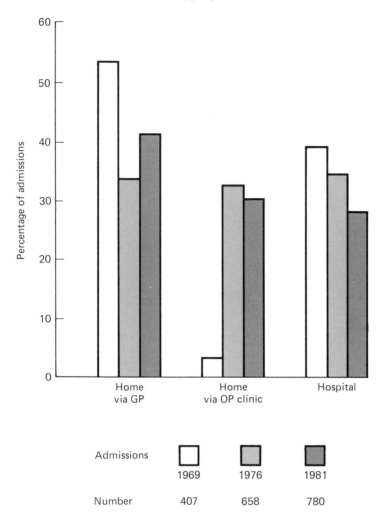

Fig. 1.2 Breakdown of admissions to St Christopher's Hospice: the effect of developing home care, 1969–81 inclusive.

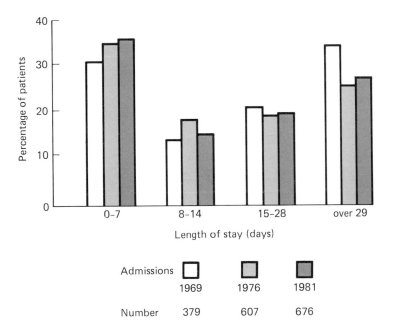

Fig. 1.3 Comparison of length of stay at St Christopher's Hospice, 1969–81 inclusive.

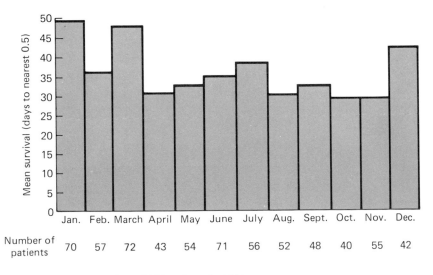

Fig. 1.4 Monthly survival of 660 patients in 1981.

Table 1.1 Primary site of malignant tumour (to nearest 0.25 per cent): admissions to St Christopher's Hospice 1976 and 1981

	1976 (%)	1981 (%)
Gastrointestinal tract	24.75	24.50
Lung/bronchus	21.50	23.25
Breast	18.25	14.75
Genitourinary tract	15.00	15.00
Central nervous system	2.75	3.50
Head and neck	4.25	2.25
Other sites*	13.50	16.75

* Includes pancreas, melanoma, sarcoma, reticular, liver, miscellaneous and unknown.

Table 1.2 Main symptoms on admission to St Christopher's Hospice

Symptom	Percentage		
	Male	Female	Total
Pain	76.5	73.1	74.7
Weight loss	71.4	69.6	70.4
Anorexia	66.2	58.9	62.3
Cough	57.9	27.4	41.4
Dyspnoea	55.0	40.8	47.3
Constipation	45.3	46.3	45.8
Nausea/vomiting	37.6	45.5	41.8
Effusion/ascites/oedema	37.6	37.5	37.6
Weakness	33.7	30.9	32.2

Table 1.3 Analgesic and adjuvant drugs in St Christopher's Hospice, 1981

Of the 676 patients with malignant disease:

106 (15.68%) received no diamorphine. Of this number:
  75 (70.75%) received oral morphine or MST with or without another analgesic
  17 (16.05%) received no morphine but were given other analgesics
  14 (13.2%) received no analgesic

570 (84.3%) received diamorphine during their stay
528 (78.1%) received morphine during their stay
263 (38.9%) of patients, 104 males and 159 females, received a non-steroidal anti-inflammatory drug
545 (80.6%) of patients, 254 males and 291 females, received a phenothiazine
105 (15.5%) of patients, 37 males and 68 females, received an antidepressant
262 (38.8%) of patients, 119 males and 143 females, received diazepam

Table 1.4 A retrospective analysis of patient records for 1979 undertaken to examine those patients who received oral morphine

Admissions	643
Oral morphine	474 (73.72%)
Oral morphine (only)	76 (11.82%)
Parenteral diamorphine	541 (84.14%)
Parenteral diamorphine (only)	119 (18.5%)
Other analgesics	292 (45.41%)
No analgesic	27 (4.20%)

2

Some pathological aspects of advanced malignant disease

R. L. Carter

'But who could tell? Even doctors, how could they detect whether the solitary, destructive cells had or hadn't stolen through the darkness like landing craft, and where they had anchored?'
(Solzhenitsyn, 1968)

Advanced malignant disease presents diverse and often complex problems in diagnosis and clinical management. A preliminary description of the underlying pathology is therefore necessary to provide a context in which such problems can be viewed.

A schematic and highly simplified representation of certain aspects of the natural history of progressive tumour growth is shown in Fig. 2.1. Three somewhat arbitrary phases may be recognized: subclinical disease, clinically early disease, and clinically advanced disease. The first phase is illustrated by a tumour comprising $\sim 10^9$ cells and weighing ~ 1 g. Unless superficially located, such a lesion will not be detectable clinically, though it may be revealed by appropriate cancer screening tests if such are available. Although the tumour may appear to be localized, there will be at least microscopic infiltration into the surrounding tissues, and the early stages of metastasis may have begun. Clinically early disease usually corresponds to a tumour of $\sim 2 \times 10^9$ cells. An unknown proportion of patients will already have occult metastases, their numbers and location depending on the type of primary tumour. Most patients present at this stage. The third phase—clinically advanced disease—is the theme of this chapter. The patient will by now have widespread cancer with perhaps a total burden of tumour amounting to $\sim 10^{12}$ cells, representing 1 kg of tumour tissue. The semi-quantitative approach adopted here serves to emphasize the sheer mass of tumour that may be present. This, in turn, throws some light on the progressive failure of radical surgery, radiotherapy and chemotherapy; it provides a rationale for the eventual change of tactics from control of disease to control of symptoms and palliation, and it gives at least an indication of the complexities of advanced malignant disease which need further investigation.

The primary tumour

In most patients the primary tumour will have been previously treated. There is often no evidence of any residual primary neoplasm, and the patient presents with disseminated disease. In certain circumstances, however, the primary

STAGE OF DISEASE   INVESTIGATIVE PROCEDURES

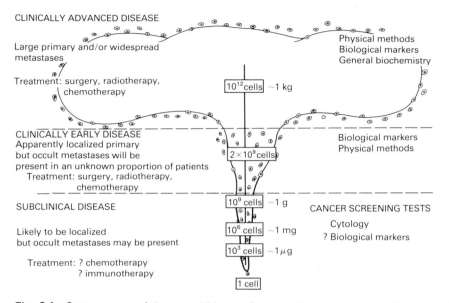

CLINICALLY ADVANCED DISEASE

Large primary and/or widespread   Physical methods
metastases   Biological markers
                                                             General biochemistry

Treatment: surgery, radiotherapy, 10^{12} cells ~1 kg
           chemotherapy

CLINICALLY EARLY DISEASE
Apparently localized primary   Biological markers
but occult metastases will be   Physical methods
present in an unknown proportion of patients 2×10^9 cells
     Treatment: surgery, radiotherapy,
                chemotherapy

SUBCLINICAL DISEASE 10^9 cells ~1 g   CANCER SCREENING TESTS

                                                                         Cytology
Likely to be localized 10^6 cells ~1 mg   ? Biological markers
but occult metastases may be present
                                             10^3 cells ~1 μg

     Treatment: ? chemotherapy
                ? immunotherapy   1 cell

Fig. 2.1   Some aspects of the natural history of progressive tumour growth. The three (arbitrary) stages of disease are illustrated, together with general comments on appropriate methods of investigation and clinical management.

The scheme is selective and oversimplified, omitting important considerations such as fluctuations in the rate of tumour cell proliferation, tumour cell loss, and effects of treatment. The approximate weights of the lesions (~1 μg, ~1 mg, ~1 g) take no account of the non-neoplastic supporting stroma. (Reproduced, with permission, from Symington and Carter, 1976.)

tumour may still be present, though almost always accompanied by regional and/or distant metastases.

1. The lesion may have been neglected and the patient has delayed seeking medical advice. Such cases, often presenting as large fungating masses, are sometimes encountered in the breast, cervix uteri, external genitalia, and skin.

2. Primary tumours may be refractory to treatment or, more frequently, they recur after treatment. Local recurrences, which in most instances can be regarded as one manifestation of more generalized metastatic disease, are most often seen in cancers of the breast and of the head and neck, less frequently at the sites of surgical scars, stomata and anastomoses, fistulae, amputation stumps and in peripherally arising melanomas and sarcomas of soft tissues and bone. Local recurrences vary in size and appearance; multiple 'satellite' lesions may occur. Local recurrence is likely if the primary tumour cannot be completely ablated. This situation is illustrated by gliomas infiltrating vital or inaccessible parts of the brain and spinal cord. Systemic metastases from primary tumours of the central nervous system are excessively rare, and patients die with *local* infiltrative disease (Fig. 2.2).

3. The primary tumour may be very small and elude detection. Despite its

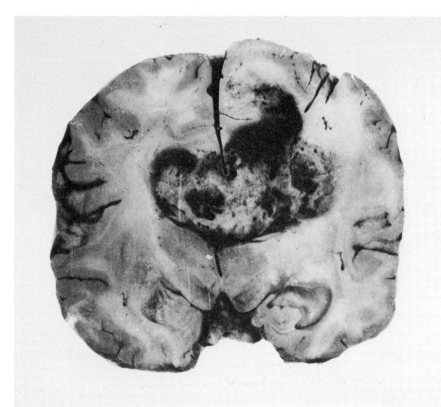

Fig. 2.2 Glioblastoma multiforme—a highly aggressive tumour which grows rapidly and infiltrates the surrounding brain substance. This tumour arose in the right parietal lobe and has spread across the midline destroying the corpus callosum, blocking and distorting the lateral ventricles, and invading the opposite cerebral hemisphere. The right cerebrum is markedly swollen and there is extensive haemorrhage in and around the tumour.

The clinical pictures accompanying a tumour of this kind can be readily inferred, with symptoms and signs initially referable to the right parietal lobe and then becoming more diffuse as the tumour spreads within the brain substance and blocks the lateral ventricles. This, combined with the associated haemorrhage and oedema, results in a progressive increase in intracranial pressure.

size, such a tumour can metastasize widely, and 'carcinomatosis, primary unknown' is a familiar problem in clinical oncology. Certain sites for minute primary tumours fall under particular suspicion in such circumstances—breast, bronchus, thyroid, testis, stomach and kidney. Efforts should be made to localize these elusive primary lesions (despite the presence of advanced disease), as such information can modify the overall clinical management. But the problem often remains and, even after a meticulous autopsy, the pathologist is sometimes unable to determine the primary focus disease.

Initial development and growth of primary tumour
↓
Invasion of adjacent tissues and direct
spread into contiguous body cavities
↓
lymphatics
Penetration of   near or within primary
tumour

blood vessels
↓
Dissemination of tumour cells in
lymphatic and blood circulations

Lymphatic spread→regional lymph nodes, then
to more distant nodes

Haematogenous spread: arrest of circulating tumour
cells; penetration of vascular
walls; entry into interstitial
compartment   of   distant
tissues
↓
Initial survival of disseminated
tumour cells in tissue spaces
Acquisition of fibrovascular stroma

progressive growth
↓
Macroscopic metastases

Fig. 2.3 A simplified scheme of the metastatic process. The emphasis here is on lymphatic and vascular spread, but several other, less important, modes of tumour dissemination also operate. The scheme emphasizes that metastasis comprises a sequence of interlocking processes, sometimes referred to as the 'metastatic cascade'. (Reproduced, with permission, from Symington and Carter, 1976).

Metastatic tumours

Most of the common fatal tumours kill because they metastasize; rarely is death directly attributable to the primary lesion itself. Metastasis is a complex and ill-understood process, the basic elements of which are summarized in Fig. 2.3.

The common sites of metastatic tumours (with particular reference to carcinomas) are illustrated in Fig. 2.4, and some of these are discussed briefly below.

Lymph nodes

Most carcinomas, and some melanomas, malignant teratomas and neuroblastomas, spread initially in the local lymphatic systems to the nearest group of lymph nodes. The lymphatic vessels are infiltrated by tumour cells, either singly or in clumps. If the invasive process is massive and accompanied by a measure of local lymphatic obstruction, it can sometimes be observed clinically—for example, in superficial malignant melanomas and in breast cancer with its 'peau d'orange' effect. The tumour cells are carried in the slowly moving lymph stream to regional lymph nodes, where they are retained. Some of them then become established, and grow out and replace normal nodal

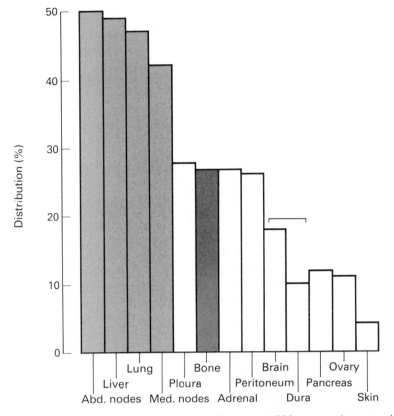

Fig. 2.4 Distribution of macroscopic metastases in 1000 consecutive autopsies on patients with carcinoma of various sites. The study was made at the Montefiore Hospital for Chronic Diseases, New York. The principal sites of metastatic tumour are intra-abdominal and me-diastinal lymph nodes, liver, lungs and pleura, and bone. (Figure based on data from Abrams *et al.*, 1950.)

structures. Afferent lymph flow falls progressively, and incoming tumour cells are diverted to fresh nodes in contiguous anatomical groups. Lymph node involvement usually follows an orderly pattern, predictable on anatomical grounds (Fig. 2.5), though anomalies in the distribution of nodal deposits are quite frequent. Lymph nodes replaced by metastatic tumour are usually enlarged, sometimes greatly so, and can cause symptoms and signs as a result of pressure on, or erosion into, adjacent structures. Large superficial lymph node metastases—in the neck, axillae, and groins—occasionally ulcerate through the skin, and discharging sinuses may form which become infected.

Lymph node metastases must be distinguished from enlarged lymph nodes due to primary malignancies of the lymphoid system—Hodgkin's disease and the non-Hodgkin's lymphomas. Patients with advanced lymphomas have multifocal tumours in other parts of the lymphoid system, often spreading to the bone marrow and to non-lymphoid structures such as the liver, the gastro-intestinal tract, soft tissues and skin. Enlarged lymph nodes may also be en-

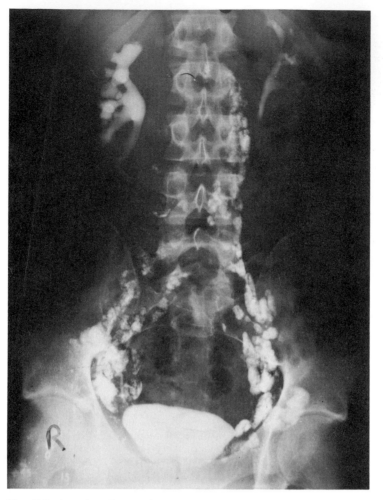

Fig. 2.5 Lymphangiogram from a 25-year-old man with a seminoma of the testis. The tumour has metastasized to the pelvic and para-aortic nodes and, on the right side, there is compression and kinking of the ureter which is giving rise to a hydronephrosis. Despite this extensive intra-abdominal metastatic disease, the tumour regressed in response to radio-therapy and chemotherapy. The patient remains well 9 years later.

countered in the leukaemias. Lymph node metastases from sarcomas are uncommon.

Liver

The liver is a major site for metastases from intra-abdominal malignancies, particularly carcinomas of the colon and rectum, stomach and pancreas. The main route of access is via the radicles of the hepatic portal venous system. Blood-borne (or lymph-borne) hepatic metastases may also be derived from primary cancers of the breast and lungs. Haematogenous spread to the liver,

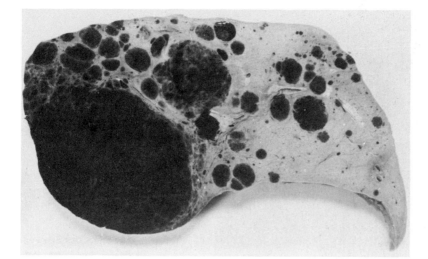

Fig. 2.6 Liver metastases. The patient, a woman of 44, developed malignant melanoma in the right eye. The orbit was cleared and she remained well for 10 years. Her liver then became tender and enlarged rapidly, and she lost weight, developed several pigmented skin nodules, and became increasingly breathless and confused. At autopsy she was found to have widespread malignant melanoma with metastases in the brain, lungs and pleura, pericardium, liver, lymph nodes, kidneys, bones and skin. The liver was enormously enlarged, weighing 9.5 kg; the figure shows the cut surface with numerous deposits of metastic melanoma. Most of the metastases contain abundant melanin pigment, but a few are amelanotic—a very old example of the functional heterogeneity of neoplastic cell populations within a single tumour.

with sometimes massive involvement, is common in disseminating malignant melanoma (Fig. 2.6).

Intrahepatic metastases are generally numerous and sometimes very large; haemorrhage and necrosis are often marked. The whole organ, studded with deposits, may fill the abdomen and weigh several kilograms. The clinical findings of a large, palpable liver, often tender and with an irregular knobbly edge, are easy to interpret. Jaundice may be due to intrahepatic metastases or, less often, to extrinsic biliary obstruction as a result of lymph node deposits in the porta hepatis. Progressive impairment of liver function is frequently observed, but it is also striking how some aspects of normal liver function still remain intact in the face of massive replacement of hepatic parenchyma by metastatic tumour.

Lungs

Most pulmonary metastases are derived from tumour cells which invade peripheral capillaries and venules in the systemic circulation. Sarcomas, in particular, metastasize to the lungs in the bloodstream (Fig. 2.7). So, too, do several carcinomas, though these may also spread to the lungs via lymphatics—for example from the breast. The overlying pleura is frequently involved, and pleural effusions are a common clinical concomitant (see later). Intrapulmonary

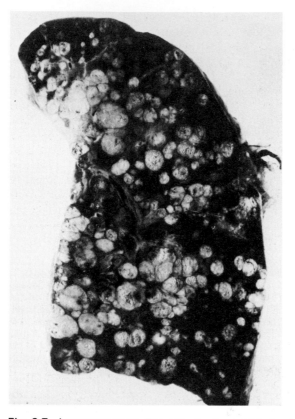

Fig. 2.7 Lung metastases. The patient, a boy of 14, developed an osteosarcoma in the right femur. The leg was disarticulated at the hip, and he received chemotherapy. Multiple lung metastases appeared at 16 months and grew rapidly. At autopsy, metastatic disease was confined to the lungs and the figure illustrates massive pulmonary involvement by metastatic osteosarcoma.

The small amount of uninvolved lung substance is dark as a result of intrapulmonary congestion and haemorrhage.

metastases are usually multiple and vary in size, the larger lesions tending to become haemorrhagic. They are associated with varying degrees of local oedema, congestion, haemorrhage and infection in the uninvolved parenchyma. Large deposits may compress and obstruct peripheral bronchi and bronchioles; obstruction of major bronchi is usually due to enlarged mediastinal lymph nodes. Varying degrees of atelectasis, with or without infection, will result. As in the liver, there may be progressive loss of normal function, with death ensuing from organ failure (see Fig. 2.9).

Bones

Skeletal metastases are almost always blood-borne. Direct invasion of bone is seen in advanced carcinomas of the head and neck, bronchus, breast and pelvic viscera. Some primary cancers show a particular predilection to metastasize to bone (breast, prostate, kidney, thyroid, and lung) and to involve particular sites (Fig. 2.8). The axial skeleton (skull, ribs and sternum, vertebrae, pelvis, upper humerus and femur) is frequently infiltrated, while more peripheral bones, lacking red marrow, are usually free of metastatic tumour. Once established within the skeleton, tumour cells evoke complex local reactions of bone destruction (osteolysis) and new bone formation (osteosclerosis). Most bone metastases are predominantly osteolytic, but some deposits, notably from prostatic carcinomas, are osteoblastic. The marrow cavities are invaded to the extent that tumour cells appear in bone marrow aspirates. Extensive destruction of bone may result in pathological fractures and compression of the spinal cord and nerve roots, giving rise to diverse neurological symptoms and signs. Local or referred pain may be severe and difficult to control, and complete paraplegia may develop. Hypercalcaemia is common, but this change (which is also encountered in cancer patients without overt bone metastases) may also reflect ectopic hormone production by the tumour (see later; also Chapter 7).

Body cavities

Invasion of the peritoneal, pleural and pericardial cavities by disseminating tumour is common in advanced malignant disease. It is usually a result of direct spread, either from the primary tumour itself or from adjacent metastases. Serosal deposits are generally multiple and tend to 'seed' throughout the involved cavity. They are frequently accompanied by effusions of protein-rich, bloodstained fluid in which tumour cells can be identified. Many litres of fluid may accumulate in the peritoneal and pleural cavities, producing intense abdominal discomfort and dyspnoea. Secondary infection may supervene, particularly in the pleura. Repeated paracenteses tend to induce fibrosis, with loculation of fluid. Peritoneal effusions (ascites, carcinomatosis peritonei) are particularly associated with carcinomas of the ovary and, to a lesser extent, stomach, large bowel and pancreas; pleural effusions with carcinomas of breast, lung and oesophagus and with pulmonary metastases from various sources. These same three primary tumours may also induce pericardial effusions resulting in low-grade pericarditis or fatal cardiac tamponade. The membranes of the brain and their associated spaces are commonly involved by cortical metastases in the cerebrum and cerebellum. Meningeal infiltration may occur alone, notably in relapsed acute leukaemias. Primary intracranial tumours occasionally seed along the spaces surrounding the neuraxis.

Some of the basic patterns of cancer dissemination have been described, and certain qualifying comments about metastasis must now be added.

1. It is a clinical commonplace that malignant tumours vary in their capacity to metastasize. It was noted earlier that gliomas kill by invading locally within the central nervous system, and that distant metastases are exceptionally rare (see Fig. 2.2). Other tumours— testicular teratomas, some melanomas, and 'oat-cell' carcinomas of the bronchus—tend to disseminate widely. The basis for this spectrum of 'metastatic potential' in different malignant tumours is unknown, but it is crucial to the understanding of the metastatic process.

2. The number, size and distribution of metastatic tumours all vary (a point

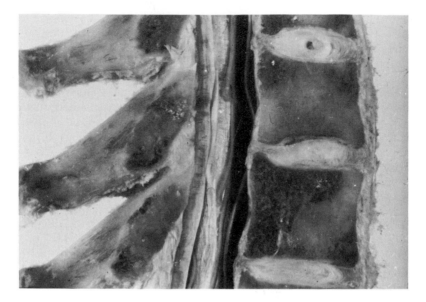

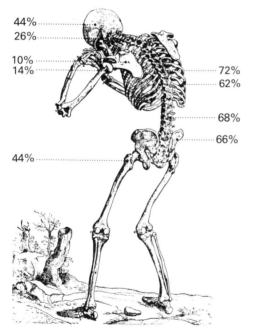

Fig. 2.8 Bone metastases. (a) Vertebral bodies infiltrated by metastasizing carcinoma of the breast. The tumour is replacing much of the marrow spaces and bone trabeculae, but the cartilaginous intervertebral discs and the periosteum are not involved. There is no evidence of extension into the spinal canal here, but compression of the cord and/or nerve roots may complicate metastatic disease in the spine. (b) The distribution of bone metastases in carcinoma of the breast. The skeleton is from Vesalius' *De humani corporis fabrica* of 1543; the superimposed figures, which show the distribution of skeletal deposits detected by scintigraphy in 50 patients, are quoted from Galasko (1972).

made clear by two of the preceding illustrations). Malignant melanoma (see Fig. 2.6) and osteosarcoma (see Fig. 2.7) are both tumours with a high metastatic potential, and both the examples quoted had metastasized, mainly by the bloodstream; but the malignant melanoma produced massive disease in many sites, whereas the osteosarcoma spread into the lungs but apparently nowhere else. Again, the amount of tumour present may vary enormously for a given neoplasm. In carcinomas of the breast or bronchus, for example, one patient may have solitary or a few scattered deposits, while another is riddled with metastases equivalent to perhaps 1 kg or more of tumour tissue (see Fig. 2.1). The distribution of metastases is *non-random* and there are definite sites of predilection. It was made clear in Fig. 2.4 that certain tissues and organs are regularly involved by mestastases while others are not. There is no mention in Fig. 2.4, for example, of the heart, spleen or skeletal muscle. Although these structures have a rich blood supply and, in the cases of skeletal muscle, comprise a large proportion of the total body mass, involvement by metastatic tumour is uncommon.

3. A variable proportion of metastatic disease in any one patient is likely to be occult and will go undetected during life. Examples include small or solitary deposits in deeply placed lymph nodes, the adrenal glands, the kidneys, or even parts of the brain. Clinical findings alone are imprecise, and more accurate appraisal of tumour spread can be made by additional investigations as diverse as radiology (including scintigraphy, arteriography, lymphangiography and computerized axial tomography), isotope and ultrasonic scans, serum enzyme level estimations, bone marrow aspiration, tissue biopsy and surgical staging procedures. Despite these techniques, however, the accurate detection of metastatic disease remains a major problem in clinical oncology. In general, most clinicians tend to underestimate the extent of metastatic tumour which is eventually found at autopsy.

4. The effects of chemotherapy and radiotherapy on the growth of metastases vary widely in different tumours. Some metastases may completely regress, while others continue to grow progressively. Examples of 'spontaneous' regression of metastatic deposits are recorded; they are exceptionally rare and the underlying mechanisms are obscure.

5. The assumption of an orderly progression of malignant disease—with an overt primary tumour followed after a while by metastases—is fallacious. Several variant patterns may be encountered. The disease may first declare itself through metastases rather than the primary tumour—an unexplained anaemia, lymphadenopathy, a pathological fracture—the primary lesions remaining occult. The interval between recognition of a primary tumour and the development of metastases is also variable and, with many tumours, clinical experience indicates that the metastatic process is often under way by the time the patient first presents with an ostensibly localized lesion. On the other hand, many years may elapse before metastases become apparent, as in some carcinomas of the breast and kidney, and malignant melanoma (see Fig. 2.6). The reasons for these protracted latent periods—perhaps 15 or 20 years—are wholly obscure.

General aspects of advanced malignant disease; the role of the limited symptom-orientated autopsy

The effects of disseminated tumour are now recognized to be both complex and subtle. Certain complications of extensive tumour growth have long been familiar, such as pressure on and distortion of normal structures resulting in obstruction, fistula formation, haemorrhage, ulceration and infection. Some of these local effects may have more extensive consequences: compression of the ureters, for example, may result in hydronephrosis (see Fig. 2.5) and progressive loss of functioning renal parenchyma. The systemic effects of extensive malignancy include metabolic derangements (cachexia, abnormal purine metabolism, hypercalcaemia, hypoglycaemia), fever, autoimmune disorders, deranged immune function, and disturbances in the skin, joints and nervous system. The underlying mechanisms involved in such changes are poorly understood. Several tumour products have been described such as ectopic hormones, oncofetal antigens, prostaglandins and angiogenesis factors; but the origin, chemical nature and biological activity of such materials are, in most instances, far from clear. Most of them are 'tumour associated' rather than 'tumour specific', and are derived from both tumour and host sources. Some products such as carcinoembryonic antigen (CEA), α-fetoprotein (αFP) and the β-subunit of human chorionic gonadotrophin (β-HCG) are useful in monitoring the course of the disease and, in some instances, in initial diagnosis.

The causes of death in advanced malignant disease are often complex (Fig. 2.9), and many of the medical problems posed by patients remain unsolved. Examples include uncontrollable pain, vomiting or dysphagia, oedema and confusion. Such symptoms are almost always multifactorial, and some of the contributory factors to each will be functional and biochemical. Others, however, can often be shown to have a clear anatomical basis. *Limited symptom-orientated autopsies* were developed at St Christopher's Hospice in 1979, and preliminary experience from some 50 cases has already justified this work. The information obtained has proved valuable retrospectively, (often clarifying hitherto puzzling features in a patient's last illness) and, more importantly, prospectively in the better identification and more effective management of similar problems when they appear again. One example may be quoted. Limited autopsies performed on 24 patients with advanced squamous carcinomas of the head and neck have revealed an apparently new dysphagia syndrome associated with cancer of the oropharynx. The clinical features suggest complete mechanical obstruction, but at autopsy the pharyngeal lumen is fully patent. The symptoms appear to be due to 'splinting' of the pharynx by local fibrosis and tumour invading *outwards* into the soft tissues of the neck, perineural spread of tumour into the ipsilateral vagal trunk (sometimes accompanied by segmental infarction), and variable infiltration of the ipsilateral sympathetic chain. These findings are far from academic because the dysphagia can be temporarily palliated with corticosteroids. Another symptom-complex which is under investigation is the ill-defined entity of 'subacute intestinal obstruction', a condition which is not uncommon in patients with advanced intra-abdominal malignancy and which has been shown (see Chapter 7) to be compatible with survival for several weeks. Fifteen examples have so far been examined and it is already clear that several different morphological and mechanical factors are involved.

Drawing on the pathological findings, the eventual aim will be to achieve a more specific clinical diagnosis and to recognize the very small numbers of patients in whom surgical intervention would be appropriate.

Close and continuing collaboration between clinicians and pathologists is essential for the planning and performance of symptom-orientated autopsies, but the time and effort are amply repaid. Combined with modern histological techniques such as immunohistochemistry, their future potential—notably in exploring some of the structural bases for intractable pain—is considerable.

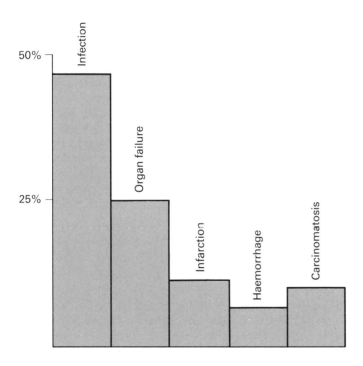

Fig. 2.9 Causes of death in 816 cancer patients at the M.D. Anderson Hospital, Tumor Institute, Houston, Texas. All patients had a complete autopsy.

Notes

Infections. Mostly septicaemia and/or major visceral infections such as pneumonia, peritonitis or pyelonephritis; Gram-negative bacteria (*Escherichia coli, Klebsiella* Spp., *Pseudomonas aeruginosa*) predominate.

Organ failure. Lungs > heart > liver > CNS > kidneys; mainly or exclusively the consequence of tumour invasion except for cardiac insufficiency.

Infarction. Lungs > heart; pulmonary emboli derived about equally from distal venous thrombosis and from tumour cells.

Haemorrhage. Gastrointestinal tract > brain > ruptured vesel > lungs; related to underlying tumour and/or to thrombocytopenia or other bleeding diathesis.

Carcinomatosis. Usually severe metabolic and/or electrolyte abnormalities with extensive disseminating disease but no other specific pathological process. Several patients will have one or more of these 'causes' of death—for example, a combination of infection and organ failure. The incidence of the various causes will in part reflect selection of patients. Fatal haemorrhage due to thrombocytopenia will be more common in units with a special interest in leukaemias and lymphomas. (Figures based on data from Inagaki *et al.,* 1974.)

Acknowledgements

I am grateful to the clinicians of the Royal Marsden Hospital for permission to quote details of cases under their care. I am also indebted to the physicians of St Christopher's Hospice for their collaboration in setting up our symptom-orientated autopsy service. Financial support from the Medical Research Council is acknowledged.

References and further reading

Abrams, H.L., Spiro, R. and Goldstein, N. (1950). *Cancer N.Y.* **3**, 74.

Becker, F.F. (Ed.) (1975). *Cancer, a Comprehensive Treatise*, Vols. 1–4. Plenum Press, New York and London.

Carter, R.L. (1982). *Journal of Clinical Pathology* **35**, 1041.

Carter, R.L., Pittam, M.R. and Tanner, N.S.B. (1982). *Journal of the Royal Society of Medicine* **75**, 598.

Holland, J.F. and Frei, E. (1973). *Cancer Medicine*. Lea and Febiger, Philadelphia.

Inagaki, J., Rodriguez, V. and Bodey, G.P. (1974). *Cancer, Philadelphia* **33**, 568.

Kefford, R.F., Cooney, N.J., Woods, R.L., Fox, R.M. and Tattersall, M.H.N. (1981). *European Journal of Cancer and Clinical Oncology* **17**, 1117.

Klastersky, J., Daneau, D. and Verhest, A. (1972). *European Journal of Cancer* **8**, 149.

Solzhenitsyn, A. (1968) *Cancer Ward*, Part II, Bodley Head, London.

Symington, T. and Carter, R.L. (Eds.) (1976). *Scientific Foundations of Oncology*, Heinemann Medical, London.

Willis, R.A. (1973) *The Spread of Tumours in the Human Body*, 3rd Edn. Butterworths, London.

3

Physical aspects

K.C. Calman and J. Welsh

'I am not so much afraid of death as ashamed thereof.'
   (Sir Thomas Browne)

'Protect me
From a body without death. Such indignity
Would be outcast, like a rock in the sea.
But with death, it can hold
More than time gives it, or the earth shows it.'
   (Fry, 1954)

Terminal illness in cancer patients occurs when such patients have been accurately diagnosed, in whom death does not seem far off and in whom medical effort has turned from the curative to the palliative. This definition carries three implications:

1. that the diagnosis has been firmly established, and that the symptoms and signs present are related to progressive malignant disease and not primarily to conditions which are not terminal;
2. that it is possible to give some prediction of the time of death;
3. that conventional anticancer therapy has been used to the full.

Although this chapter is concerned with physical aspects of terminal care, the importance of all other aspects of care should not be forgotten.

What are the main symptoms and signs?

Both should emerge from a careful clinical history and examination, the importance of which cannot be overemphasized.

The history

Close attention must be paid to the clinical history. Only when a patient's problems have been adequately described (and understood) can there be a rational approach to treatment. Traditionally, the clinical history is pieced together in a system-by-system enquiry; but while this has the merit of thoroughness, it is often more useful to adopt a problem-orientated approach with the terminally ill patient. Each symptom—pain, nausea and breathlessness—is described and, after examination, a clinical diagnosis is made. The various findings are then collated, specific investigations are undertaken where neces-

sary, and treatment is arranged. The response to treatment is carefully documented and any subsequent modifications necessary for more effective symptom
control are made.

Certain specific questions should be asked, including the following.

Pain. What is the site of pain? How long does it last and what is the time-
intensity relationship? How severe is it? What makes it better or worse? The
management of pain is fully discussed in Chapter 5; the more information
available, the easier it should be to determine the underlying aetiology and
begin appropriate pain-controlling measures.

Mouth problems. Are there ulcers, soreness, dysphagia, thirst, changes in taste?

Appetite. How much and what type of food is taken? Does anorexia occur at
the thought of food? Does anything alleviate this anorexia?

Nausea and vomiting. When does it occur? What provokes or improves it?

Breathlessness. What are the provoking causes, particularly in relation to movement and posture? What are the time relationships? It is associated with coughing? What makes it better or worse?

Episodes of bleeding. Is there haemoptysis, haematemesis and melaena, haematuria, vaginal and rectal bleeding?

Disturbances in bowel and bladder function. Is there incontinence, dysuria, discharge? Are surgical stomata functioning adequately? Constipation must not be
forgotten.

Sleeplessness. What, in particular, are its time relationships? Is it linked to pain
or breathlessness or urinary frequency?

The quantification of symptoms, though difficult, is often useful in the assessment of treatment. Symptoms such as pain, anorexia or vomiting may be scored
as mild, moderate or severe, or by a series of pluses: +, + +, + + +. Alternatively, a linear analogue scale may be used in which a 10-cm line is drawn.
At each end of the scale the extremes of the symptoms are noted, for example:
no pain—pain unbearable; unable to eat at all—eating normally; no vomiting—
vomiting continuously. The patient is then asked to mark the point on the scale
which corresponds to the severity of his own symptom. Although this method
remains subjective, it is simple and has been widely used to document the course
of the disease.

The general activity of the patient must be assessed, and limiting factors such
as pain, breathlessness and weakness need to be carefully documented. It is
often useful to know how the patient passes the day. How much is he in bed or
in a chair? Can he manage at home, and how much help does he need to do
so? Can he see to read, work with his hands, write? Such factors can be expressed semi-quantitatively by the Karnovsky index (Table 3.1) and the Eastern
Co-operative Oncology Group (ECOG) score (Table 3.2); schemes of this kind
add little to a thorough clinical assessment, but they may be useful in comparing
patients when some new therapeutic procedure is being evalutated. They may
also be useful in assessing some aspects of the quality of life. This is particularly
the case in relation to physical problems and side-effects of treatment.

It is important to obtain a full list of drugs being taken, together with their
frequency of administration and their effectiveness for the patient. Inadequate
relief of symptoms is sometimes due to appropriate drugs inappropriately prescribed. When, towards the end of the interview, a rapport has been established,

Table 3.1 Karnovsky index of performance status

Normal	100
Minor signs or symptoms	90
Normal activity with effort	80
Unable to carry on normal activity, but cares for self	70
Requires occasional assistance with personal needs	60
Requires considerable assistance and medical care	50
Disabled	40
Severely disabled and hospitalized	30
Very sick: active supportive treatment necessary	20
Moribund	10
Death	0

Table 3.2 ECOG performance status

Grade 0	Fully active, able to carry on all pre-disease performance without restrictions
Grade 1	Restricted in strenuous activity but ambulatory and able to carry out work of a light and sedentary nature, e.g. light housework or office work
Grade 2	Ambulatory and capable of all self-care but unable to carry out any work activity; up and about more than 50% of waking hours
Grade 3	Capable of only limited self-care, confined to bed or chair more than 50% of waking hours
Grade 4	Completely disabled, cannot carry out any self-care, and totally confined to bed or chair

the patient should be encouraged to discuss what he himself knows, thinks and fears about his condition (see Chapter 4). Talking to the patient's relatives is essential to corroborate and extend these findings and to provide further information.

The physical examination

Although this will concentrate on the points raised in the preceding history, it must be sufficiently general to reveal any problem not mentioned by the patient. The following points are particularly important.

1. The entire skin surface should be examined to exclude superficial recurrent or metastatic tumour. Pressure sores and breaks in the skin—over the vertebral spines, sacrum, ischial tuberosities, ankles, and elbows—must be recorded. Examination of the skin also provides evidence of the degree of hydration.

2. Examination of the mouth, tongue and pharynx will indicate the state of hydration and the presence of local lesions such as ulceration and fungal infections, notably by *Candida*. It is important to examine the mouth with the dentures removed.

3. In the alimentary system, the examiner should concentrate on gastric distension, incipient bowel obstruction, abdominal masses, ascites, functioning of surgical stomata, and hepatomegaly. A rectal examination is essential in all patients to check for faecal impaction and perianal infection.

4. Examination of the lungs, heart, blood pressure and peripheral pulses may clarify the breathlessness and chest pain of which patients often complain.

5. Careful neurological examination may establish the basis for local symptoms such as pain or impending paraplegia. The distinction between widespread intracranial metastatic disease and neuropsychiatric disorders can be extremely difficult. Restlessness in a confused patient may be due to bladder distension. Careful palpation of the skeleton may reveal specific tender areas due to bony metastases.

The history and physical examination of the patient have been discussed here in some detail, but their importance is worth repeating: without an adequate description and identification of a patient's symptoms and signs, treatment cannot be effectively planned and no valid assessment can be made of therapeutic responses.

Is the diagnosis correct?

The question must now be asked: are the symptoms and signs elicited attributable to malignant disease, or do they reflect some unrelated disease progress which is occurring coincidentally in a patient with cancer? In such patients, sinister symptoms are sometimes simple. An accurate history and physical examination may be sufficient to decide the point, but additional simple investigations are sometimes required. The following patients provide some examples.

1. A 55-year-old male with inoperable gastric carcinoma, diagnosed six months previously and treated by chemotherapy. His general practitioner telephoned to say that the patient had developed pulmonary metastases and that he would be cared for at home in what was described as a terminal phase. The patient was, however, admitted to hospital, where he was found to have a cough and purulent sputum; a chest x-ray showed changes of chronic bronchitis only. He was treated with antibiotics and was well enough to return home after five days. He lived for 15 months.

2. A 50-year-old male with advanced non-Hodgkin's lymphoma of the stomach which had been successfully treated by chemotherapy. The abdominal mass disappeared, the patient was free of tumour on investigation, and treatment was stopped. The general practitioner telephoned to say that the patient had developed severe backache; he assumed that the patient now had disseminated tumour and would require no further active treatment. The patient was, however, seen at the out-patient clinic. He was still clinically tumour free, and the history and physical signs suggested a prolapsed intervertebral disc. Bone scan and skeletal surveys were negative and the disc lesion was treated conservatively. The patient remained well for a further two and a half years.

3. A 60-year-old female with bilateral breast carcinoma and evidence of secondary spread, presented with jaundice and right upper abdominal pain. The initial diagnosis was of liver metastases, but further investigations revealed gall-stones and the patient had a cholecystectomy. She remained pain free until her death from disseminated cancer nine months later.

4. Male, aged 60, with oesophageal carcinoma which had been resected two months previously. The patient presented with dysphagia, suggesting locally recurrent tumour. Endoscopy showed a non-absorbable suture in the lumen at the site of the anastomosis. This material was removed, the dysphagia was relieved, and he remained well for a further 14 months.

These four patients illustrate a number of points. Their symptoms, though not related directly to their malignant disease, were serious and required prompt treatment in their own right. The relief of these symptoms improved the quality of the patients' lives even though the underlying malignant disease continued to advance. They illustrate certain attitudes of doctors to patients with advanced malignancy. There is a sharp contrast between the clinician who says merely that a patient has advanced disease and requires sedation, and the clinician who says that a patient has advanced disease and requires symptom control—and at the same time recognizes the need for the nature of that symptom to be explored in more detail.

Investigative procedures in the terminally ill

This is a debatable topic. Some clinicians argue that such patients should be treated on a purely symptomatic basis. In many instances, access to laboratory or radiological facilities may be difficult or impossible. Within a few days of death, investigative procedures might be regarded as positively unethical.

At some point the clinician must surely ask himself: 'Why has my patient developed this symptom? And if I understood it more fully, could it not be treated more effectively?' Two points must, however, be clearly stated. Investigative procedures should never be used as grounds for delaying symptomatic treatment, and the investigations chosen should be directed specifically to particular symptoms.

It is obvious that the type of investigation will be determined by the place where the patient is being treated; but some examples of simple, readily available procedures and their applications are given below.

1. *Haemoglobin estimation.* Breathlessness, weakness and fatigue in some severely anaemic patients may be relieved by blood transfusion (see later; also Chapter 7). Such relief will be transitory, but it may be suitable for a particular patient at a particular time in his illness.

2. *Characterization of infections.* Asymptomatic infections require no investigation. Infection causing severe symptoms should usually be treated: isolation of organisms and determination of their antibiotic sensitivities will be carried out in the usual way. It is improbable that the treatment of serious intercurrent infections materially prolongs life, but the patient will be more comfortable. Major infections occurring as an obvious terminal event should be treated symptomatically (see Chapter 7).

3. *Measurement of serum electrolytes* may be useful in a few instances. Hypercalcaemia, in particular, is worth detecting and correcting (see later; also Chapters 5 and 7).

4. *Radiological investigations* may be considered when appropriate. They should not be carried out routinely.

In general, the investigation and treatment of symptoms may well be justifiable if this action leads to an improvement in the quality of life.

The value of research in patients with terminal illness

It is only by asking questions and attempting to solve them, that advances can be made in the practical management of advanced malignant disease. In many instances we still lack basic information on the mechanisms of symptom production and their control (see Chapter 2). It is possible to justify clinical research on these grounds alone, but two questions are paramount: are unnecessary investigations being performed, and are patients suffering needlessly?

Controlled clinical trials

For symptoms such as nausea or anorexia, it is still not clear which mode of therapy is most appropriate; it may be necessary to carry out a study to determine optimal therapy. (This topic is discussed further in Chapter 7.)

Problem-orientated research

Many specific symptoms, such as pain, still need to be studied in depth. The form of investigation may involve a patient in procedures which do not contribute directly to his management. It is thus essential that he is fully aware of the purpose of the study and gives his informed consent, and that he receives effective symptomatic therapy at all times.

Investigations involving particular scientific disciplines

The clinician may, for example, have a special interest in biochemical aspects of malignant disease and he may wish to look further into mechanisms of (say) hypercalcaemia or ectopic hormone secretion. The pharmacologist may be interested in drug interactions, an extremely important area when so many patients have multiple drug therapy. Again, such investigations may not directly benefit individual patients, but if carried out in an ethical way they may contribute to a greater understanding of the underlying processes of advanced malignant diseases and their possible palliation.

Has conventional therapy been used to the full?

Surgery, radiotherapy, chemotherapy and hormone therapy

These are all discussed elsewhere (see Chapters 8-10), but it is worth noting here that there is an essential difference between the use of conventional methods of anticancer therapy in patients with early disease and in those with terminal disease. In the first circumstance, treatment is used to eradicate tumour in the hope of cure; in the latter it is used for palliation. As modes of treatment become more effective, particularly in the use of combined methods, the point at which there is a change of tactic—from active anticancer therapy to active symptomatic care—becomes less easy to define. It is essential not to regard the 'care' or 'cure' situation in too rigid a manner; the important thing to establish is that the patient is in the appropriate category at each stage of the disease.

Has the time for terminal care been reached?

This fundamental question must be answered for each individual patient after an assessment of some or all of the following factors:

symptomatology;

evidence for advanced, progressing disease;

inability to treat the disease by conventional means or the failure to respond to therapy;

psychological attitude of the patient.

Great difficulties may be encountered in assessing individual cases. As Basil Stoll has written, 'For the physician to communicate to the patient a finite figure of months or years as the prognosis is to deny hope, apart from showing ignorance of the vagaries of cancer behaviour.' (Stoll, 1982). A patient may complain of severe, incapacitating pain and yet not have rapidly progressive disease or evidence of clinical deterioration. Conversely, a patient may have advanced, progressive disease and yet remain reasonably well, able to work and to function normally. It must be emphasized that advanced metastatic disease is not, in itself, a reliable index of terminal illness. Indeed, some patients, regarded as having far-advanced terminal disease, may remain stable for long periods of time. It is essential that such cases are reviewed regularly, the diagnosis confirmed and more intensive antitumour measures reinstituted where appropriate: continued assessment is the key to appropriate care. It is also essential at times that the clinician seek a second opinion. This is in no sense a gesture of defeat, but rather an acknowledgement of the difficulty of the problem and the fluidity, in individual cases, of the 'cure'/'care' situations—which can be summarized as cure $\rightleftharpoons$ care (see Chapter 1).

Some systemic changes in patients with terminal cancer

The patient with terminal malignant disease often presents an extremely complex clinical picture. The major symptoms are discussed in Chapter 7; here, we shall stress some of the underlying systemic changes associated with terminal illness which may make management of such symptoms more difficult (see Chapter 2).

Cachexia

This common symptom complex is associated with loss of weight, decreases in body fat, protein and carbohydrate, increased basal metabolic rate and abnormal iron metabolism. Cachexia is not simply starvation, but a more profound metabolic problem.

The patient presents clinically with weakness and tiredness associated with weight loss. The aetiology is complex. Cachexia may be consequent upon anorexia, nausea or vomiting, or on gastrointestinal obstruction. It may be compounded by loss of body fluids in association with bleeding or malignant ulcers. Intestinal malabsorption may be involved (see below). The tumour itself may play a part, either by its increased demand for essential nutrients or, more subtly, by synthesizing and releasing products which cause the metabolic changes (see Chapter 2).

Apart from the weakness and tiredness associated with cachexia, there are other serious problems. Such patients are metabolically and nutritionally abnormal, and they may metabolize drugs in a different way from normal individuals; drug efficacy may therefore be modified (see later).

Malabsorption

Malabsorption has frequently been described in patients with cancer, either as a primary event or as a consequence of previous treatment. Repeated courses of chemotherapy or radiotherapy to the abdomen may, for example, induce villous atrophy. Previous surgical treatment of intra-abdominal neoplasms may have been performed with bypass or resection of segments of small bowel.

Malabsorption has serious consequences for the patient. He may develop impaired absorption of essential nutrients, including vitamins. Vitamin deficiency may be associated with skin and mucosal lesions, anaemia, cardiac failure and neurological impairment. Correction of such deficiencies will be symptomatically beneficial. Several of the vitamins are involved in drug metabolism, and vitamin deficiencies will modify drug efficacy. In addition, absorption of drugs may be delayed or actually impaired. When patients do not respond as expected to drug therapy (for example, in pain control), attention should be given to malabsorption and the drug given parenterally for a trial period.

Influence of previous treatment

Previous surgery of the tumour may result in residual anatomical or functional impairment to adjacent normal tissues. Such damage may be unimportant when a patient is tolerably well, but it becomes more significant when he is terminally ill. Radiotherapy and cytotoxic drugs may also induce tissue damage which declares itself at a later stage. Fibrosis is a particular example of this and may effect several organs, such as the skin, lungs and lymphatics. Radiation-induced cystitis and proctitis may occur.

Drug therapy may be associated with severe bone marrow toxicity and immune depression, thus favouring infections (see later). Many side-effects may be encountered in patients treated with high doses of corticosteroids, particularly weakness, glycosuria, osteoporosis and peptic ulceration.

Renal problems in advanced cancer

These are associated with direct involvement of the kidneys or lower urinary tract by tumour or, in a small percentage of cases, with deposition of immune complexes in the glomerular basement membrane. There is deterioration of renal function with rising blood urea and serum creatinine levels. Drug excretion in such patients may be delayed, and consideration should always be given to this possibility when severe and unexplained side-effects of drugs occur. Hepatorenal syndrome, due to failing renal perfusion, is a frequent late terminal finding.

Hepatic involvement in advanced cancer

Liver metastases, often massive, are common in many patients with advanced cancer. In addition to causing the specific symptoms and signs of jaundice, itch, nausea and sometimes profound anorexia, more general consequences may ensue. Protein synthesis is decreased with widespread liver involvement. There is a fall in serum albumin levels, which may be associated with peripheral oedema. Drug metabolism may be altered. The synthesis of components of the blood coagulation system, including fibrinogen, may be affected. Rapid hepatic enlargement or bleeding within liver metastases is often associated with severe local pain.

Haematological problems in the terminally ill

Patients with advanced malignant disease are frequently anaemic. Mild asymptomatic anaemias require no investigation or treatment, but severe symptomatic anaemia may require therapy. The cause is usually obvious—for example bleeding from a tumour or marrow invasion—and little investigation is needed. Blood transfusion is likely to improve symptoms for only a short time before the anaemia recurs. This short time can, however, mean the difference between a patient being treated at home or in hospital, and there are individual occasions when even one weekend at home, made possible by blood transfusion, is justified for some domestic or social occasion.

Coagulation abnormalities, involving either bleeding or disseminated intravascular coagulation, may be encountered in terminal illness. They do not require active management. Intramuscular injections should be avoided in these circumstances in case they cause painful bleeding.

Other biochemical changes

Hypercalcaemia occurs more frequently in advanced malignant disease than is often supposed. Its symptoms include confusion, abdominal pain, constipation, restlessness and irritability, progressing to drowsiness and coma. Adequate hydration will control this symptom complex in about half the cases. Where this is not successful, prednisolone or cortisol may be used together with oral phosphate. In the small number of patients who do not respond to these methods, intravenous mithramycin may be successful. Calcitonin is rarely required. Hypercalcaemia can simulate intracranial metastases and, as it is a treatable condition, it should not be overlooked.

Hyperuricaemia may occur, caused by anticancer therapy. As it can result in painful gouty tophi, it may merit active management. Phenylbutazone is given in the acute situation and allopurinol as a preventive measure.

Electrolyte imbalance is common in patients with repeated vomiting or excessive fluid loss, and such patients are often severely dehydrated. Where it occurs shortly before death, intravenous fluid replacement is inappropriate. Regular mouth care is essential, and saliva substitutes may be useful. But it may be necessary to consider such measures in patients in whom the acute problem can be resolved—for example by palliative surgery (see Chapter 10).

Peripheral oedema in the cancer patient has a complex aetiology. It may be related to low serum albumin levels, electrolyte abnormalities, tumour involvment of lymph nodes and lymphatic obstruction, hepatic failure, renal failure or myocardial failure. Oedema of this type is often resistant to therapy; treatment with diuretics or cardiac glycosides may bring undesirable side-effects, and the possibilities of deleterious drug interactions should not be forgotten.

cially some carcinomas of the lung. Ectopic ACTH secretion is associated with the symptoms of Cushing's syndrome. Excessive secretion of antidiuretic hormone (ADH) results in electrolyte abnormalities associated with water intoxication: serum sodium levels fall and the patient becomes weak, confused and inco-ordinated. Coma and convulsions may occur. The condition can be corrected by fluid restriction and occasionally by the use of hypertonic solutions. More recently, lithium and demeclocycline have been used successfully. Excess parathyroid hormone secretion may result in hypercalcaemia (see above).

The importance of these somewhat esoteric biochemical problems does not, in the present context, lie in the elucidation of the underlying abnormality; rather, it lies in the exploitation of this knowledge to improve the quality of care given to patients with advanced malignant disease. Confusion, restlessness, nausea and vomiting may all result from these biochemical abnormalities; if they are corrected, the patient will feel better and the quality of his remaining life will be improved. By the simple expedient of measuring the serum electrolytes, calcium and uric acid, any abnormalities noted can often be treated.

Confusion in the patient with terminal cancer

The patient with advanced cancer may be confused and restless in the end stages of disease as a result of several factors.

Intracerebral metastases. These are a common cause of confusion, usually associated with neurological signs and an abnormal EEG or brain scan. Temporary benefit may result from the use of dexamethasone (see Chapters 5 and 7).

Drug overdosage. It is essential to review the drug history of the confused patient. He may be suffering from excess sedation or the inappropriate use of tranquillizers.

Biochemical disturbances. Some of these have already been discussed. It is worth considering whether the confused, restless patient has an acute vitamin deficiency, particularly of the B group. Wernicke's encephalopathy, which may be confused with cerebral metastases, responds well to intravenous vitamin therapy.

Other physical problems. These include pain, bladder dysfunction and retention of urine.

Psychological problems and psychiatric disturbances. These may also occur and be associated with confusion.

Infection and the immune response

It is now well established that patients with advanced cancer often have depressed immunological responses involving cell-mediated immunity, antibody production, or both. Such patients are more prone to infection, sometimes by unusual micro-organisms or organisms which are usually of only minimal pathogenicity.

Drug metabolism and drug interactions

Throughout this chapter, reference has been made to anomalies of drug metabolism consequent upon malabsorption, metabolic abnormalities, or renal and liver failure.

Drugs used in the patient with terminal illness include a wide variety of analgesics, antiemetics and sedatives. The use of such drugs, in combination, may result in significant interactions. Metoclopramide, for example, enhances gastric emptying and may alter the affect of other drugs. Monamine oxidase inhibitors interact with pethidine and the tricylic antidepressants and they should be used together only with the greatest care. Aspirin may interact with probenecid and methotrexate. Many of the drug combinations used in clinical practice have unknown interactions and the clinician must always be on the watch for adverse results.

Physical aspects of terminal care in children

The plan of management outlined in this chapter applies equally well to children as to adults. The metabolic problems which occur in children are often more acute, but their remarkable resilience makes them able to withstand these more readily. Inevitably, the decision that a child has reached a terminal state is made more reluctantly. There is a tendency to 'treat till the last' in the hope that something will work; consequently, the time during which symptomatic care only is given may be relatively short (Chapter 14).

Nevertheless, whatever the patient's age, the overriding requirement is attention to detail—to the causes behind the symptoms and, above all, to a continual assessment which ceases only with the patient's death.

References and further reading

Browne, Sir Thomas (1672). *Religio medici pti*, p. 39.
Calman, K.C. and Welsh, J. (1983). Acute problems in cancer management. In *Recent Advances in Critical Care Medicine*, 2, pp. 161–74. Ed. by I. McA. Ledingham and C.D. Hanning. Churchill Livingstone, Edinburgh.
Fry, Christopher (1954). *The Dark is Light Enough*. Oxford University Press, London.
Stoll, Basil (Ed.) (1982). *Prolonged Arrest of Cancer*. John Willey, Chichester.

Cachexia and nutritional problems

Calman, K.C. (1982). Cancer cachexia. *British Journal of Hospital Medicine* **26**, 28.
Strain, A.J. (1979). Cancer cachexia in man: a review. *Investigative Cell Pathology* **2**, 181.

Ectopic hormones

Ratcliffe, J.G. and Rees, L.H. (1974). Clinical manifestations of ectopic hormone production. *British Journal of Hospital Medicine* **11**, 685.
Ross, E.J. (1972). Endocrine and metabolic manifestations of cancer. *British Medical Journal* **1**, 735.

Hypercalcaemia

Coombes, R.C., Ward, M.K., Greenberg, P.B., Hillyard, C.J., Tullich, B.R., Morrision, R. and Joplin, G.F. (1976). Calcium metabolism in cancer. *Cancer* **38**, 2111.
Symposium (1977). Hypercalcaemia in malignant disease. *Proceedings of the Royal Society of Medicine* **70**, 191.

Haematological problems

Alvares. A.P., Anderson, K.E., Conney, A.H. and Kappas, A. (1976). Interactions between nutritional factors and drug biotransformations in man. *Proceedings of the National Academy of Sciences of the USA* **73**, 2501.
Rumach, B.H., Holtzman, J. and Chase, H.P. (1973). Hepatic drug metabolism and protein malnutrition. *Journal of Pharmacology and Experimental Therapeutics* **186**, 441.
Zannoni, V.G. and Rikans, L.E. (1976). Ascorbic acid and drug detoxification. *Trends in Biochemical Sciences* **1**, 126.

Immunological problems

Currie, G.A. (1980). *Cancer and the Immune Response*. 2nd edn. Edward Arnold, London.

4

Psychological aspects

C. Murray Parkes

'How little the real sufferings of illness are known and understood. How little does anyone in good health fancy him or even herself into the life of a sick person.'
(Nightingale, 1946)

Time to live

A knowledge of the psychosocial aspects of dying is as important to those who care for people approaching death as is a knowledge of anatomy to the surgeon. In a sense, a cancer can extend beyond the person who harbours it, and any approach to understanding must embrace the entire social unit.

One could say the same of any other potentially fatal illness, but cancer has one great advantage over most of the rest—it gives us time. In one study of people who died from cancer in two London boroughs, 18 per cent were still under investigation or active treatment at the time of death. The rest were known by their relatives to have come to the end of active curative treatment *before* they died (Parkes, 1978). They had received a period of care, much of it at home, during which the patient, the family and care-givers had an opportunity to come to terms with the realities of the illness and to prepare themselves for the changes in the family which would come about when the patient died. In this chapter we shall examine how it is possible to do this and how doctors, nurses and others can help.

Both clinical experience and systematic studies confirm the importance of time in enabling people to prepare for disasters. The Harvard Bereavement Study showed that the death of a husband or wife under the age of 45 had a much more devastating effect if it was sudden and unexpected than if it had been gradual and anticipated. The diagnosis of malignant disease, as opposed to other causes of death, was significantly correlated with better adjustment to bereavement in the spouse a year later (Glick *et al.*, 1974; Parkes and Weiss, 1983).

Time is of little use if it is not properly employed. For the family and for the patient, the period of terminal care can be a time of growth and shared preparation, or it can be a time of defeat and mutual destruction. Used well, it can see the fulfilment and completion of a marriage. Used badly, it can mar the memory of good relationships and undermine the health of the survivors for years to come.

This was demonstrated by Cameron and Parkes (1983) in a comparison of 20 spouses of cancer patients who died in the Palliative Care Unit in Montreal, with 20 spouses of cancer patients who died in other wards of the same hospital.

43

The former had a great deal of support from professional staff and volunteers before and after bereavement. Their grief was measurably less severe and protracted and there was strikingly less anger and bitterness reported by the palliative care group than by the comparison group.

It is clearly imperative for us, the care-givers, to try to help patient and family to make the best use of the time that remains to them. This is the main aim of terminal care and the most important single service which we have to offer. If we fail to recognize the opportunity which terminal care represents in terms of family growth and development, we have nothing to offer but palliation, the mitigation of suffering by symptom relief alone. This type of palliative care (Latin *palliare*, to cloak) is of very limited value.

The starting point of any positive approach to terminal care must lie in the care-givers' ability to understand the nature of the problems confronting the family. The family (which includes the patient) is the unit of care, and the fact that it may be the patient who has sought our help gives us no excuse for ignoring the rest of the social unit which has been invaded by cancer. It would seem that the traditional injunction to young doctors to 'treat the whole patient' should be expanded to 'treat the whole family'. This implies that we must meet the family, or at least those members who are most closely involved, and attempt to open an effective channel of communication with them.

Traditional psychiatric diagnosis is of little value in this field. It will be of no help to a dying man to label him as suffering from 'a depression', nor will his wife benefit from being told she is suffering from 'an anxiety state'. Similarly, in deciding how to help a dying man, it is more appropriate to attempt to understand the problems to which his illness has given rise and to work out a way of helping him with these problems than to prescribe a 'treatment' as if the problems were themselves an illness.

Occasionally, malignant disease, or its medical or surgical consequences, may damage the brain and there is then a need to differentiate the symptoms of organic mental disorder from the emotional accompaniments of the disease. However, the symptoms of the organic disorder produced by malignant disease are no different from those of organic disorder arising from other causes; both are described in textbooks of neurology and psychiatry.

In considering the psychological aspects of malignant disease, a different frame of reference is required. This has emerged from studies of bereavements and other major life changes in recent years. Two main components have been identified as regular occurrences whenever a person is faced with the need to abandon one set of assumptions about the world and develop another. On the one hand, there is fear, apprehension and attempts to ward off the dangers which may yet be averted; on the other hand, there is grief, mourning and a tendency to move towards the realization of the new situation which is emerging.

In the face of advancing malignant disease, these two components are seen in family members as well as patients, and they influence all the interactions between care-givers and cared-for. For convenience we shall consider first how they affect the patient, and then move on to consider the other members of the patient's family before looking at some of the implications for the organization of the care-giving team.

Fear and the patient

Effective communication about matters of life and death is often hedged round with difficulties, most of them caused by the fear which such communication evokes in the patient, the family and the care-givers themselves. Our starting point for the understanding of this situation must therefore be to examine the fear.

Fear is a natural reaction to danger and it is easy to understand why it occurs when a family member is threatened with death. We are familiar with the neurophysiological accompaniments of fear and can appreciate their biological function in the fight/flight responses classically described by Cannon (1929). What is less generally recognized is the extent to which the expression of fear often becomes blocked, distorted or denied in a patient faced with the prospect of incurable disease.

This distortion of fear was illustrated clearly by a woman in her middle 50s. She was proud of the fact that she had forced her doctor to tell her that she had cancer and that she had no fear of dying. Her only complaint at the time of her admission to St Christopher's Hospice was concerned with her eyes. Every time she looked in the mirror she was upset by the expression on her face. This expression contrasted with her protested lack of fear, for her upper eyelids were retracted and she gave the appearance of being terrified. The ward staff tried to reassure her and give her the support which she needed, but within 24 hours she ran away by discharging herself home. During the ensuing weeks her medical attendants and her family found it hard to support her and cope with the continued deterioration in her physical condition. However, patience and concerned care paid off, and before long she was accepting help from the home-care nurses from the hospice. As her physical status became worse, her mental status improved, and eventually she asked to return to the hospice. On readmission, her frightened stare had passed and she was relaxed and seemed delighted to be back. The ward staff were struck by the change in her demeanour which remained friendly and serene until she died peacefully a few weeks later.

This case illustrates clearly the way in which fear can be intellectually denied but remain physiologically active. It also illustrates the interesting paradox that as death comes closer and more inescapable, the fear may grow less. This progression can never be taken for granted but, if circumstances of care are good, it occurs with sufficient frequency to encourage the nurses and doctors to do all in their power to further it.

In this example it was the existence of fear which was denied. In other cases, fear is accepted but its cause is denied or displaced. Thus a person may admit to feeling generally anxious but be unable to recognize any cause for his anxiety. Alternatively, the fear may be focused on a particular symptom or circumstance which has little to do with its real cause. Some people can feel fear on behalf of somebody else, a husband or wife whose life is affected by their illness, but deny any fear on their own behalf. Others attempt to control their fear by avoiding any thought or utterance which will evoke it; they restrict communication to trivialities and pointedly ignore any opportunity which doctors or others may give them to talk about their illness.

These defence mechanisms are not confined to the patients. Family members and even doctors and nurses regularly avoid or deny recognition of the danger which the patient is in as if, by so doing, they could thereby avoid the danger itself. Such avoidance of reality is assumed to be justified on the grounds that there is no point in upsetting people. 'Recognizing the danger will not make it go away. Why not pretend it isn't there?'

This may lead to a conspiracy between the family and the medical attendants to deceive the patient into thinking that he is getting better—a benevolent conspiracy often upset by the disease process itself. Faced with increasing evidence of his physical deterioration, the patient may eventually conclude that, if everybody is trying to deny the facts, then the facts must be truly terrible. This only increases his fear. As one patient sardonically remarked, 'I'm relieved to hear that I'm not dying of anything serious!'

Responding to the patient's fear and anxiety

When a person has an illness likely to prove fatal, it is too easy for us to imagine that we understand his anxiety and to discourage further communication about this distressing topic. He may say, 'I am frightened of dying,' and we hastily murmur, 'Yes, I understand,' and change to some more cheerful subject. Yet the dying patient can fear many things, and a more appropriate response may be, 'Are you? Well tell me just what you mean by that.' Encouraged to talk further, the patient will then express fears, some of which may be quite needless.

Five common fears were expressed to the writer by 61 patients who had been referred for psychological support at St Christopher's Hospice (Parkes, 1973). In that setting the commonest fears, expressed by 38 per cent of these patients, was of separation from loved people, homes or jobs. This separation fear is likely whenever people enter hospital and is, of course, a reasonable cause for distress among those who are dying. If the patient can find the courage to face up to the prospect of his death, the fear is transformed into grief with the prospect of resolution which this entails. The grief can be mitigated, if it is shared with others, and patients often express gratitude when permitted to 'break down'.

Separation anxiety will also be reduced if members of the family are encouraged to stay close to the patient and no restrictions are placed upon them visiting him in hospital. Likewise, every opportunity should be given to patients in hospital to visit their homes, if only for a few hours at a time. But in the end the grief of separation must be borne.

Second in frequency was the fear of becoming dependent on others, of losing control of physical faculties, of 'being a nuisance'. Fears of this type were experienced by 23 per cent of patients, many of them autonomous, self-reliant people who, throughout their lives, had preferred to look after others rather than be looked after themselves. It was most important for staff to respect their independence, to avoid patronizing or 'matronizing' attitudes, and to convey to the patients the fact that our service to them is a privilege rather than a chore.

Twenty per cent expressed fears of what would become of spouses, children or others who had been dependent on them in the past. Mothers, in particular, find it hard to believe that their children can survive without them, and it is often better for the family to face that fact squarely and to attempt to find a solution rather than postponing decision in the vain hope that the mother will recover. One very capable wife, who had coddled her husband throughout their married life, took just pride in the way she weaned him to a more autonomous life in the course of her final illness. After her death her husband continued to look after himself and his household 'Because that is the way my wife would have expected me to behave'. Caring staff may be able to help family members to make plans and to provide positive reassurance that help in bereavement will be available if it is needed.

Less common, experienced by 10 per cent, were fears of failing to complete some life task or fulfil some obligation. People who had spent years working to achieve some end which would now never be accomplished, or couples who had been staying together in the hope that a difficult relationship would one day improve, found it hard to accept the fact that their hopes would not be realized. In such instances, as in many others, anger is an understandable reaction and the patient might need to rage against God and man before he can take stock of the value of the life which remains to him. Any attempt on our part to combat the patient's rage by rational argument or reassurance is likely to fail and be taken as a rejection. It is better to 'bow before the storm' and wait until the patient is ready to take a more positive view.

Finally, there was a minority (7 per cent) whose main fear was of pain or mutilation. Most of these patients had already suffered severe pain at an earlier stage of the illness and they were fearful that it would return. The public image of cancer as a terrible disease which inevitably causes agonizing pain and physical mutilation is often reinforced by horror stories of patients who have died in agony. One Maltese lady assured me that she had known a person with cancer whose 'eyes dropped out', and it is always advisable to ask patients if they have ever known or heard of anybody who had a condition similar to their own. In most such cases it is possible to reassure them that they do not have *that* kind of cancer.

Some patients view themselves as having been made hideous by the disease, and it is important that we indicate by our behaviour that we can ignore any physical manifestation and continue to relate positively to the person regardless of his disabilities.

Linked with this is the fear of illness or death as a punishment. It seems to me that the concept of death as something done to a person which can be viewed as fair or unfair according to his deserts is the modern equivalent of the fear of judgment which played so large a part at the deathbeds of earlier times. This is sometimes expressed as a fear of the unknown. But if we have faith in the known, we have less need to fear the unknown. Not many people today express a fear of hell or a hope of heaven, but there are still many who find it easier to approach death because of some belief in an ultimate purpose which they may or may not call God.

Less easy to assess is the fear which is a reflection of that which patients see in the eyes of those around them. This was seldom reported but it was very evident whan it had led to avoidance of communication with family members or medical attendants who should have been the first people to be turned to for information and support.

These examples hardly do justice to the complexity of the problems which are encountered in our day-to-day work with people who are near to the ending of their lives, but we do not need to feel pessimistic. If the fear is unrealistic, we must provide reassurance; if it is realistic, we must be prepared to help the patient to confront the losses which are impending and to express the grief which is appropriate to each loss. By demonstrating our willingness to share the patient's grief we make it easier for him to accept it himself. Thus we gently help the patient to move from a position of avoidance towards a position of acceptance.

Grief and the patient

The strongest argument against benevolent conspiracies is not that they do not work (they sometimes do), but that they are rarely necessary. Experience has repeatedly shown that if a person is given the opportunity to learn the facts of his case, little by little, at his own pace, and provided he is encouraged to share with others the feelings which these facts evoke, and provided that others are not constantly feeding back to him their own fears, he will move progressively closer to a full realization of the situation without suffering overwhelming panic or despair.

The process of realization

This follows much the same pattern as the process of realization (grief) which follows any major loss (Parkes, 1972a). Grief arises in any situation in which a person is forced by circumstances to give up one constellation of attachments and accept another for which he is not prepared. The people and things we love are not encapsulated objects tied to us by individual strings. Each of them is the origin of a thousand strings. A loss can invalidate in one moment a great number of assumptions about the world. Hopes, plans, personal identity, the meaning of 'I' and 'we', habits of thought, ways of solving problems or obtaining comfort, all must change. For a while nothing can be taken for granted. The familiar world seems to have become unfamiliar, and a painful and exhausting process of revision must begin. The griever moves progressively from (i) a state of incomprehension or numbness ('I can't believe it's true'), to (ii) a period of intense inner struggle in which awareness of the reality of death conflicts with a strong impulse to recover the lost person or world in some form or other. This is followed by (iii) a phase of dejection and hopelessness in which the grieving person is aware of the discrepancy between his assumptions about the world and the world which now exists. Finally, (iv) little by little a new set of assumptions is built up to replace those that are now redundant. The widow begins to think of herself as a widow, the man who has a disabling illness stops thinking of himself as a provider. Both of them have to discover a new identity.

The transition is by no means smooth and people tend to go repeatedly through each of these phases of grief. For a long time, anything which brings the person or world which has been lost strongly to mind has the power to evoke another pang of grief, an episode of acute pining in which the urge to recover the lost person or world returns yet again. Hence people will say, 'It doesn't end'. On the other hand, the frequency and intensity of the pangs of grief grow gradually less. Most people who have suffered a major loss eventually experience a regaining of strength which encourages them to use words such as 'recovery' as if they had been through some kind of sickness; other terms which are equally appropriate are 'reintegration' or 'acceptance'.

The dying patient's grief

For the patient who is approaching the end of his life, the sickness of grief can complicate the physical sickness from which he is suffering; we have all heard of people who, on learning that their situation was 'hopeless', turned their face to the wall and died after a rapid decline. It would seem from anecdotes of this kind that psychological factors can play a part in determining the length of survival. Confirmation of this fact comes from an important study by Weisman and Worden (1975). These investigators calculated the average survival time of patients with various types of incurable cancer. They then compared a group of patients who survived longer than average with another group who died in a shorter period.

> 'Longevity ... was significantly correlated with patients who maintain active and mutually responsive relationships, provided that the intensity of demands was not so extreme as to alienate people responsible for the patients' care.'

On the other hand:

> 'Shorter survival was found among cancer patients who reflected long-stand-ing alienation, deprivation, depression and destructive relationships, which extended into the terminal stage of life. These attitudes of patients were expressed in despondency, desire to die, contemplation of suicide, inordinate complaints, all of which heaped more self-defeat and isolation upon them-selves.'

Clearly, the interaction between staff and patients is likely to play a major part in survival. More important, the quality of the life of the patient will be better if he has the opportunity to come to terms with his illness a little at a time. The question is not 'Should the doctor tell?', but 'How much is this patient ready to be told at this point in this illness?' We want to avoid the situation in which a person who is unprepared for bad news is told that he must lose everything he values. This situation is more likely to arise if doctors mislead their patients than if they admit from the start that the illness may be serious.

In the usual, and most desirable, course of events, the cancer patient is not faced with one massive loss but with a series of disappointments, each of which, with proper guidance, he can master before he is confronted with the next. He may need, at first, to realize that his symptoms are going to cause some major disruption in his life. After his first surgical operation he may be faced with lasting disability. If the disease recurs, he will probably come to recognize that he is unlikely to return to work, and eventually that his long-term plans will need revision. As the illness progresses, it may become appropriate for him to face the fact that he is unlikely to live for as long as he had hoped. If he can do this, it will then become easier for him to accept a shorter and shorter prognosis. When, at last, the final stage of the illness is reached, increasing disability seems to reduce the appetite not only for food but for life itself. The last episode is often more peaceful and less distressing than any previous phase.

Elizabeth Kubler Ross, in her classical study of the emotional reactions to dying, describes five stages which correspond fairly closely to the phases of realization which are found after bereavement (Ross, 1970). Other writers have criticized this classification on the grounds that many patients do not seem to follow the stages as described (Schulz and Aderman, 1974).

In fairness to Ross, she never claimed that all of her stages must be passed through by every patient, but the fact that she terms them 'stages' leads us to expect a sequence. Ross's stages are: (1) denial and isolation; (2) anger; (3) bargaining; (4) depression; and (5) acceptance. They describe a process of realization with the later stages reflecting a greater recognition of the facts of death. One of the reasons why this progression is seldom seen clearly among cancer patients is the irregular and unpredictable character of the disease itself. There is seldom one particular moment when doctors and patient become aware that the patient has a certain limited time to live; even when we think we can guess how long our patients are likely to survive we are usually wrong—to judge from a study of predictions of survival at St Christopher's Hospice (Parkes, 1972b). More often, the patient is faced with a number of disappointments, each of which must be grieved before the person is ready to move on to the next. Thus, the course of the emotional reaction to the illness is likely to take a step-wise pattern, with episodes of anxiety leading to episodes of grief followed by relatively peaceful periods of acceptance until the next turning point is reached. Weisman and Worden (1977, personal communication) call these 'crisis points', and are currently mapping out the 'crisis points' which characterize each major type of cancer. Some of these disappointments may be overcome quite easily while others may severely tax the patient's resources of courage and hope.

A relaxed and contented patient is a great source of reassurance to the family, particularly if he is being nursed at home. Conversely, the patient who is suffering unrelieved distress may place an intolerable burden on the family who may be quite unable to cope with his rage and despair. I have known relationships to break down because of the irritability and anger evoked by severe physical distress.

Fear and the family

The period of terminal care enables family members to prepare for the patient's death and to make restitution to him for the fact of their own survival and for any failures or ambivalence which have previously impaired the relationship. The term 'anticipatory grieving' has been used to describe this process, but this is usually a misnomer. A wife whose husband is about to die may experience a great deal of fear and anticipatory anxiety, but her grief will seldom proceed to the point of detachment and she will not make serious plans for her future life. The reasons are twofold. One is that far from encouraging detachment, the presence of a sick person strengthens attachment; we tend to come closer to the helpless and weak. The other is that a plan is psychologically so close to a wish that any plan for life after the patient's death can become a wish. The person who has wished another one dead eventually feels that it was the wish which caused the death and he may even come to see himself as a murderer.

A dying patient may want to make plans for his nearest relatives and this may be something which they will respect. The dying know, of course, that their wishes are likely to be respected and this gives them a power which may be abused. More appropriately, a person who is close to death can attempt to influence those whom he expects to survive him, not by prescribing what they should or should not do, but by releasing them from any sense of continued obligation to him.

Both patients and family members have their own fears and griefs to face and they may choose to avoid communication with each other about them. Even then, however, each continues to influence the other, and any attempt to understand the situation must take this into account. A wife, for instance, may deliberately avoid discussing her husband's illness with a doctor for fear that she will be unable to conceal from her husband any distress to which this communication gives rise. She may, therefore, fail to understand the nature or seriousness of his condition and be unprepared for its outcome. Similarly, a patient may imagine that he is protecting his spouse by concealing from her his awareness of the true state of affairs. The spouse, on the other hand, may be under considerable strain because she is attempting to conceal the same facts from him. In this way both parties are deprived of the chance to share their feelings and to create something positive out of the last chapter of their marriage.

More often than not, patient and family are 'out of step' because the patient is given a more optimistic view of his situation than are his family. One might expect this to make the family members more distressed than the patient since they have a fuller knowledge of the danger, but in fact family members regularly adopt the psychological defence of postponement as a means of coping with the situation. In order to fulfil their obligations to the patient and provide him with proper care, they repress their own grief, adopt a rigorous policy of self-control and behave as if their understanding of illness was the same as the patient's. This inhibition of realization is bought at a price and many family members are aware of a strong sense of rising inner tension which may be expressed as a fear that they will 'break down'. They may show many of the physiological accompaniments of severe anxiety—eating little, losing weight and sleeping poorly—and it is sometimes necessary to take the patient into hospital simply to give his nearest relatives a rest. A minor tranquillizer such as diazepam by day or nitrazepam at night will often enable a spouse to continue his or her care for the patient, but doctors should be wary of encouraging dependence on these and other drugs.

The sad fact is that much of this defensiveness is unnecessary. If only the patient and the family can be helped to share the truth instead of avoiding it, the general level of tension will often be reduced and the need for drugs to reduce emotional tension artificially will diminish. Unfortunately, doctors and nurses usually find it easier to administer the drugs than to take the time to talk with patients and family members in the hope of resolving rather than repressing their problems.

During the terminal stage the primary focus of care is inevitably the patient rather than the family, and family members should not be discouraged from the self-sacrifice which may be their last gift to the patient. It is easy for doctors and nurses to reassure them that their help is not needed—'Don't you worry, leave everything to us'. But in doing so we may simply confirm a relative in the belief that he or she is unable to care for the dying person at this most critical time in his life. The wife, who after nursing her husband at home finally realizes that she cannot cope, will feel doubly guilty if the ward staff make her feel an intruder at his bedside and restrict the time which she can spend with him in hospital.

Relatives and patients are usually grateful for the efficient way in which hospital staff take over responsibility for a situation which has become increasingly frightening, but we should not let their gratitude blind us to the important role which each of them will continue to play in the life of the other. At this time it is we, not they, who are the intruders and we should make our intervention as gentle as possible. In a terminal care ward the patient's family are not intruders, nor are they honoured guests; they are an intimate part of the network of care. They are both care-givers and cared-for. They belong in the hospital as of right and their needs must be of paramount importance to us. The patient's troubles are likely soon to be over but the family's may be just beginning.

Research has shown that family members tend to spend more time at the patient's bedside in St Christopher's Hospice than at other hospitals in the vicinity and they play a larger part in caring for the patient. In other hospitals the care is characterized by the term, 'Leave it to us'; at St Christopher's the preferred phrase is, 'The hospital is a family' (Parkes and Parkes, 1983).

Counselling the family

There are few forms of therapy more exacting than counselling a family which includes a dying patient. But it is inspiring to see how family members can grow together at such times. The method of counselling is too personal for a general description to be appropriate, but there are a few simple rules which apply whether it is a patient or close family member who needs our help. Non-verbal communication is as important as verbal—the touch of a hand or a smile at the right moment which implies 'It's all right, you don't need to feel afraid,' or the sensitive awareness that this is the moment to remain silent and wait for the truth to sink in and for the next question to emerge.

Confidence in our ability to cope with the situation in our own way and confidence in the other person's abilities will increase with experience. Awareness of the right moment to lower tension by smiling or encouraging someone to 'cheer up' and the right moment to remain serious when the other is offering you an escape ('You didn't come here to listen to my moaning') will grow if we observe carefully the outcome of our attempts to help. One important component is a philosophical or a religious attitude in the counsellor which enables him or her to indicate that although the final phase of life may be 'awful' in the old meaning of the word (filled with awe), it need not be approached with pessimism. If we can see the life which precedes death as a positive time with a meaning to be discovered, then patients and their families will find it easier to do the same. We must, however, allow them to discover their own meanings—we cannot impose our own, however valid they may seem to us. People of a religious faith are in a minority today, and for most of us the search for meaning is not expressed in 'religious' language. Even so, one can justifiably regard the search as a 'religious' activity since it is concerned with the attempt to relate the significance of an individual life to that of some wider reality.

'Involvement' and 'distancing'

Although the counselling of the family at times of death is exacting, I do not think it is too difficult to be attempted by the majority of people who have chosen to join the care-giving professions. There are, however, certain peculiarities about the circumstances in which death now takes place and certain aspects of the training of doctors and nurses which militate against this. It is almost as if the health care system, by dedicating itself to the saving of life, had ruled death out of order. Or, as Eric Cassell (1974) put it, 'Death is now a failure of technology'. The doctor's basic medical training teaches him to see the human body as a series of mechanisms which are liable to disorder. The case-demonstration method of teaching at the bedside educates the young doctor to see his fellow human beings as 'the cancer in the end bed' and teaches him how to communicate with his colleagues *about* the patient without communicating *with* the patient at all. The dying patient is commonly omitted from discussion altogether.

Nurses learn that it is not permitted for them to discuss serious issues with a patient, and they are encouraged to model themselves on the brisk, efficient senior who sees it as a virtue not to get 'emotionally involved'. Unlike trainee nurses, medical students seldom see 'emotional involvement' as a problem, probably because they rarely get to know a patient well enough for it to become a risk. However, for the nurse or social worker whose work brings her closer to her patients for longer periods of time, there is always the 'danger' of a relationship developing.

We cannot avoid this issue; human relationships are dangerous. When we get attached to our patients we begin to suffer with them and we may even become involved to the point where we are overwhelmed by our own distress and become useless to them. Although this is true, it does not justify the extreme distancing which is encouraged in many teaching hospitals.

In all social situations the question of 'appropriate distance' arises. We are constantly monitoring the physical and mental distance which governs effective and useful communication. Some people are bad at distancing—either they stand too close and assume an intimacy which does not exist, or they put up barriers and repel attempts to 'make contact'.

In general the person who is feeling frightened or insecure has a greater need of close physical contact with people he can trust than the person who is strong and independent. If we are to support a family through the hard times of terminal illness, it will usually be necessary for us to achieve a closeness which is unusual outside the family. We may need to hold a hand or to put an arm round a person who is in deep distress and give them the same kind of non-verbal assurance which a mother can give to her child. Nevertheless, even a mother who is comforting a child must remain in control. We must remain close but at the same time capable of taking a detached view of what is going on.

Difficult patients and difficult staff

A well-organized network of care will deal with most of the problems which emerge with sufficient success for morale to be maintained among patients, families and staff for most of the time, but there are some situations of particular difficulty. The person whose insecurity causes him to panic, or cling or make angry and unreasonable demands, is likely to be labelled as 'attention seeking'. This label may be justified, but it will only make the person more insecure if we get angry in return. If we recognize the underlying reason for such be-haviour, we can usually succeed in supporting the person in the manner which suits him best. For some a firm line which says 'I know what I'm doing and you're going to learn to trust me' is best; for others a full explanation of the nature of the treatments which are being prescribed, and for others positive reassurance will be needed. In all cases, a listening ear and the opportunity to express feelings are prerequisites to successful care.

We shall often meet bravado in the compulsively self-reliant person who has never trusted anybody but himself—an attitude which often reflects deep-seated insecurity which may have been present from childhood. Such people need to believe that it is they who control us and not we who control them.

It is hard for a relf-reliant person to accept the restrictions of illness and it often helps to show him that you realize how hard it is by discussing the problem. Staff members of a controlling disposition are likely to get at odds with this type of person. The doctor or nurse may be provoked to make dispro-portionate use of his or her power, and in the end nobody emerges with credit. The care of the self-reliant requires patience, flexibility and not a little humility.

Paradoxically, it is often those who are most afraid of dying who demand euthanasia. They seem to be saying, 'Since I cannot avert the thing that I dread I will at least control it by choosing it for myself.' Again, the basic problem is lack of trust. Sometimes requests for euthanasia are reasonable re-quests for a way out of intolerable pain or physical distress. In such circum-stances the obvious answer is to provide proper care so that the distress is relieved. Likewise, the relief of psychological distress will usually bring about a change in attitude to euthanasia. Among those who do not change their minds one often has the feeling that if one said, 'Do you want it now?' the patient would reply, 'No, but I would like to have it available in case I need it.' Similarly, one sometimes meets a depressed patient who keeps the means of suicide to hand as a source of reassurance.

Despite the prominence given to recent debates on euthanasia, it is rare for a patient with incurable cancer to commit suicide. Nevertheless, suicides do occasionally occur and there is evidence from statistical studies of an increased risk of suicide after bereavement (Sainsbury, 1982). We should be aware of that risk when assessing the mental state of any severely agitated or depressed person. The question, 'Has it been so bad that you have wanted to kill yourself?' will nearly always get an honest answer and we should never be afraid to ask. Once the risk is recognized, it is usually possible to provide the physical and emotional care which will remove it.

Family members are often afraid that revealing the facts of his illness to the patient will cause him to kill himself. They may even try to force us to agree to a policy of concealment. Such fears are usually unrealistic and reflect the family's own fears of the situation. It follows that we should respond, not by colluding with the family or by ignoring their wishes, but by exploring with them their feelings about the situation and giving them the emotional support which they need.

Finding time

Of all the problems which we are faced with in the care of the dying patient, the greatest and one of the commonest is lack of time, either because the illness is progressing rapidly or because we are ourselves over-committed. In the latter case it should be possible to call on the help of others: a busy family doctor, for instance, may find that a health visitor or district nurse can spend time talking with patient and family, local clergy can be asked to provide pastoral care, neighbours or friends or the members of various voluntary organizations can be involved.

The problem resolves ultimately into one of priorities. How important is the contribution which doctors and nurses can make to the conscious life of a dying man or a bereaved relative? How does this compared with the importance of other demands upon our time?

If it is the patient who lacks time or is caught in a mesh of fear, denial or depression, it may still be possible to achieve a lot with the judicious use of drugs. Drugs such as diazepam 5 mg four-hourly are usually safe and often effective. If a more powerful agent is needed, a phenothiazine such as chlorpromazine 12.5-25 mg four- to six-hourly will reduce agitation. This has the advantage that phenothiazines potentiate the analgesic effects of morphine or diamorphine and can conveniently be added as a syrup to the narcotic mixture (see Chapter 7).

For the depressed patient who is inaccessible because he 'has given up' or who is failing to respond to our efforts to help, tricyclic antidepressants such as amitriptyline (which also help to reduce anxiety) 25 mg three times daily or 50-75 mg at night may help to make life worth living. But we should expect to have to wait five to ten days for these drugs to become fully effective. The monoamine oxidase inhibitors should not be prescribed because they are incompatible with opiates and many of the other drugs which are likely to be needed in the terminal stage. On the other hand, I have known a few cancer patients with psychotic levels of depression and psychomotor retardation who failed to respond to tricyclic antidepressants but made a rapid response to modified electric convulsive therapy.

The use of morphine and diamorphine is discussed elsewhere (Chapter 5), but it is worth noting at this point that they are themselves tranquillizers and are particularly effective when unpleasant physical symptoms are producing distress. Patients who are in severe physical distress are unlikely to make progress in tackling the psychological implications of their situation. But drugs should never be used as a substitute for personal attention and support. Drugs are not a way of relieving the care-givers of the responsibility of caring or of providing a 'happy ending' by 'knocking the patient out' ('She's asking questions—double the Largactil'). It is rarely necessary to render a patient unconscious in order to relieve distress, although many patients will become drowsy and at times a little confused in the last few hours or days of life.

Grief and the family

The use of drugs is much more controversial when we come to consider the needs of the relatives. As long as the patient is alive, they need to remain fully competent and to support him; clearly, medication should be kept to a minimum. We should also be very wary of using drugs after bereavement. Grief needs to be expressed and clinical experience suggests that drugs inhibit such expression. There are no grounds for prescribing tranquillizers or antidepressants to bereaved relatives as a routine. Such drugs should be reserved for the potentially suicidal and for those who, despite all efforts to help, remain in states of chronic agitation or depression for abnormally long periods.

Vulnerability

At St Christopher's Hospice we have identified as needing support in bereavement members of one family in four by using a screening procedure derived from the Harvard Bereavement Study (Parkes, 1981). There is evidence from our follow-up studies that certain individuals are at greater risk than others (to a statistically significant degree), but the results are not so clear-cut that we can say for sure that others should *not* be followed up.

Whether the screening procedure is used as a means of deciding who should be visited by a counsellor or simply as a way of alerting counsellors to the need to give rather more support to some than to others, it is suggested that attempts should be made to assess the risk to the person most affected by the patient's death whenever sufficient evidence is available.

The following people were found to be at special risk after bereavement,

1. Persons of low socio-economic status.
2. Housewives without employment outside the home.
3. Those with young children at home (who may themselves be at risk).
4. Those without a supportive family or with a family which actively discourages the expression of grief.
5. Those who show a strong tendency to cling to the patient before his death and/or to pine intensely for him afterwards.
6. Those who express strong feelings of anger or bitterness before or after the patient's death.
7. Those who express strong feelings of self-reproach.

All these criteria can be assessed by hospice staff in about 90 per cent of the families of patients who die at St Christopher's. Other evidence of risk may emerge in a few cases. For instance, we may occasionally learn that a family member has a history of previous suicidal threats or psychiatric illness. Even if none of these criteria is satisfied, it should always be possible for staff members to request a follow-up visit.

It is still uncertain whether a formal screening procedure is necessary in order to identify those at risk. We have developed a questionnaire based on the above questions, and have demonstrated that it does have predictive value (Fig. 4.1). But there is still much room for improvement, further research is necessary before any definitive statement can be made and another form is currently being tested. Any assessment of this kind must be treated as highly confidential, and it is particularly important to avoid stigmatizing the bereaved people who are visited or indicating to them that they are expected to collapse under the strain of bereavement.

The effectiveness of the bereavement counselling practised at St Christopher's

CONFIDENTIAL   Case Note

Name of patient   Age   Number:

(surname first in capitals)

                              Date of admission   Date of death

---

Surname of   First
key person   Name:
Address: Telephone

Relationship to patient   O.P. Yes/No

Do you think key person would object to follow up?   Yes/No/Not known

Staff members(s) most closely involved:

Other family members in need of help:

Comments (include details of help already being given):

FSP   Signed: p.t.o

Questionnaire (Ring one item in each section. Leave blank if not known: CONFIDENTIAL

...... Tick here if key person not well enough known to enable these questions to be answered.

A.	B. Occupation of principal wage earner of key person's family**	C.	D.	E.
Children under 14 at home		**Employment of K.P. outside home**	**Clinging or pining**	**Anger**
0. None	1. Profs. & Exec.	0 Works FT	1. Never	1. None (or normal)
1. One	2. Semi-profes.	1. Works PT	2. Seldom	2. Mild irritation
2. Two	3. Office & clerical	3. Retired	3. Moderate	3. Moderate occasional outbursts
3. Three	4. Skilled manual	4. Housewife only	4. Frequent	4. Severe spoiling relationships
4. Four	5. Semi-skilled manual	5. Unemployed	5. Constant	5. Extreme always bitter
5. Five or more	6. Unskilled manual		6. Constant intense	
	** If in doubt, guess			

F.	G.	H.
Self-reproach	**Relationship now**	**How will key person cope?***
1. None	0. Close intimate relat. with another	1. **Well.** Normal grief and recovery without special help
2. Mild vague and general	2. Warm supportive family permitting expression of feeling	2. **Fair,** probably get by without special help
3. Moderate—some clear self-reproach	3. Family supportive but live at distance	3. **Doubtful,** may need special help.
4. Severe—preoc. self blame	4. Doubtful	4. **Badly,** requires special help.
5. Extreme—major problem	5. None of these	5. **Very badly,** requires urgent help.
		* All scoring 4–5 on H will be followed up.

Fig. 4.1 'Key person' card.

Hospice over the last eight years has been evaluated in a random allocation study. This showed that counselling of 'high-risk' widows and widowers was associated with a level of adjustment 20 months after bereavement, which was equivalent to that of low-risk widows and widowers who had not been counselled. Unsupported 'high-risk' widows and widowers described more symptoms reflecting persisting anxiety and tension and significantly greater consumption of drugs, alcohol and tobacco than the counselled group (Parkes, 1981). Further confirmation of the value of bereavement counselling has been reported by Raphael in a similar study using a comparable method of selecting widows at special risk (Raphael, 1977), but some other bereavement services, which make no attempt to identify 'high-risk' bereaved or which expect the bereaved to come to an office rather than visiting them in their homes, have proved less satisfactory.

The St Christopher's service uses volunteer counsellors who visit in their home people thought to be at risk. Visitors may be specially recruited or selected by the volunteer organizer from among the local volunteers who offer help to the hospice. An exhaustive programme of further selection and training is currently being piloted by a psychologist, Susan Le Poidevin. Those thought suitable take part in a training programme which aims to teach them basic interviewing skills as well as acquainting them with the special problems of bereavement. Role play forms a large part of the training and helps to make familiar the kinds of situation which the visitors will meet in counselling the bereaved. It also helps them to understand what it feels like to suffer a family bereavement, and they soon become more 'expert' at bereavement visiting than many of the 'professionals'.

The initial visit is usually made 10–14 days after death. By this time the family members, who have usually converged during the week of the funeral, have dispersed, and the bereaved have come through the initial stage of shock or numbness. Grief is at its height and someone who calls at this time will usually find the bereaved glad of the opportunity to talk. Although the visitors have been warned never to press themselves on any person who seems reluctant to see them, it is rare for them to be treated as intruders. Bereaved people today often seem afraid of expressing their grief to their family for fear of upsetting them. Their friends, they think, will drop them if they embarrass them by crying, and the professionals, be they doctors, lawyers or bank managers, are thought to be too busy. Consequently, the visitor who has called 'Because I know what it is like and I thought you might like to talk about it' will be very welcome and will be meeting an important need.

The psychological reaction to bereavement usually follows the pattern described on page 48. Apart from permitting the expression of grief and, in most cases, reassuring the bereaved that the violent emotions and physical sensations they are experiencing are normal, visitors are able to assess the need for additional support. They can find out how much reliance the bereaved can place upon family members and how many others rely on them. Some idea can also be obtained of the ways in which the other members of the family are reacting to the loss and whether any of them are likely to need help. If there are health problems or there seems to be any danger of suicide, visitors urge the bereaved to obtain medical help, and themselves report without delay to the doctor in charge of the visiting scheme so that he can contact the family doctor.

The help of social workers, lawyers, clergy and others may be needed and the initial visit may reveal that full support is already being provided and no further visits will be needed. But in most cases several visits will be necessary, if only to ensure that the support which was anticipated is being given.

As the intensity and frequency of the pangs of grief grow less, a different set of problems emerges. At this time it is more likely that the bereaved will need permission to stop grieving rather than to express grief. They may need to be helped to find new opportunities for personal development. It takes courage to recommit oneself in a world in which one has suffered a great loss. The bereaved have discovered that grief is the price they pay for love, and they hesitate to run the risk that they will have to pay that price again—'It's safer not to fall in love'. And yet in time they may also find that they have survived the pain of grief and that death has left them more willing to recognize the full range of meanings—good and bad—which life offers to us.

Many of the people who seek help in their bereavement win through to greater maturity and a richer life. And we too can benefit from their experience. Just as close relationships with the dying help to reduce our fears of death, so counselling the bereaved makes it easier to see bereavement as an acceptable part of life.

Some special problems

Every bereavement is different and we can never know how a person will emerge. People who deny the need to grieve by filling their lives with activities or by getting rid of all reminders of the lost person are only storing up trouble. In these instances it is important to reassure them that it is safe to grieve and to seek for 'linking objects' (mementoes, photographs and the like) which help to trigger repressed grief. Once grief has been expressed it will tend to follow a more normal course.

Anger and guilt

The expression of anger or guilt after bereavement is one of the most difficult problems. At this stage it is too late to say to the dead person, 'I'm sorry', and the bereaved are sometimes tempted to punish themselves or those around them by endless and embittered grieving ('grief' and 'aggrieved' have a common origin). Yet many bereaved people discover ways of expressing their discontent which are creative rather than destructive (St Christopher's Hospice is itself the consequence of one such creative endeavour). The role of the counsellor is to provide a sounding board, a patient and understanding person who will accept the contradictions of ambivalence without criticism or rejection. But the function of the sounding board is not just to absorb; when the right note is struck it can resound and respond with encouragement and hope. The bereavement counsellor is not passive, but alert to all that is passing and ready to give praise and comfort when they are due.

Suicide

During the years 1969–74, no less than six relatives of patients who had died at St Christopher's Hospice are known to have killed themselves within two years of bereavement. Between 1975 and 1982, when the Family Service was offering bereavement counselling to all family members thought to be at risk, only two suicides are known to have occurred.

The importance of assessing suicidal risk cannot be overstressed and we should never hesitate to ask direct questions on this topic. Bereavement is one of the commonest causes of suicide, and much needless loss of life could be prevented if we faced up to the implications of this fact (Sainsbury, 1972)).

Several studies have shown that the majority of suicidal people talk about their plans before a suicidal attempt is made. The person who is a serious suicidal risk may not mention the fact unless directly questioned, but will then be found to have a well-thought-out plan. On the other hand, remarks such as 'I wouldn't care if I died tomorrow' seldom indicate a true suicidal intent.

Those tempted to suicide are often isolated from their families and it is important to draw in the support of someone who can keep a close eye on them until the danger is past. In some cases the family doctor may need to arrange admission to psychiatric care, in others he may decide that the situation can be contained at home. In either case he will be well advised to encourage visitors to continue their support. Given the choice between taking an overdose and phoning the friend who has left a telephone number 'which you can ring at any time if things get unbearable', the potential suicide will often choose the latter course.

Withdrawal from life

For those who lack confidence to begin again, either because they have always had a low opinion of themselves or because there is little inducement to look forward, it is tempting to use grief as an excuse to withdraw from life. In such cases the counsellor may be misused as a means of validating this withdrawal ('You understand how much I loved him, you tell them that I can't cope without him'). Like the physically disabled patient who clings on to the 'sick role' after the illness is past, so the mourner may demand endorsement of the 'mourning role'.

Those who are particularly lonely or lacking in confidence can easily come to rely too much on the visitor. In such cases the time will come for the counsellor to prepare a plan for his or her own withdrawal. This is not done in an abrupt or rejecting way, but the usual rule of medical care (the sicker the patient, the more care he gets) must be reversed. Continued support becomes conditional upon the bereaved person moving toward the accomplishment of a new set of goals. It sounds brutal to say 'Ring me again when you have gone out of the house on your own', but this is sometimes necessary and, provided our expectations are not unrealistic, will usually produce results. Often a small initial success leads to a greater one. If this policy is adopted, the danger of the bereaved becoming perpetually dependent on the counsellor is lessened.

The care-givers

In the brief compass of this chapter it has been impossible to do more than touch on the range of problems which are as numerous and as varied as the people who suffer from them. In offering guidelines, I have inevitably oversimplified in the interests of clarity. Not all the people we set out to help will benefit from our ministrations, and we must be prepared to admit and understand our own failures.

The risk of failure should not deter us from trying. There is no such thing as a 'hopeless case' and no excuse for ignoring the psychological needs of the dying and the bereaved. If we accept that fact, we should provide as wide a range as possible of skilled people to meet these needs. There is a place for volunteers and others with little training in psychological medicine, but we should not conclude that more sophisticated approaches are never needed. The needs of the dying and the bereaved will sometimes tax the skills of the most experienced social workers and psychiatrists, and it is important that these are available as a source of additional help.

Support to the supporters

The capacity of the care-givers to cope with the emotional needs of patients and families is fostered by any formal or informal network of support which allows them to put into words and share with each other their perceptions of the life situations which they encounter. The members of the network, be it a ward team, home-care team or other work group, should be sufficiently open with each other for it to be possible for them to talk, not only about the emotional problems of the patients and families whom they are trying to help, but also about the feelings which these people evoke in the team members themselves. Regular team meetings at which problems arising in the care of particular families can be discussed in more depth are an important source of support for patients' families and the caring team. A well-functioning support group will know when one of its members is becoming too closely involved and will move at once to support him or her—either by taking over some of the care or by pointing out what the care-giver is doing in the hope that, with insight, he or she will behave more appropriately. Similarly, members of a group may help each other to understand why a particular patient evokes anger or makes them feel guilty; in doing so, the group will learn to take a more objective view of a painful situation.

It is, of course, important for team members to be able to trust each other, and a support group is no place for scoring points off each other or undermining confidence. The senior member of the group carries particular responsibility for ensuring that the group is truly supportive, and it follows that the leaders will need their own support. How this is organized will depend on the size and circumstances of the institution.

There will always be some who, for one reason or another, are not adequately helped by their own work team. Hierarchial struggles within the team or fear of censure from above may reduce the effectiveness of such a group. For this reason it is important to ensure that there are a number of alternative sources of support available to staff who are working in emotionally charged situations. The visiting psychiatrist has an important role to play here, but not everyone wants to talk to a psychiatrist; a range of nurse advisers, visiting clergy, social workers and others should be accessible and able to provide individual or group support. A terminal care service or team should be a community—a network in which nobody need feel isolated.

Much support will be informal and take place outside staff meetings. There are no rigid roles; at times we shall all be care-givers and at other times cared-for. The senior staff must keep a close watch for sources of strain within a particular part of the organization—a spate of deaths on one ward, the absence on leave of a key member of staff, the effects of an influenza epidemic on staffing levels, or the approaching death of a favourite patient should all alert the seniors to give extra support to a particular part of the network. It is essential to have sufficient numbers and flexibility of staff to ensure that this support is available.

The psychiatrist should take final responsibility for the most difficult or intractable psychological problems. Experience at St Christopher's Hospice indicates that these are comparatively few. Much more important is the role of the psychiatrist as a support to the front-line care-givers. He should play a part in organizing and maintaining high standards of psychosocial care; teaching the medical and nursing staff, consulting regularly with staff about the patients and family members under their care and, at times, providing individual support to staff members who have problems of their own (although it is advisable to refer them to other places if long-term therapy is required).

The sharing of information within the care-giving team is a necessary activity in any therapeutic community in which the responsibility for care is shared by a number of people. It implies that the team as a whole will exercise professional standards of discretion and will not gossip outside the work group or otherwise misuse the information at their disposal. Within the team, a free and frequent interchange of ideas and observations should be encouraged. At problem-focused meetings, a group of nurses on a ward can piece together the information which each of them has picked up in day-to-day interaction with a family to make a picture of the whole which immediately explains why a particular patient or family member is in difficulties. Apart from the value of this exercise to the person they are trying to help, the sharing of information in this way alerts the staff to the importance of listening and fosters their interest in psychosocial aspects of care.

Terminal care is a matter of human relationships. There are skills to be learned and insights which can be gained from reading books, but the challenge and the reward of terminal care arise from the fact that it demands that we use the whole of ourselves to relate to fellow human beings who are in trouble. This can only be learned by experience in a community in which relationships are valued and fostered.

> "'Mourning is not forgetting,' he said gently, his helplessness vanishing and his voice becoming wise. "It is an undoing. Every minute tie has to be untied and something permanent and valuable recovered and assimilated from the knot. The end is gain, of course. Blessed are they that mourn, for they shall be made strong, in fact. But the process is like all other human births, painful and long and dangerous."'
>
> (Allingham, 1957)

References

Allingham, Margery (1957). *The Tiger in the Smoke*. Penguin, Harmondsworth.

Cameron, J. and Parkes, C.M. (1983). Terminal care: Evaluation of effects on surviving family of care before and after bereavement. *Postgraduate Medical Journal* **59**, 1.

Cannon, W.B. (1929). *Bodily Changes in Pain, Hunger, Fear and Rage*. Appleton, London and New York.

Cassell, E. (1974). Dying in a technological society. In *Death Inside Out*, p.43. Ed by P. Steinfels and R.M. Veatch. Harper & Row, New York.

Glick, I.O., Weiss, R.S. and Parkes, C.M. (1974). *The First Year of Bereavement*. Wiley, New York.

Nightingale, F. (1946). *The Art of Nursing*. Claud Morris, London.

Parkes, C.M. (1972a). *Bereavement: Studies of Grief in Adult Life*. Tavistock and Pelican, London; International Universities Press, New York.

Parkes, C.M. (1972b). Accuracy of predictions of survival in later stages of cancer. *British Medical Journal* **2**, 29.

Parkes, C.M. (1973). Attachment and autonomy at the end of life. In *Support, Innovation and Autonomy*, pp. 151–66. Ed. by R. Gosling, Tavistock, London.

Parkes, C.M. (1978). Home or hospital? Patterns of care for the terminally ill cancer patient as seen by surviving spouses. *Journal of the Royal College of General Practitioners* **28**, 19.

Parkes, C.M. (1981). Evaluation of a bereavement service. *Preventive Psychiatry* **1**, 179.

Parkes, C.M. and Parkes, J. (1984). 'Hospice' versus 'Hospital' care; re-evaluation after ten years as seen by surviving spouses. *Postgraduate Medical Journal* **60**, 38.

Parkes, C.M. and Weis, R.S. (1983). *Recovery from Bereavement*. Basic Books, New York.

Raphael, B. (1977). Preventive intervention with the recently bereaved. *Archives of General Psychiatry* **34**, 1450.

Ross, E.K. (1970). *On Death and Dying*. Tavistock, London.

Sainsbury, P. (1972). The social relation of suicide: the value of combined epidemiologial and case study approach. *Social Science and Medicine* **6**, 189.

Schulz, R. and Aderman, D. (1974). Clinical research and the stages of dying. *Omega* **5**, 137.

Weisman, A.D. and Worden, J. (1975). Psychosocial analysis of cancer deaths. *Omega* **6**, 61.

Weisman, A.D. and Worden, J. (1977). Personal communication.

5

Relief of pain

Robert G. Twycross

'Among the remedies which it has pleased Almighty God to give to man to relieve his sufferings, none is so universal and so efficacious as opium.'
(Thomas Sydenham, 1680)

'He was far too humble and indeed, too experienced, to expect that the Almighty's more quixotic benefits should ever prove to be unadulterated jam.'
(Allingham, 1957)

To many people, incurable cancer means a painful progressive illness ending in an agonizing death. In fact only about two-thirds of patients with far-advanced cancer experience significant pain in the weeks or months prior to death, and satisfactory relief is obtained in the majority (Twycross and Lack, 1983). There are still, however, too many patients for whom comfort is denied. This may be temporary because of a long latent period between the onset of pain and the initiation of treatment. Alternatively, unrelieved pain may continue to be a problem until death, largely because of a failure to apply the well-established principles of cancer pain management (Hunt *et al.*, 1977).

The nature of pain

Perhaps one of the most important reasons for unrelieved pain is a failure by doctors and nurses to appreciate fully that pain is not simply a physical sensation. It is a dual phenomenon: one part being the perception of the sensation, and the other the patient's emotional reaction to it. It follows that a person's pain threshold will vary according to mood and morale, and intensity of pain likewise. Attention must therefore be paid to non-pharmacological factors which modulate pain threshold as well as to the correct use of analgesic and other drugs (Table 5.1).

Death is probably the loneliest experience any of us will ever have to face. Most patients fear the process of dying—'Will it hurt?', 'Will I suffocate?'—and many fear death itself. Many of these fears will remain unspoken unless the patient is given the opportunity to express them. The doctor needs to give time and opportunity for the patient to talk about his progress or lack of it. To quote from the experience of one group of general practitioners: 'As the doctor-patient relationship improved, many doctors found they could reduce the drugs. As the true diagnosis of the patient's pain became clear and the patient was helped to deal with the pain of dying, there was less need for sedatives, tranquillizers and analgesics' (Harte, J.D. (1975), personal communication).

Table 5.1 Factors affecting pain threshold

Threshold lowered	Threshold raised
Discomfort	Relief of symptoms
Insomnia	Sleep
Fatigue	Rest
Anxiety	Sympathy
Fear	Understanding
Anger	Companionship
Sadness	Diversional activity
Depression	Reduction in anxiety
Boredom	Elevation of mood
Introversion	Analgesics
Mental isolation	Anxiolytics
Social abandonment	Antidepressants

Moreover, it is all too easy for a doctor to forget that acute (transient) and chronic (persistent) pains are as different from one another as acute and chronic renal failure. A doctor's understanding of pain is usually taken from his own experience of acute pain—toothache, headache, bruise or sprain—all of which pass relatively quickly. On the other hand, chronic pain is a situation rather than an event and it:

(a) is impossible to predict when it will end;
(b) usually gets worse rather than better;
(c) lacks positive meaning;
(d) frequently expands to occupy the patient's whole attention—and when this happens, life is no longer worth living.

Assessment of pain

It is necessary to be as systematic in assessing pain in far-advanced cancer as it is in the case of a patient with, for example, acute abdominal pain. A diagnosis of cancer does not necessarily mean that the malignant process is the cause of pain. Pain in cancer may be:

(a) caused by the cancer itself;
(b) caused by treatment;
(c) associated with debilitating disease;
(d) unrelated to either the disease or treatment.

When the pain is due to the cancer, it is important also to determine the mechanism underlying it as the treatment is often dependent on the cause.

Diagnostic probabilities

A prospective survey of 100 cancer patients with pain admitted consecutively to Sir Michael Sobell House, Oxford, illustrated the pattern of pain in advanced cancer (Twycross and Fairfield, 1982). The number of anatomically distinct pains in individual patients ranged from one to eight. Eighty had more than one pain; 34 four or more. The total number of pains experienced was 303. In only 41 patients was all the pain caused by the cancer itself. In 9, no pain came into this category.

Of the pains caused by cancer, bone and nerve compression were the most common. Soft tissue infiltration and visceral pains also occurred frequently. Pain caused by muscle spasm secondary to underlying bone disease occurred in 11 patients. Postoperative scar pain was the commonest type related to treatment, and constipation the most common debility-associated pain.

Twenty-seven patients recorded a total of 43 musculoskeletal pains. The most common type was myofascial. This occurred in 12 patients and accounted for 24 pains. Miscellaneous unrelated pains included tension headache, pain in one or both pinna, several abdominal complaints, urinary retention, coccydynia, restless legs syndrome, and artherosclerotic claudication.

Site and intensity

Each site where pain is experienced should be recorded on a body image (Fig. 5.1). A body chart is readily available in most hospitals as part of the standard stationery for use in clinical notes. The pictorial record acts as a baseline for future reference, and helps in the consideration of underlying mechanisms.

Intensity of pain is assessed both by the patient's description and also by discovering which drugs have failed to relieve, whether sleep is disturbed, and in what way activity is limited—'How long is it since you went out?', 'What are you doing around the house?' In addition, the patient's spouse should be interviewed. Usually one finds that the patient has made light of his suffering. A patient can be in severe pain without looking distressed.

Any pain that fails to respond to weak narcotics such as codeine or dextro-propoxyphene is, by definition, severe. If it significantly limits activity, the pain is very severe/incapacitating. Detailed assessment is difficult when pain is overwhelming, and one is faced with a distressed, exhausted patient who says or implies, 'It's all pain, doctor'. This, together with a catalogue of failed remedies, is, however, sufficient to allow treatment with a strong narcotic in combination with diazepam or chlorpromazine.

Quality

Patients often find it difficult to describe the quality of pain, though if adjectives are used, or agreed with, it helps in deciding the mechanism of the pain (Duboisson and Melzack, 1976). 'Like raving toothache' or 'sharp, shooting pain, especially on movement' suggests nerve compression and will influence the course of treatment should analgesics alone fail to relieve.

Variation

Intensity of pain may vary considerably during the day. There are undoubtedly several reasons for this (Glynn et al., 1976), but the use of medication which eases pain for an hour or two is often a major factor. Diurnal variation in pain intensity should be carefully recorded because such information helps in the choice of analgesic, dose and frequency of administration. In some patients,

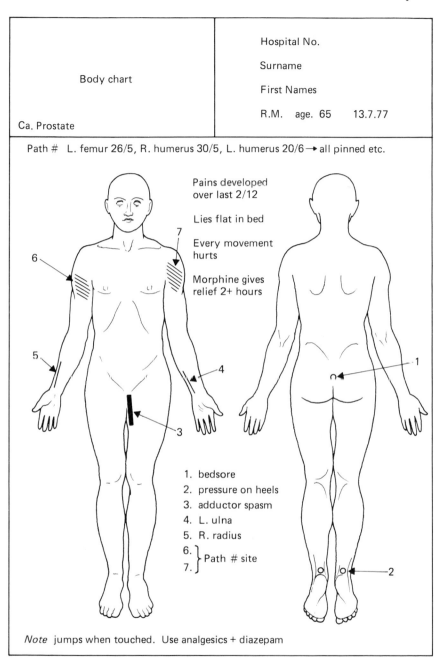

Body chart	Hospital No.
	Surname
	First Names
	R.M. age. 65 13.7.77
Ca. Prostate	

Path #   L. femur 26/5, R. humerus 30/5, L. humerus 20/6 → all pinned etc.

Pains developed
over last 2/12

Lies flat in bed

Every movement
hurts

Morphine gives
relief 2+ hours

1. bedsore
2. pressure on heels
3. adductor spasm
4. L. ulna
5. R. radius
6. ⎫
   ⎬ Path # site
7. ⎭

Note jumps when touched. Use analgesics + diazepam

Fig. 5.1 Pain chart of 65-year-old male with carcinoma of the prostate. Note that adductor spasm is usually protective, i.e. secondary to involvement of the pubis; treatment is as for bone pain, although sometimes diazepam also may be necessary.

pain is minimal at rest but intolerable on movement or when walking. Relationship to micturition, defaecation, eating, breathing, coughing or posture should also be noted.

Reassessment

The probability that the initial prescription will be inadequate increases with the intensity of pain. Patients should therefore be reassessed within hours if the pain is overwhelming, or after one or two days if severe or moderate. If troublesome or unacceptable side-effects result, treatment may need to be modified. In addition, the relief of the major pain may allow a second, less severe, pain to become apparent.

Pain relief

There is always more to analgesia than analgesics. To obtain the best results a 'broad-spectrum' approach is generally necessary, often using several different methods at that same time, rather than adopting a sequential pattern.

Explanation

Explanation of the cause(s) of pain is fundamental to success. The patient needs to understand, to make sense of what is happening. Severe pain that does not make sense or, worse, is seen as a threat to one's way of life or existence is always more intense than pain which is understandable. In advanced cancer, several pains may merge into a diffuse pattern of increasing discomfort. There is need to help the patient discriminate between his various pains and so make better sense of them.

Although pain may continue to serve as a reminder of the underlying presence and progression of the disease, explanation by the doctor as to its cause takes much of the mystery and uncertainty from it. Whatever negative attributes continue to surround the pain, explanation cuts it down to size psychologically. For the patient whose pain is all non-malignant in origin, the relief will be even greater. It is folly to initiate other pain-control measures without preliminary and repeated explanations about the underlying mechanisms, and it reduces the likelihood of a beneficial response to treatment.

Use of analgesics

1. *Persistent pain requires prophylactic (preventive) therapy.* To allow pain to re-emerge before administering the next dose not only causes unnecessary suffering but encourages tolerance. 'Four-hourly as required' (p.r.n. medication) has no place in the treatment of persistent pain (Fig. 5.2). Whatever its aetiology, continuous pain requires regular preventive therapy. The aim is to titrate the dose of the analgesic against the patient's pain, gradually increasing the dose until the patient is painfree. The next dose is given before the effect of the previous one has worn off and, therefore, before the patient may think it necessary. In this way it is possible to erase the memory and fear of pain (Table 5.2).

If the pain is completely relieved but returns in less than four hours either:

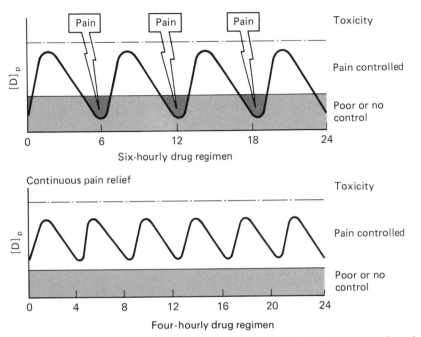

Fig. 5.2 Diagram to illustrate the results of (a) 'as required' and over-spaced regular medi-cation, compared with (b) regular 4-hourly morphine sulphate. $[D]_p$ =plasma concentration of drug.

Table 5.2 Comparison of analgesic use—acute versus cancer pain

	Acute	*Cancer*
Aim	Pain relief	Pain relief
Sedation	Often desirable	Usually undesirable
Desired duration of effect	2–4 hours	As long as possible
Timing	As required (on demand)	Regularly (in anticipation)
Dose	Usually standard	Individually determined
Route	Injection	By mouth
Adjuvant medication	Uncommon	Common

(a) increase the regular dose, or
(b) decrease the time interval to three hours.

The correct course of action can be ascertained by asking the patient the following questions:

'Does the medicine ever take the pain away completely?'
'Does the pain return before it is time for the next dose of medicine?'

If the answer to the first question is no, then the dose should be increased. If the answer to the second question is yes, the dose should also be increased; on most occasions this will correct the deficit in pain relief. Should it not, the time interval should be decreased. In practice, however, it is *rarely* necessary to use a three-hourly regimen.

If a strong analgesic other than morphine is used, the physician must be familiar with its pharmacology. For example, pethidine (meperidine) is effective for an average of two to three hours. Yet, it is commonly charted to be given 'every four hours or every six hours'. This is clearly insufficient, and forces the patient to be in pain for at least three out of every six hours.

2. *Use oral medication whenever possible.* The route of administration is a significant consideration because it has substantial impact on the patient's way of life. The patient taking oral medication is free to move around, travel in a car and, most important, be at home. Injections promote dependence on the person administering the drug. Oral administration eliminates muscle trauma, enables the patient to maintain control over his own drug administration, and helps to retain his options over where to spend his last days.

3. *Doses should be determined on an individual basis.* The effective analgesic dose varies considerably from patient to patient. The right dose of an analgesic is that which gives adequate relief for at least three and preferably four or more hours. 'Maximum' or 'recommended' doses, derived mainly from postoperative parenteral single-dose studies, are not applicable in cancer. The dose of morphine and other strong narcotic agonists can be increased almost indefinitely. On the other hand, the non-narcotics, weak narcotic agonists and narcotic agonist-antagonists all reach a plateau of maximum effect after two or three upward dose adjustments. Thus, if the upper effective does has been reached with one of these agents, the dose should *not* be increased further but a stronger drug should be prescribed.

4. *Keep it simple.* The three basic analgesics are aspirin, codeine and morphine. The rest should all be considered alternatives of fashion or convenience. Appreciating this helps to prevent the doctor 'kangarooing' from analgesic to analgesic in a desperate search for some drug that will suit his patient better. In a non-narcotic–weak narcotic preparation such as aspirin–codeine or paracetamol–dextropropoxyphene fails to relieve, it is usually best to move directly to a small dose of oral morphine sulphate.

It is, of course, necessary to be familiar with one or two alternatives for use in patients who cannot tolerate the standard preparation. Aspirin has two alternatives. Paracetamol (acetaminophen), which has no anti-inflammatory effect, is one; nonsteroidal anti-inflammatory drugs, as a group, are the other. Which alternative is appropriate depends on whether there is need for a peripheral anti-inflammatory effect. The individual doctor's basic analgesic ladder, with alternatives, should comprise no more than nine or ten drugs in total (Table 5.3). It is better to know and understand a few drugs well than to have a passing acquaintance with the whole range. The following should be noted.

(a) With mild or moderate pain, use a non-narcotic in the first instance.

(b) It may be appropriate to continue to prescribe aspirin despite the use of a narcotic, especially in patients with bone pain.

(c) it is logical to combine analgesics that act via different mechanisms, for example:
aspirin and paracetamol,
paracetemol and codeine,
aspirin and morphine.

Table 5.3 A basic analgesic ladder

Category	Parent drug	Alternatives
1. Non-narcotic	Aspirin	Paracetamol (acetaminophen) Flurbiprofen (Britain) Naproxen
2. Weak narcotic	Codeine	Dextropropoxyphene Oxycodone (USA)
3. Strong narcotic	Morphine	Papaveretum Phenazocine (Britain) Levorphanol Hydromorphone (USA)

However, it is not always wise to do so from the point of view of patient compliance, nor is it always therapeutically necessary.

(d) It is pharmacological nonsense to prescribe two weak narcotics simultaneously; likewise, two strong narcotics.

(e) It is sometimes justifiable for a patient on a strong narcotic to have another narcotic (weak or strong) as a second 'as required' analgesic for occasional, troublesome pain. Generally, though, patients should be advised to take an extra dose of their regular medication if breakthrough pain occurs.

(f) If one weak narcotic preparation does not control the pain, do not waste time by prescribing an alternative; move to something definitely stronger.

(g) Morphine or an alternative strong narcotic should be used when non-narcotics and weak narcotics fail to control the pain.

(h) 'Morphine exists to be given, not merely to be withheld': the severity of the pain determines the choice of analgesic, not the doctor's estimate of life expectancy, which is often wrong. A patient should not be made to wait in pain until the last days of life.

(i) The top of the analgesic ladder is not reached simply by prescribing morphine. Morphine may be given in a wide range of doses from as little as 2.5 mg to more than 200 mg.

(j) Do not prescribe a narcotic agonist-antagonist (e.g. pentazocine, buprenorphine) with a narcotic agonist (i.e. codeine, morphine, etc).

5. *Adjuvant medication is generally necessary.* Laxatives are almost always necessary, especially with patients receiving a narcotic. Unless fairly experienced, an antiemetic should be prescribed routinely with morphine or other strong narcotic. There are many situations in which a better result is obtained by adding a second drug rather than increasing the dose of, say, morphine indefinitely (Table 5.4).

6. *Do not use mixtures routinely.* At some centres, morphine is always prescribed with a second drug, either cocaine (a stimulant) or a phenothiazine (a tranquillizer). Sometimes both are added. In these circumstances, increasing the dose of morphine can be hazardous if, by increasing the *volume* of the mixture taken, the dose of the adjunctive medication is automatically increased also, regardless of need. Depending on the adjunctive drug, this can lead to agitation and restlessness or to somnolence. It is far better to give adjunctive medication

Table 5.4 Co-analgesics in the relief of cancer pain

Types of pain	Co-analgesic
Bone pain	Aspirin 600 mg 4-hourly *or* flurbiprofen 50–100 mg b.i.d. *or* naproxen 500 mg b.i.d
Raised intracranial pressure	Dexamethasone 2–4 mg t.i.d.–q.i.d. diuretic (?)
Nerve pressure pain	Dexamethasone 2–4 mg daily—b.i.d. prednisolone 5–10 mg t.i.d.
Superficial dysaesthetic pain	Amitriptyline 25–100 mg *nocte*
Intermittent stabbing pain	Valproate 200 mg b.i.d.–t.i.d. *or* carbamazepine 200 mg t.i.d.–q.i.d.
Gastric distension pain	Anti-flatulent 10 ml p.ċ. and *nocte*; metoclopramide 10 mg 4-hourly
Rectal tenesmoid pain	Chlorpromazine 10–25 mg 8–4-hourly, *or* rectal belladonna alkaloids 0.2 mg*
Muscle spasm pain	Diazepam 5 mg b.i.d. *or* baclofen 10 mg t.i.d.
Lymphoedema	Diuretic and corticosteroid (?)
Infected malignant ulcer	Metronidazole 400 mg b.i.d. *or* clindamycin 300 mg q.i.d.

* Can be pre-injected into standard morphine suppositories (Britain) or administered as B & O supprettes (USA).

separately, either as a syrup or tablet/capsule. The dose of each pharmacologically active substance can then be adjusted individually against patient need.

7. *Psychotropic drugs should not be used routinely.* If the patient is very anxious, an anxiolytic should be prescribed. If a patient remains depressed after several days of much improved pain relief, an antidepressant may be necessary.

8. *Insomnia must be treated vigorously.* Discomfort is worse at night when the patient is alone with his pain and his fears. The cumulative effect of many sleepless, pain-filled nights is a substantial lowering of the patient's pain threshold with a concomitant increase in pain intensity.

Non-drug treatments

Many patients derive greatest benefit from a combination of drug and non-drug treatments. Radiotherapy gives partial or complete relief in 90 per cent of patients with bone pain (Allen *et al.*, 1976) and sometimes can be administered in a single non-fractionated dose (see Chapter 8). A nerve block may be necessary when the pain is caused by compression or infiltration of a nerve, though the use of morphine and a corticosteroid in combination may obviate the need for this. Moreover, the fact that a patient is receiving radiotherapy, for example, does not mean that analgesics should be withheld. A combined approach should be employed. When the patient is pain free, the analgesic regimen can be modified—the existing medication reduced, or tailed off completely or a weaker analgesic prescribed.

Attention to detail

Analgesic regimens should be simple to understand and easy to administer. It is only necessary to adopt a four-hourly regimen if morphine or a comparable analgesic is being used. With other patients, 'with meals and at bedtime' will cover all other drug requirements. Variations include: 'on waking, after lunch and tea, and bedtime', and 'after breakfast and at bedtime'.

If some drugs are best given before meals and others after, it is usually advisable to forsake pharmacological purity and to opt for one or other time so as to avoid an impossibly complex schedule. It is necessary to look at boxes and other containers to check that the pharmacist has not given the patient contrary or complicating advice.

When a four-hourly regimen is adopted, the first and last doses are linked to the patient's waking and bedtimes. The best additional times during the day are usually 10 a.m., 2 p.m. and 6 p.m., unless the patient wakes exceptionally late. The list of drugs and doses for the patient (and family) to work from should be written out clearly. It is useful to add what the different preparations are for, even if this seems obvious to the doctor.

Capsules should be described as capsules and tablets as tablets, not *vice versa*. Doses should not be described simply as 'spoonfuls'. Patients have been known to use a tablespoon (15 ml) instead of a teaspoon (3.5–5 ml). A plastic beaker or cup with each 5 ml clearly marked is generally the best way for the patient to self-administer liquid preparations. Sometimes, if the above recommendations are carried out, the patient can cope immediately with a new regimen. Not infrequently, however, the patient is found to be in confusion when visited the next day.

Expectations

Relief is obtained within two or three days in some patients, but in others, particularly those whose pain is made worse by movement and in the very anxious and depressed, it may take three to four weeks of in-patient treatment to achieve satisfactory control. Even so, it should be possible to achieve some improvement within 24–48 hours in all patients. Although the ultimate aim is complete freedom from pain, we will be less disappointed but, paradoxically, more successful if in practice we aim at 'graded relief'.

As some pains respond more readily than others, improvement should be assessed in relation to each pain. The initial target should be a pain-free, sleep-full night. Many patients have not had a good night's rest for weeks or months and are exhausted and demoralized. To sleep through the night pain free and wake refreshed is a boost to both the doctor's and the patient's morale. Next, one aims for relief at rest in bed or chair during the day; finally, for freedom from pain on movement. The former is always eventually possible; *the latter is not*. Even so, the encouragement brought by relief at night, and when resting during the day, gives the patient new hope and incentive and enables him to begin to live again despite limited mobility. Freed from the day- and nightmare of constant pain, his last weeks or months take on a new look.

With cancer one is dealing with a progressive pathological process. This means that new pains may develop or an old pain re-emerge. A fresh complaint of pain does not merely call for an increase in a previously satisfactory analgesic regimen; it demands reassessment, explanation to the patient, and, only then, modification of drug therapy or other intervention.

Aspirin and bone pain

In recent years, the role of aspirin in the management of cancer pain has assumed greater importance because of discoveries about osteolytic factors produced by osseous metastases. The growth of an osseous metastasis appears to be linked with induced bone resorption. Initially, this is mediated via osteoclastic activity but, subsequently, an osteolytic agent is produced by the tumour itself (Galasko, 1981). Most studies relating to solid tumours implicate prostaglandin E_2 (PGE_2) as the principal factor involved. Other work has shown that prostaglandins of the E series cause pain when injected subdermally at high concentrations (Ferreira, 1972). In lower concentrations, the same prostaglandins exacerbate pain, probably by sensitizing free nerve endings. Aspirin (in high dosage) and other non-steroidal anti-inflammatory drugs (NSAID) are known to be potent inhibitors of prostaglandin synthesis. This suggests that, compared with morphine, NSAID should be relatively more efficacious in bone pain caused by soft tissue infiltration. Our experience in Oxford would support such a hypothesis.

Response to prostaglandin inhibitors is, however, variable—a fact which can be explained if certain cancer cell types synthesize osteolytic agents other than or in addition to PGE_2. It has been shown, for example, in patients with hypercalcaemia in association with multiple myeloma or a reticulosis, that the urinary excretion of prostaglandin metabolites is normal and that bone resorption appears to be due to secretion of 'osteoclast-activating factor' by tumour cells (Mundy and Spiro, 1981). Other candidates include ectopic parathyroid hormone and active vitamin D metabolites or related sterols. Although complex, as further research elucidates the relative importance of these substances, the ability to relieve bone pain by pharmacological means should steadily improve.

Despite the introduction of many novel NSAID, the humble aspirin still has much to commend it. If this is not well tolerated, one of the following may be used:

aspirin–glycine (Paynocil)	600 mg 4-hrly
benorylate suspension	10 ml b.i.d.
flurbiprofen	100 mg b.i.d.
naproxen	500 mg b.i.d.

Flurbiprofen is used as the alternative NSAID of choice at Sir Michael Sobell House, Oxford. It does, however, cause dyspepsia and vomiting in a significant minority of patients. When this is the case, one of the other NSAID should be tried. Side-effect liability is not necessarily transferable.

The NSAID have been described as '40–50%' drugs, a reminder that they relieve only that proportion of the pain related to the production of prostaglandins. It is possible, however, that elevation of the peripheral pain threshold by administration of a NSAID may be enough to raise the patient's total pain threshold to a degree sufficient to relieve the pain completely. When aspirin is used, this is more likely because of its suggested multifocal action; the same will be true of benorylate. A decision to use a NSAID alone or in combination with a narcotic will, in practice, depend on the intensity of pain. If severe, a combination should be used, at least initially.

Strong narcotic analgesics

In the majority of patients requiring a strong narcotic, morphine is both efficacious and acceptable (Table 5.5). If a patient appears to have persistent intolerance to morphine, an alternative that is chemically distinct should be used in the hope that this does not cause the unwanted effect (Table 5.6).

Table 5.5 Twenty points on the use of morphine sulphate solution

1. Strong narcotic of choice at most hospices
2. Administered in simple aqueous solution (e.g. 10 mg in 10 ml)
3. No advantage in giving as 'Brompton Cocktail'
4. Usual starting dose 10 mg every 4 hours
5. If patient has previously only had a weak narcotic analgesic, 5 mg may be adequate
6. With frail elderly patients, if may be wise to start on suboptimal dose in order to reduce likelihood of initial drowsiness and unsteadiness
7. If changing to morphine from alternative strong narcotic (such as dextromoramide, levorphanol, methadone), a considerably higher dose may be needed
8. Adjust upwards after first dose if not more effective than previous medication
9. Adjust after 24 hours 'if pain not 90% controlled'
10. Most patients are satisfactorily controlled on dose of between 5 mg and 30 mg 4-hourly; however, some patients need higher doses, occasionally up to 500 mg
11. Giving a larger dose at bedtime (1.5 or 2 × daytime dose) may enable a patient to go through the night without waking in pain
12. Use co-analgesic medication as appropriate
13. Either prescribe an antiemetic concurrently or supply (in anticipation) for regular use should nausea or vomiting develop
14. Prescribe laxative, e.g. Dorbanex, Peri-Colace; adjust dose according to response; suppositories may be necessary
    Unless carefully monitored, constipation may be more difficult to control than the pain
15. Write out regimen in detail with times to be taken, names of drugs and amount to be taken
16. Warn patient of possibility of initial drowsiness
17. Arrange for close liaison and follow-up
18. For the patient who cannot cope with a 4-hourly regimen or liquid medication, controlled release morphine sulphate 10, 30, 60 and 100 mg tablets (MST-Continus) b.i.d.–t.i.d. should be considered
19. It is almost never necessary to resort to parenteral administration for pain control *per se*. If swallowing becomes very difficult or vomiting persists, give one-third of previously satisfactory dose of morphine as diamorphine hydrochloride (Britain) or one-half of previous dose as morphine sulphate (elsewhere) by subcutaneous/intramuscular injection
20. Suppositories of morphine sulphate are also available in Britain (10, 15, 20, 30 and 60 mg); elsewhere these can be made by any helpful pharmacist

Diamorphine

Diamorphine (diacetylmorphine, heroin) is a semi-synthetic derivative of morphine. Its pharmacological profile is almost identical to that of morphine. Diamorphine is readily absorbed by all routes of administration. The oral-to-intramuscular potency ratio is approximately 1 : 2.5. Given intravenously, it acts faster than morphine and causes less vomiting but more sedation (Loan *et al.*, 1969). By mouth, because of relatively rapid *in vivo* deacetylation (Way *et al.*, 1965), diamorphine is essentially a pro-drug for morphine. The plasma half-life of diamorphine, and its pharmacologically active metabolites monoacetylmorphine and morphine, is comparable to that of morphine. The duration of useful

Table 5.6 Strong narcotic analgesics: approximate oral equivalents to morphine sulphate

Analgesic		Proprietary name	Potency ratio with morphine sulphate[2]		Duration of action (hours)[3]
Pethidine/ meperidine		Demerol	1/8	(1/12)[1]	2–3
*Dipipanone	in	Diconal	1/2	(1/3)	
Papaveretum		Omnopon, Pantopon	2/3	(1/2)	3–5
†Oxycodone[4]	in	Percodan Percocet Tylox (capsule)	1	(2/3)	3–5
*Dextromoramide		Palfium	(2)[5]	(1.5)	2–4
Methadone		Physeptone, Dolophine	(3–4)[6]	(2–3)	6–8
Levorphanol		Dromoran, Levo- dromoran	5	(3)	4–6
*Phenazocine		Narphen	5	(3)	4–6
†Hydromorphone		Dilaudid	6	(4)	3–4

* Not available in USA.
† Not available in Britain.
[1] Column of figures in parentheses refer to approximate potency ratio with diamorphine (heroin).
[2] *Multiply* dose of stated drug by the potency ratio to determine the equivalent dose of morphine sulphate.
[3] Dependent to a certain extent on dose, often longer lasting in very elderly and those with considerable liver dysfunction.
[4] Oxycodone is available in Britain only as Oxycodone pectinate suppositories (q.v.).
[5] Dextromoramide single 5-mg dose is equivalent to morphine 15 mg (diamorphine 10 mg) in terms of **peak** effect but is generally shorter acting; overall potency rate adjusted accordingly.
[6] Methadone single 5–mg dose is equivalent to morphine 7.5 mg (diamorphine 5 mg). Has a prolonged plasma half-life which leads to cumulation when given repeatedly. This means it is several times more potent when given regularly.

analgesic is four to five hours. Because diamorphine is more lipid soluble, it is more readily absorbed than morphine. This accounts for the greater potency (though not efficacy) noted even when taken orally. By mouth, diamorphine is 1.5 times more potent, i.e. 10 mg of diamorphine hydrochloride is equi-analgesic to 15 mg of morphine sulphate (Twycross, 1977a). Parenterally, the potency ratio is greater (Beaver *et al.*, 1981; Kaiko *et al.*, 1981).

Diamorphine hydrochloride is, however, considerably more soluble than the commonly available morphine salts: 100mg will dissolve in 0.2 ml. For this reason alone, diamorphine hydrochloride is still used as the parenteral strong analgesic of choice in many centres in Britain. The volume injected need never be large (Table 5.7). This is an important consideration when repeated injections have to be given to a cachetic cancer patient. Most patients can, however, be maintained on oral medication. The main indication for parenteral administration, apart from the last few hours of life, is intractable nausea and vomiting despite the prescription of an antiemetic. The need for injections can, of course, be circumvented by using morphine sulphate suppositories.

Debate continues as to whether diamorphine is 'necessary' for the manage-

Table 5.7 Volume of injection of equi-analgesic doses of diamorphine hydrochloride and morphine sulphate*

Dose of drug (mg)		Volume of injection (ml)		
Diamorphine	Morphine	Diamorphine	Morphine	
		freeze-dried	15 mg/ml†	30 mg/ml‡
5	12.5	0.1	1	0.5
10	25	0.1	2	1
20	50	0.1	4	2
30	75	0.1	5	2.5
60	150	0.1	10	5
90	225	0.15	15	7.5
120	300	0.2	20	10

* Using a potency ratio of 2.5:1 (Beaver *et al.*, 1981). If the potency ratio is taken to be 2:1 (Kaiko *et al.*, 1981), the volumes given should be reduced by 1/5.
† Maximum strength available in USA.
‡ Maximum strength available in Britain.

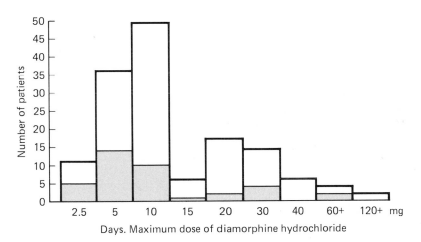

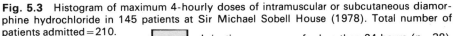

Days. Maximum dose of diamorphine hydrochloride

Fig. 5.3 Histogram of maximum 4-hourly doses of intramuscular or subcutaneous diamorphine hydrochloride in 145 patients at Sir Michael Sobell House (1978). Total number of patients admitted = 210.

▨ Injections necessary for less than 24 hours (n = 38)

☐ Injections given for more than 24 hours (n = 107)

Median dose = 10 mg. *Note:* '60 +' includes one patient who received 80 mg; '120 +' includes one patient who received 140 mg.

ment of pain in a proportion of patients with cancer (Lasagna, 1981; Tattersall, 1981). Details of injections of diamorphine hydrochloride at one British hospice are shown in Fig. 5.3. If a 2-ml injection of morphine sulphate is considered acceptable (3 ml with an antiemetic), then only those patients who received 30 mg of diamorphine or more 'needed' it; the rest could readily have received morphine instead. If 1 ml (2 ml with an antiemetic) is considered the upper acceptable volume limit, all patients needing more than 10 mg would remain in the 'diamorphine necessary' group. Excluding patients who received diamorphine for less than 24 hours, this gives the percentage of patients at Sir Michael Sobell House 'needing' diamorphine as 9.5 per cent using the 2 + 1 ml formula and 19 per cent using 1 + 1 ml.

Is 9.5 per cent sufficient to warrant the medical profession in countries without diamorphine to campaign for its re-introduction? Some feel the answer is 'yes', while others continue to say 'no'. For those who say yes, the following should be noted.

1. Hospices in North America are not campaigning for medicinal diamorphine; they are content to use morphine.

2. Syringe drivers for continuous subcutaneous infusion are now available.

3. Morphine acetate is almost as soluble as diamorphine and, if freeze-dried, could substitute readily for patients who 'need' diamorphine.

4. Hydromorphone hydrochloride (see below), although half as soluble, is some two or three times more potent than diamorphine. The time-action characteristics of intramuscular hydromorphone are comparable to those of diamorphine. This makes it an ideal alternative (Kaiko et al., 1981). As with morphine acetate, a freeze-dried preparation would be needed to maximize its benefits.

A first step in the right direction would, however, be the immediate introduction of an ampoule in the USA containing 30 mg of morphine sulphate in 1 ml.

Pethidine

Pethidine (meperidine) is a synthetic narcotic analgesic which also has atropine-like effects. It is about one-third as potent by mouth as by injection. It is about one-eighth as potent as morphine. It cannot relieve such severe pain as morphine, but in higher doses is considerably more effective than codeine. Pethidine differs from morphine in a number of ways.

1. Shorter duration of action.
2. Ceiling effect.
3. Not antitussive.
4. Less constipating.
5. Less smooth muscle spasm.
6. Pupils not constricted.

Pethidine causes vomiting about as often as morphine. Equi-analgesic doses depress the respiratory centre to a similar extent.

Used correctly, orally administered pethidine can substitute for up to 30 mg of morphine sulphate four-hourly. Unfortunately, pethidine is often prescribed with little regard for its pharmacokinetics (Marks and Sachar, 1973). It usually needs to be given every two to three hours because of the short duration of its action. An order for four- to six-hourly administration condemns the average patient to pain for a total of 12 out of every 24 hours.

It is difficult to persuade a patient to take more than 200 mg of pethidine three-hourly because of the number of 50 mg tablets required. This is not such a problem in the patient who cannot take morphine and who is strongly motivated by the prospect of pain relief without unacceptable side-effects. However, with pethidine the incidence of unwanted CNS effects, namely tremor, twitching, agitation and convulsions, increases considerably at doses above 200–300 mg three-hourly. These are caused by cumulation of the toxic metabolite norpethidine. This, together with the problem of compliance, means that there is, in practice, a ceiling to its efficacy. In this way pethidine resembles a weak rather than a strong narcotic. It is not a complete alternative to morphine.

Pethidine should be used with caution in patients with impaired renal function because of the increased likelihood of norpethidine side-effects (Szeto et al., 1977). Phenobarbitone and chlorpromazine enhance the production of norpethidine (Stambaugh et al., 1977; Stambaugh and Wainer, 1981).

Pethidine should not be given to a patient receiving a monoamine oxidase inhibitor, as this may cause respiratory depression, restlessness, hypotension, and even coma—effects possibly related to the inhibition of the hepatic enzyme that demethylates pethidine.

Methadone

Methadone is absorbed well from all routes of administration. Orally it is about one-half as potent as by subcutaneous or intramuscular injection. The plasma half-life of a single oral dose is about 15 hours (Inturrisi and Verebely, 1972b), though when given regularly the half-life increases considerably, up to two to three days in some patients (Inturrisi and Verebely, 1972a). This implies that problems from cumulation are likely to occur, especially in the debilitated and elderly. The plasma concentration may not reach a steady state for two to three weeks in some patients. Given in a single dose, methadone is marginally more potent than morphine but, in repeated dosage, it is several times more potent. Its effective analgesic range is the same as that of morphine. It is generally longer acting than morphine, useful analgesia lasting some six to eight hours. Methadone, like morphine, has no obvious ceiling effect. It is used by a number of centres as the strong analgesic of choice for severe cancer pain. It is perhaps the strong narcotic of choice for children (Martinson et al., 1978). A number of important interactions between methadone and other drugs have been reported. Cimetidine inhibits the metabolism of methadone: this may lead to increasing drowsiness, or even coma. Rifampicin, an antibiotic, speeds up methadone metabolism and may, on occasion, precipitate withdrawal symptoms (Kreek et al., 1976).

Other strong narcotic agonists

Oxymorphone (Numorphan) 1 mg is equi-analgesic with 10 mg of subcutaneous morphine (Swerdlow, 1967). It is at least as likely to produce unwanted effects, possibly more so. It is not available in an oral preparation. A 5-mg rectal suppository is manufactured in the USA. A dose of 10 mg of oxymorphone per rectum is equivalent to only 20 mg of oral morphine sulphate.

Hydromorphone (Dilaudid) is available in the USA as 1-, 2-, 3- and 4-mg tablets, in ampoules containing 1, 2, 3 and 4 mg, and as 3-mg rectal suppositories. The mean plasma half-life is about four hours. Intramuscularly, 1.5 mg is equivalent to 10 mg of morphine. The oral potency ratio is of the same order.

Hydromorphone is possibly less constipating than morphine. It is slightly shorter acting.

Levorphanol causes less nausea and vomiting than morphine and will often provide relief for six hours. The longer duration of action relates in part to lipid solubility and cumulation of the drug in body fat. As with methadone, this may result in excessive sedation in the elderly.

Phenazocine (Narphen) is as potent as levorphanol but, for oral use, is available in Britain only in 5-mg tablets. This is equivalent to 20–25 mg of oral morphine sulphate. The tablets are scored, though it is not easy for a patient to break them. They dissolve readily and are effective sublingually. Like other narcotics, phenazocine is bitter in taste. The incidence of vomiting with sublingual phenazocine is 5 per cent.

Dipipanone is available for oral use in Britain as Diconal. This contains dipipanone 10 mg and cyclizine 30 mg. On a weight-for-weight basis, it is approximately half as potent as morphine sulphate. In patients requiring more than two tablets, the anticholinergic and sedative effects of cyclizine tend to be troublesome, notably blurring of vision, dry mouth, and drowsiness.

Dextromoramide by mouth is more potent than morphine on a weight-for-weight basis. Pharmacokinetic data are scanty. Published data of a study involving one subject are available (Caddy and Idowu, 1979). This study primarily concerned assay techniques for the analytical detection of drugs *in vivo* rather than pharmacokinetics in a clinical context. After a single 5-mg dose to one subject, a biphasic plasma half-life was found for dextromoramide of approximately seven hours for the first phase and over 60 hours for the second phase. These results do not give sufficient information to draw general conclusions regarding plasma half-life in the therapeutic situation (Judd *et al.*, 1981). In any case, as with methadone, the plasma half-life of dextromoramide does not correlate closely with its duration of analgesic effect: a number of studies quote four to six hours (Kay, 1973). Many doctors, however, have a strong clinical impression that for severe pain, the modal duration of action is only some two to three hours.

Buprenorphine

Buprenorphine is a strong narcotic analgesic with antagonist properties. It should not be used in conjunction with other narcotic analgesics as a variable degree of antagonism may occur. The doses–response curve for subjective effects is bell shaped; in one study, does of 1.2 mg produced less effect than 0.6 mg (Heel *et al.*, 1979). Morphine-like effects are maximal at a dose of about 1 mg subcutaneously. The plasma half-life is about three hours after intramuscular injection. Onset of action is about 30 minutes, and peak effect after three hours (morphine = one hour). The duration of useful effect is some six to nine hours (morphine = three to five hours). Most patients are satisfactorily controlled on an eight-hourly regimen. It is readily absorbed when taken sublingually. Subjective and physiological effects are generally similar to morphine, including drowsiness when used postoperatively or during the first few days of chronic use. *Naloxone does not reverse the effects of buprenorphine when used in doses of 0.4–0.8mg intravenously.* It is generally considered to have a low abuse potential and is not a controlled drug in countries where it is available.

Sublingual administration allows absorption directly into the systemic circulation. The 'first-pass' effect (hepatic metabolism) seen after ingestion from the stomach or intestine is avoided. As a result, buprenorphine is relatively more potent sublingually than are other narcotics when ingested orally. Sublingually, 0.4 mg is equipotent, with 0.3 mg intramuscularly.

By injection, buprenorphine is 30–40 times more potent than morphine—and longer lasting. It would seem reasonable to assume that, compared with orally administered morphine, sublingual buprenorphine is some 60–80 times more potent. Thus, when changing from an unsatisfactory buprenorphine regimen to oral morphine sulphate, as a rule of thumb, the total daily dose of buprenorphine should be *multiplied by 100* and converted to a convenient four-hourly regimen. Fortunately, although adding buprenorphine to morphine may lead to perceptible antagonism of the latter, changing from buprenorphine to high-dose morphine does not result in a period of uncontrolled pain. The buprenorphine is already firmly attached to the opiate receptors, and morphine substitutes for this as and when the buprenorphine becomes detached and is metabolized.

The maximum effective dose for subjective effects is 1 mg when given parenterally; higher doses are *less* effective. Although a comparable bell-shaped dose–response curve has not been clearly demonstrated for analgesia, this remains a possibility and poses a number of practical questions.

1. What is the maximum effective *single* sublingual dose?
2. What is the maximum effective *daily* sublingual dose?
3. What is the optimum time interval between doses?
4. What do patients on maximum, or near maximum, doses do if they get breakthrough pain or a sudden severe new pain?

Adjuvant medication

Most patients with advanced cancer have more than one symptom, often necessitating the prescription of several drugs at the same time. Moreover, use of narcotic analgesics is frequently complicated by constipation and/or nausea and vomiting. Any discussion of analgesics in advanced cancer must therefore include adjuvant medication.

Corticosteroids

The use of a corticosteroid as a 'co-analgesic' should be considered whenever there is a large tumour mass within a relatively confined space. There is often an oedematous area around a tumour, and pressure on neighbouring veins and lymphatics may lead to further local or regional swelling. In other words, the total tumour mass = neoplasm + surrounding hyperaemic oedema. Corticosteroids reduce this oedema, thereby reducing the total tumour mass.

The classic situation is that of headache caused by raised intracranial pressure in association with cerebral neoplasm. There may be other central nervous symptoms or signs and patients often show improvement for weeks or months after starting treatment. When headache is the main symptom, analgesics, a diuretic, and elevating the head of the bed also may help to relieve pain.

Corticosteroids also relieve the pain of nerve compression by reducing oedema of the nerve. About 50 per cent of nerve compression pains respond to analgesics alone, and most of the rest respond to the combined use of analgesics and a corticosteroid. Only a minority of patients with nerve compression pain fail to respond to pharmacological measures, and thereby become candidates for neurolytic block.

Amiphenazole

It has been claimed that the use of amiphenazole (Daptazole), a respiratory stimulant, permits more rapid adjustment of morphine dosage as it antagonizes the respiratory depressant effect of the opiate (Shaw and Shulman, 1955). However, in a controlled trial of morphine with and without amiphenazole, it was demonstrated in non-tolerant, ex-addict volunteers that the addition of amiphenazole (1.2 mg for each milligram of morphine) had no demonstrable effect on respiratory rate or volume. Injections of up to 120 mg of morphine were used four times a day (Fraser *et al.*, 1957).

In fact, significant respiratory depression is rarely a problem when narcotics are used by mouth in individually determined doses (Walsh *et al.*, 1981). Patients with tachypnoea often feel considerably better if, for example, the respiratory rate is reduced from 40 to 25 a minute. With this observation in mind, one should consider raising the dose of morphine, even if pain is controlled, in order to ease dyspnoea. In general, though, the dose of morphine in the management of dyspnoea alone is smaller than that used to relieve severe pain. It is wise to start with a dose of 2.5 mg, increasing to 5 mg the next day. Further increments of 2.5 mg or 5 mg may be made at two- to three-day intervals up to 15–20 mg. The aim is to produce maximum benefit without respiratory failure (cyanosis) or confusional symptoms.

In patients with a normal respiratory rate, it is unusual for this to fall below about 12 a minute when receiving morphine orally. Individuals most at risk include the elderly and those who require an above-average dose of morphine together with diazepam or methotrimeprazine (see below). In these patients, the rate may drop as low as 4–6 breaths/minute when the patient is asleep, a fact which naturally concerns the nurses. Occasionally, in an elderly patient, the medication may need to be modified if poor oxygenation precipitates or aggravates confusion; the need to do this is, however, uncommon.

Cocaine

More than 80 years ago, Herbert Snow (1896) began to prescribe cocaine with opium or morphine for patients with advanced cancer. He maintained that cocaine helped to 'sustain vitality', though subsequently he had to stop using it because of the cost. It was re-introduced in the 1920s by J.E.H. Roberts, a surgeon at the Brompton Hospital, who used a morphine–cocaine elixir as a post-thoracotomy analgesic (Kerrane, 1975). The mixture subsequently became known as the Brompton Cocktail. Since 1973, the British Pharmaceutical Codex has included a standard formulation for both morphine–cocaine and diamorphine–cocaine elixirs.

The addition of cocaine is said to enhance the mood of the patient: 'The euphoria renders the patient comparatively cheerful, and relieves his mental and physical distress' (Love, 1962). Only recently, however, has the effect of a standard 10-mg dose of cocaine hydrochloride been evaluated (Twycross, 1976). In this study, patients were stabilized on morphine–cocaine, or diamorphine–cocaine, or morphine alone or diamorphine alone. After two weeks, patients receiving cocaine stopped receiving it, and *vice versa*. Stopping cocaine appeared to have no effect, though starting it resulted in a small but definite improvement in feeling of alertness and strength. This observation suggested that when cocaine is given in a small fixed dose, tolerance develops after a few days. Cocaine would thus be of benefit during the initiation of treatment with morphine or diamorphine, but thereafter would be relatively ineffective.

Many physicians have, however, had experience of patients—usually elderly—who have become restless, agitated, confused and/or hallucinated when prescribed an opiate–cocaine mixture and whose symptoms have persisted until the cocaine was withdrawn. In view of this, and the equivocal nature of the trial results, the author no longer prescribes cocaine concomitantly. Instead, the patient is told that he may feel drowsy for two or three days following the start of treatment, but subsequently the drowsiness will become less. If the drowsiness persists, dexamphetamine 5 mg or methylphenidate (Ritalin) 10 mg may be prescribed once or twice daily. In practice, this is virtually *never* necessary.

Phenothiazines

Patients prescribed a narcotic analgesic should be questioned about nausea and vomiting, and either have an antiemetic such as prochlorperazine prescribed simultaneously, or the need for such reviewed after one or two days. A patient will not continue to take an analgesic if it results in nausea or vomiting. In patients with an appreciable psychological component to their plan—for example, the patient who fears death by suffocation, or the women who feels that her fungating breast cancer is jeopardizing her relationship with her husband—promazine or chlorpromazine should be used instead. If the latter causes troublesome anticholinergic side-effects, it may be necessary to use prochlorperazine with diazepam; in the absence of nausea and vomiting the latter can, of course, be used alone. Promazine and chlorpromazine are also used to control confusion, delirium, or psychotic manifestations.

Whereas promazine and chlorpromazine merely reduce anxiety, and thereby indirectly enhance analgesia, methotrimeprazine (Veractil, Nozinan) possesses analgesic properties *per se* (Lasagna, 1965). By injection, methotrimeprazine 15 mg and morphine 10 mg are equipotent (Bonica and Halpern, 1972). The oral potency ratio has not been determined, but when allowance is made for differences between absorption and plasma half-time, it is possible that methotrimeprazine is at least as potent as morphine on a weight-for-weight basis. Its use in terminal pain is, however, limited because it is too sedative for most patients, causing unacceptable drowsiness. Methotrimeprazine also commonly causes marked orthostatic hypotension; because of this effect, some would restrict its use to nonambulant patients. However, provided one is aware of the problem, this is unnecessary. Its use should be considered in the younger, anxious patient, requiring above-average amounts of a narcotic and in those who experience marked vestibular disturbances when given a morphine-like drug. In those aged under 40, it would be reasonable to prescribe 25 mg four-to six-hourly with 50–100 mg at night; in older patients, the dose should be about half this. It is generally wise to reduce the dose of morphine when prescribing methotrimeprazine for the first time.

Benzodiazepines

Many patients appear to be psychologically dependent on nitrazepam as a night hypnotic, and it may be necessary to continue this 'for old times' sake'. Diazepam is a useful alternative to promazine and chlorpromazine, if side-effects make their use less attractive or if response is inadequate. It is also useful as a co-analgesic in muscle spasm pain and for urethral pain associated with an indwelling catheter.

Antidepressants

The need for an antidepressant increases the longer a patient is maintained on a narcotic analgesic (Twycross and Wald, 1976). Whether the onset of depression is precipitated by the protracted terminal illness itself or is a side-effect of long-continued treatment with a narcotic and a phenothiazine is not clear. It is important to be aware that depression not only can, but frequently does, supervene in patients receiving so-called 'euphoriant' drugs, and to initiate a trial of therapy when it does. Treatment should be started with half the usual adult dose, as experience has shown that debilitated patients commonly become confused and disorientated if a higher dose is given initially, particularly if they are receiving other psychotropic drugs.

Addiction

Although the term 'drug addiction' has been replaced officially by 'drug dependence', unofficially it continues to be used. Drug dependence is currently defined as:

> 'A state, psychic and sometimes also physical, resulting from the interaction between a living organism and a drug, characterized by behavioural and other responses that always include a compulsion to take the drug on a continuous or periodic basis in order to experience its psychic effects, and sometimes to avoid the discomfort of its absence. Tolerance may or may not be present' (World Health Organisation, 1969).

This is a broader definition than an earlier one which emphasized the need for both tolerance and an early development of physical dependence in addition to strong psychological dependence (World Health Organization, 1964). The term 'drug dependence' now more closely approximates to the popular conception of addiction: a compulsion or overpowering drive to take the drug in order to experience its psychological effects. Occasionally, a patient is admitted who appears to be addicted, demanding 'an injection' every two or three hours. Typically, such a patient has a long history of poor pain control and will for several weeks have been receiving fairly regular ('four-hourly as required') but inadequate injections of one or more narcotic analgesics. Given time, it is usually possible to control the pain adequately, prevent clock-watching and demanding behaviour, and, sometimes, transfer the patient to an oral preparation. But even here, it cannot be said that the patient is addicted as he is not demanding the narcotic in order to experience its psychological effect but to be relieved from pain for at least an hour or two.

Even so, many doctors are reluctant to use narcotic analgesics, particularly diamorphine or morphine, because they assume that tolerance will result in the medication becoming ineffective (Milton, 1972). This is understandable, as hitherto little information has been available concerning the long-term effects of narcotic analgesics when administered regularly to relieve persistent pain. The lack of data resulted in predictions being made on the basis of animal and human volunteer studies. For example, in a review article on narcotic analgesics (Martin, 1973), comments about tolerance in patients were supported by reference, on the one hand, to a short-term infusion study in pain-free dogs and, on

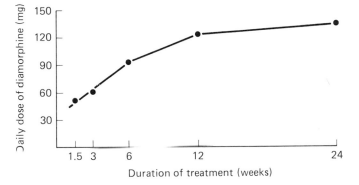

Fig. 5.4 418 patients admitted consecutively with advanced cancer were grouped according to survival following the start of treatment with diamorphine: group median final daily dose of diamorphine is shown plotted against group median duration of treatment.

the other hand, to ex-addicts. However, in studies using ex-addicts at the Addiction Research Centre in Lexington, the emphasis has been on inducing tolerance and physical dependence as rapidly as possible by using maximum tolerated doses rather than administering the drugs in doses and at intervals comparable to a clinical regimen (Isbell, 1948). Although such studies have been useful in predicting abuse liability, their relevance to clinical practice is questionable.

To allow predictions to be made on the basis of clinical experience, some ten years ago the notes of 500 patients admitted consecutively to St Christopher's Hospice were reviewed (Twycross, 1974). A total of 218 patients received diamorphine regularly for at least one week. By grouping the patients according to survival after commencing diamorphine, it was demonstrated that the longer the duration of treatment, the slower the rate of rise in dose (Fig. 5.4). In a second review (Twycross and Wald, 1976), 115 patients who had received diamorphine regularly for at least 12 weeks were selected from some 3000 patients admitted over seven years. Dose-time charts were prepared (Fig. 5.5). Visual analysis indicated that in many there was an initial phase when the dose

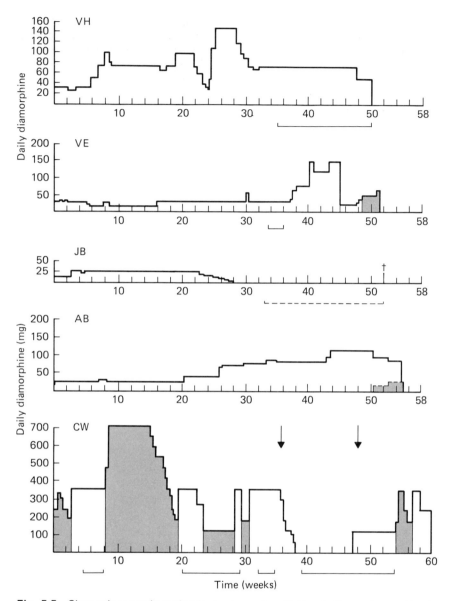

Fig. 5.5 Change in narcotic analgesic requirements with time in five patients with advanced cancer. Open areas: diamorphine by mouth; hatched areas: diamorphine by injection; dotted areas: other narcotic analgesic (V.E., C.W.): arrow: phenol-in-glycerine nerve block; horizontal bar: time spent at home. V.H., V.E., and A.B. received diamorphine up to the time of death; C.W. is still alive. Similar patterns are seen with morphine.

was increased several times within one or two weeks followed by a prolonged phase when the dose was increased less often or not at all. It was also clearly demonstrated that the longer a patient survived after prescription of diamorphine, the greater the likelihood of a reduction in dose.

Dose reductions were made on a trial-and-error basis in patients who had improved generally over a number of weeks and who had had no recent episodes of 'breakthrough' pain. Reductions were also made after successful intrathecal nerve blocks in five patients, and after treatment with a cytotoxic agent or radiation in a number of others. A total of nine patients, all in group 5, stopped receiving diamorphine; three stopped taking diamorphine altogether; four patients stopped for more than four months; and two stopped for approximately three weeks.

It was concluded that, when used as part of a pattern of total care, diamorphine may be used for long periods without concern about tolerance. Moreover, although physical dependence probably develops in most patients after several weeks of continuous treatment (Eddy *et al.*, 1959), this does not prevent the downward adjustment of dose when considered clinically feasible. Experience with methadone (Nathan, 1952), levorphanol and phenazocine suggests that the 'natural history' of their long-term use for patients in pain is similar to that of diamorphine and morphine.

Pathological fracture

Pathological fracture of a long bone occurs in under 1 per cent of patients with advanced carcinoma but, when it does, it usually inflicts a considerable burden on a patient. All but 1 per cent of such fractures occur proximal to the knee or elbow (Galasko, 1974). Internal fixation or the insertion of a prosthesis should always be considered, particularly in the case of a femur, as these measures obviate the need for prolonged bedrest. In addition, pain is either completely relieved or much reduced.

The decision whether to treat surgically depends to a large extent on the patient's general condition. In carcinoma of the bronchus or malignant melanoma, pathological fracture often presages death. This is generally not so in breast cancer, particularly if the tumour is hormone sensitive. The results of several published series indicate that the median survival after the first or only pathological fracture associated with breast cancer is about six months, ranging from two months to four years (Twycross, 1977b).

Internal fixation should always be followed by irradiation, otherwise the fracture does not unite. Radiotherapy is commonly delayed until the wound has healed and the stitches have been removed, but this is not essential. Transcervical and subcapital fractures of the femur, however, do not unite, even when treated in this way. With these, the treatment of choice is replacement arthroplasty. This controls the pain and the patient can expect to be mobile again within days.

Consideration should sometimes be given to prophylactic nailing. It is easier than the internal fixation of an established, displaced fracture and is less disturbing for the patient. Moreover, when more than half of the cortex has been destroyed, deformity takes place on weight-bearing and this causes pain. Prophylactic nailing also facilitates nursing and, should a fracture subsequently occur, it is often symptomless.

Fracture is unlikely when less than 25 per cent of the cortex of a long bone has been eroded but, when erosion is more than 75 per cent, the bone is so weak as often to fracture spontaneously (Fidler, 1973). The indications for prophylactic internal fixation of a long bone are, therefore:

(a) increasing pain,
(b) destruction of more than half the cortex radiologically.

Local irradiation of a long-bone metastases has been considered a further indication because of an increased risk of fracture (Editorial, 1981). Our experience in Oxford, however, indicates that irradiation commonly both reduces pain and results in significant recalcification. In other words, irradiation frequently modifies both the above criteria for surgery, and renders such intervention unnecessary.

A more elaborate technique has been described for use when bone destruction is widespread or when the fracture is close to the end of the bone and adequate fixation is not possible by a nail (Yablon and Paul, 1976). Lesions are first treated by excision and curettage, and then by appropriate internal fixation with the simultaneous insertion of an acrylic cement into the bone defect. By moulding the cement around the metal device, the shape of the bone can be restored. Although this probably has an adverse effect on fracture healing, fixation is adequate. In patients with advanced disease, any risk of local or general spread of the tumour as a result of curettage is outweighed by the benefits of the procedure. In one series of 73 patients, only four failed to regain function in the affected limb (Yablon and Paul, 1976).

Hypercalcaemia

Hypercalcaemia occurs in 10–20 per cent of all patients with advanced malignant disease. The figure is higher in cancer of the breast and bronchus (Watson, 1966). In addition to causing nausea, vomiting, constipation, weakness and depression, hypercalcaemia appears to precipitate or exacerbate pain by modifying the patient's pain threshold. Several reports have been published in which hypercalcaemia in malignant disease has been reduced by either subcutaneous calcitonin or intravenous mithramycin (Parsons et al., 1974; Coombes et al., 1979; Davies et al., 1979). Each report includes examples of patients who have experienced a definite reduction in bone pain, or complete relief, when the plasma calcium concentration returned to normal. Relief was noted in over half of the patients treated. Lack of response may relate to differences in the mechanisms responsible for the pain. For example, in some the pain may relate to rapid bone resorption, whereas in others, deformity on weight-bearing could be responsible. In the former, benefit from calcitonin or mithramycin might be expected, but not in the latter. Whatever the explanation for the inconsistency of benefit, steps should be taken to correct hypercalcaemia if a patient has pain which is not readily relieved by analgesics.

'Pain is the resultant of the conflict between the stimulus and the whole individual.' (Leriche, 1939)

Acknowledgements

Figures 4.1–4.3 are reproduced with permission of Pitman Books, London; Fig. 4.5 with permission of Raven Press, New York.

References

Allen, K.L., Johnson, T.W. and Hibbs, G.G. (1976). *Cancer* **37**, 984.

Beaver, W., Schein, P.S. and Hext, M. (1981). *Clinical Pharmacology and Therapeutics* **29**, 232.

Bonica, J.J. and Halpern, L.M. (1972). Analgesics. In *Drugs of Choice 1972–73*, pp. 185–217. Ed. by W. Modell. Mosby, St Louis.

Caddy, B. and Idowu, R. (1979). *Analyst* **104**, 328.

Coombes, R.C., Neville, A.M., Gazet, J.C., Ford, H.T., Nash, A.G., Bajer, J.W. and Powles, T.J. (1979). *Cancer Chemotherapy and Pharmacology* **3**, 41.

Davies, J., Trask, C. and Souhami, R.L. (1979). *Cancer Treatment Reports* **63**, 1835.

Duboisson, D. and Melzack, R. (1976). *Experimental Neurology* **51**, 480.

Eddy, N.B., Lee, L.E. and Harris, C.A. (1959). *Bulletin on Narcotics* **11**, (No. 1), 3.

Editorial (1981). *British Medical Journal* **283**, 748.

Ferreira, S.H. (1972). *Nature New Biology* **240**, 200.

Fidler, M. (1973). *British Medical Journal* **1**, 341.

Fraser, H.F., Isbell, H., and Van Horn, G.D. (1957). *Anesthiology* **18**, 531.

Galasko, C.S.B. (1974). *Journal of the Royal College of Surgeons of Edinburgh* **19**, 351.

Galasko, C.S.B. (1981). The development of skeletal metastases. In *Bone Metastasis*, p. 83. Ed. by L. Weiss and H.A. Gilbert. G.K. Hall, Boston, Mass.

Glynn, C.G., Lloyd, J.W. and Folkard, S. (1976). *Proceedings of the Royal Society of Medicine* **69**, 369.

Heel, R.C., Brogden, T.M., Speight, T.M. and Avery, G.S. (1979). *Drugs* **17**, 81.

Hunt, J.M., Stollar, T.D., Littlejohns, D.W., Twycross, R.G. and Vere, D.W. (1977). *Journal of Medical Ethics* **3**, 61.

Inturrisi, C.E. and Vereboly, K. (1972a). *Clinical Pharmacology and Therapeutics* **13**, 633.

Inturrisi, C.E. and Verebely, K. (1972b). *Clinical Pharmacology and Therapeutics* **13**, 923.

Isbell, H. (1948). *Annals of New York Academy of Science* **51**, 108.

Judd, A.T., Tempest, S.M. and Clarke, I.M.C. (1981). *British Medical Journal* **282**, 75.

Kaiko, R.F., Wallenstein, S.L., Rogers, A.G., Grabinski, P.Y. and Houde, R.W. (1981). *New England Journal of Medicine* **304**, 1501.

Kay, B. (1973). *British Journal of Anaesthesia* **45**, 623.

Kerrane, T.A. (1975). *Nursing Mirror* **140**, 59.

Kreek, M.J., Garfield, J.W., Gutjahr, C.L. and Guisti, L.M. (1976). *New England Journal of Medicine* **294**, 1104.

Lasagna, L. (1965). *Proceedings of the Royal Society of Medicine* **58**, 978.

Lasagna, L. (1981). *New England Journal of Medicine* **304**, 1539.

Leriche, R. (1939). *The Surgery of Pain*. Translated by A. Young. Baillière Tindall and Cox, London.

Loan, W.B., Morrison, D.J., Dundee, J.W., Clarke, R.S.J. Hamilton, R.C. and Brown, S.S. (1969). *British Journal of Anaesthesia* **41**, 57.

Love, M. (1962). *British Medical Journal* **2**, 1192.

Marks, R.H. and Sachar, E.J. (1973). *Annals of International Medicine* **78**, 173.

Martin, W.R. (1973). *British Journal of Hospital Medicine* **10**, 173.

Martinson, I.M., Armstrong, G.D., Geis, D.P., Anglim, M.A., Gronseth, E.C., Macinnis, H., Cersey, J.H. and Nesbit, M.E. (1978). *Pediatrics* **62**, 106.

Milton, G.W. (1972). *Medical Journal of Australia* **2**, 177.

Mundy, G.R. and Spiro, T.P. (1981). The mechanism of bone metastasis and bone destruction by tumour cells. In *Bone Metastasis*, p. 64. Ed. by L. Weiss and H.A. Gilbert, G.K. Hall, Boston, Mass.

Nathan, P.W. (1952). *British Medical Journal* **2**, 903.

Parsons, V., Dalley, V., Brinkley, D., Davies, C. and Vernon, A. (1974). *Acta Endocrinologica* **76**, 286.

Shaw, F.H. and Shulman, A. (1955). *British Medical Journal* **1**, 1367.

Snow, H. (1896). *British Medical Journal* **2**, 718.

Stambaugh, J.E. and Wainer, I.W. (1981). *Journal of Clinical Pharmacology* **21**, 140.

Stambaugh, J.E., Wainer, I.W., Hemphill, D.M. and Scwartz, I. (1977). *Lancet* **1**, 398.

Swerdlow, M. (1967). *British Journal of Anaesthesia* **39**, 699.

Szeto, H.H., Inturrisi, C.E., Houde, R.W., Saal, S., Cheigh, J. and Reidenberg, M. (1977). *Annals of Internal Medicine* **86**, 738.

Tattersall, M.H.N. (1981). *Medical Journal of Australia* **1**, 492.

Twycross, R.G. (1974). *International Journal of Clinical Pharmacology, Therapy & Toxicology* **9**, 184.

Twycross, R.G. (1976). *Studies on the Use of Diamorphine in Advanced Malignant Disease.* DM Thesis (Oxford).

Twycross, R.G. (1977a). *Pain* **3**, 93.

Twycross, R.G. (1977b). Care of the terminal patient. In *Breast Cancer Management—Early and Late*, p. 157. Ed. by B.A. Stoll, Heinemann Medical, London.

Twycross, R.G. and Fairfield, S. (1982). *Pain* **14**, 303.

Twycross, R.G. and Lack, S.A. (1983). *Symptom Control in Far-advanced Cancer. Pain Relief.* Pitman, London.

Twycross, R.G. and Wald, S.J. (1976). The long-term use of diamorphine in advanced cancer. In *Advances in Pain Research and Therapy*, Vol. 1, p. 653. Ed. by J.J. Bonica and D. Albe-Fessard. Raven Press, New York.

Walsh, T.D., Baxter, R., Bowman, K. and Leber, B. (1981). *Pain* **1**, 39.

Watson, L. (1966). *Australian Annals of Medicine* **15**, 359.

Way, E.L., Young, J.M. and Kemp, J.W. (1965). *Bulletin on: Narcotics* **17** (No. 1), 25.

World Health Organization (1964). *Expert Committee on Drug Dependence, 13th Report*, Technical Report Series No. 287. WHO, Geneva.

World Health Organization (1969). *Expert Committee on Drug Dependence, 16th Report*, Technical Report Series No. 407, Who, Geneva.

Yablon, I.G. and Paul, G.R. (1976). *Surgery, Gynaecology and Obstetrics* **143**, 177.

6

Specialized techniques for the relief of pain

Robert Baxter

Adequate pain control can be obtained in 90 per cent of patients with cancer by judicious pharmacology. In some cases, however, side-effects (nausea, excessive drowsiness, blurring of vision, etc.) may make the patients reluctant to take the dose of analgesic required. Other patients have a strong aversion to regular medication, while a few have such severe pain that no sublethal dose of analgesic would provide full control.

These groups of patients require further measures, and the purpose of this chapter is to examine the range of procedures available for the relief of pain. Such procedures are often not intended to render the patient completely pain free; they may do so but are commonly intended to reduce a specific component of an overall pain pattern, e.g. in the patient with extensive bony secondaries whose pain is controlled at rest but is locally severe on movement.

Anatomy and physiology

A sound anatomical knowledge of sensory nerve distribution is required for the planning of pain-relieving procedures. The routes of the sensory nerves from the tissues and skeleton to the cord are well described in standard anatomy texts, as are the anatomical pathways of visceral sensation.

In the dorsal horn of the spinal cord is a complex network of neurons, into which enter the afferent sensory fibres and out of which come the ascending sensory pathways. The vast majority of pain fibres have their synapses in the two most dorsal laminae of the dorsal horn—the substantia gelatinosa. Extensive modification of the sensory impulses takes place, with both inhibitory and excitatory neurons being present.

Much work is still needed before the physiology of the dorsal horn is clarified, but it is clear that modification of pain transmission at this level is practicable. Pain can be reduced by stimulation of large fibre afferents (probably A_β fibres from low-threshold mechanoreceptors), or by direct application of opiate, as well as by interruption of the anatomical pain pathway distal to, at, or proximal to the substantia gelatinosa.

Selection of nerve block

A full assessment of the patient is essential, including a normal history and examination as well as the details of the terminal condition. The assessor will find it useful to have prior knowledge of the information given to the patient about the illness. It is, for example, difficult to offer nerve blocks carrying a risk of motor dysfunction to a patient who has been led to believe that full recovery is only a matter of time.

The site and character of the pain, with knowledge of the underlying pathology, will allow the possibilities for intervention to be listed. From this, the likelihood of undesirable side-effects (bladder dysfunction, motor loss, areas of numbness, etc.) can be assessed, and the probable effects of the procedure on the patient can be considered. This will involve some functional assessment, psychological considerations, the opinions of patient and relatives regarding active treatment, annd consideration of the probable pattern of disease progression in terms of patient function.

The nerve block specialist will often find it useful to discuss the case fully with the patient's usual medical and nursing attendants before examining the patient. Discussion with the patient can then be undertaken with full knowledge of the probabilities of disease progression and of any positive or negative attitudes displayed towards therapy. Some patients are reluctant to make decisions without discussing things with a spouse or child, and advance knowledge of this fact can avoid misunderstanding if the patient appears unduly hesitant.

Once the most promising procedures have been selected, they must be discussed with the patient, and, if necessary, the relatives. The patient should be warned of any possible side-effects and this fact recorded in the notes to avoid repercussions at a later date. If at a future date the procedure is repeated, it is advisable to repeat and document the warning.

Before undertaking a neurolytic nerve block which will produce motor loss or extensive sensory deficit, it is sensible to perform the block with local anaesthetic to enable the patient to balance benefits against disability produced. Some patients find that loss of sensation is as unpleasant as pain, while others feel that loss of even a small amount of residual motor function in a nearly useless limb is unacceptable. In such cases it often transpires that the patients still have strong hopes for recovery of function, even though they appear to have come to terms with the inevitability of their disease's progression. Other patients will reject the possibility of loss of function because they have been led to believe that they will recover from their illness.

Patients should never be allowed to feel under pressure to accept a procedure, nor should they be allowed to form a false impression of the success rate or incidence of side-effects. Repeated, careful explanations may be needed and the block specialist must be prepared to fit the procedure into the patient's wishes (visiting arrangements, weekend outings etc.).

Performance of nerve block

Procedures should be planned, rather than 'spur of the moment'. Although some simple nerve blocks can be carried out in seconds with minimal assistance, many require careful positioning of the patient with more than one assistant needed to maintain the positioning for several minutes. The optimum time for these blocks is during the overlap of nursing shifts in the early afternoon. Appropriate sedation should be given (intravenous Diazemuls—a preparation of diazepam in a lipid emulsion—is ideal, as it causes minimal irritation to veins, and the dosage is easily titratable), and facilities for treatment of adverse reactions and other side-effects should be available.

There is considerable debate over both the desirability and the necessity of use of radiological screening to aid the nerve blocker. Screening can increase the accuracy of many procedures and is essential to the performance of a few. It is an excellent medicolegal safeguard, it is very satisfying to do nerve blocks under the direct vision it affords, and it is an invaluable teaching aid. It is easy, in a general hospital, to take the patient to the screening room, or to use portable screening equipment in theatre. Such equipment is unlikely to be available in a hospice, community unit or patient's home.

In these cases, the benefits of screening must be balanced against the potential ill-effects the patient may suffer from transfer to the general hospital. The adverse effects of moving ill patients are well known. Delays in waiting for transport can upset drug routines, the patient's stable drug regime may not fit with the routines and prejudices of a hospital ward, and the suspension of most ambulances is that of a commercial van designed to carry inert packages rather than fragile and pain-wracked flesh. If the nerve block specialist feels that these problems are offset by the improved safety gain afforded by screening for the particular procedure, then so be it. If, however, the screening is designed either to boost the operator's confidence or to provide medicolegal cover, rather than being an essential aid to the procedure, then the transport of the patient is difficult to justify. Some patients will not accept procedures requiring their transport from the hospice, and some will refuse anything that cannot be performed in their own homes. The problems of domiciliary nerve blocks will be considered later.

Unless there are special complicating features, my own view is that screening is only essential for radiofrequency cordotomy, rhizotomy or cranial transforaminal procedures, and for pituitary ablations and subdural, extra-arachnoid injections.

Procedures available

A book of this nature is not the proper place to give detailed instructions on the techniques of performing procedures. An outline of the variety of nerve blocks and other methods available for treating pain will be given, with a list of references from which more detailed information may be sought.

Nerve blocks

Upper limb
Analgesia for upper limb pain is often difficult to achieve by neural blockade and carries a high risk to motor function. Pain in the arm is most commonly caused by carcinoma of the breast, with axillary lesions from tumour, radiotherapy or surgery affecting the brachial plexus, or with a grossly distended painful arm from lymphoedema. Less common causes are Pancoast tumour (superior pulmonary sulcus syndrome), and secondary deposits in the cervical vertebrae or bones of the arm.

The dermatome distribution will determine whether the pain is from brachial or cervical plexus involvement, and the site of origin of the pain is usually easy to locate. Nerve block must be performed between the site of nerve involvement and the spinal cord.

Brachial plexus block is rarely possible by the axillary approach in these cases and the supraclavicular or interscalene approaches are normally required. Complete block of both cervical and brachial plexuses is possible by a single interscalene injection. Spread of solution to phrenic, vagus, recurrent laryngeal or cervical sympathetic nerves has been reported.

Blockade of major nerve plexuses supplying the upper limb should be performed initially with local anaesthetic to enable patient and operator to evaluate the likely relief of pain against probable motor and sensory loss If a neurolytic block is required, injection of local anaesthetic to confirm needle placement is a useful method of increasing success rate and minimizing side-effects. Alcohol should not be used, as the incidence of neuritis is high with this agent. Phenol is the drug of choice.

The supraclavicular approach to the plexus is less likely to produce unwanted spread to other nerves, but this advantage is offset by an incidence of pneumothorax which varies from 0.5 per cent to 6 per cent in various series.

Subdural, extra-arachnoid injection may be of value; this technique is discussed below.

Lower limb
Pain in the leg may be due to lesions in the limb itself, in the pelvic region or in the lumbosacral spine. If there is any doubt as to the origin of the pain, or the nerve blocks most suitable to its relief, trial injections with local anaesthetic, starting at the most peripheral site, may be needed in patients with multiple malignant deposits to determine the best site for 'permanent' block.

Pain from lesions below the knee is controllable by sciatic nerve block provided motor function is not a consideration. Paravertebral lumbar root block, or sacral transforaminal block, may be useful for isolated lesions in the femur and pelvis, but motor loss is a limiting factor. Hip block, performed by local anaesthetic blockade of the obturator nerve and the nerve to quadratus femoris may have surprisingly prolonged effects in patients with acetubular or upper femoral lesions.

Intrathecal blockade is an extremely useful procedure for pain related to lumbosacral nerve root distribution. The incidence of motor paresis varies from 1 per cent to 14 per cent, and of bladder or rectal dysfunction from 0.7 per cent to 26 per cent in various series. Useful analgesia may be expected in about 70 per cent of cases. Obsessional care in patient positioning and adequate number of assistants to maintain positioning will enable side-effects to be minimized.

Head and neck
Unilateral cervical pain may be helped by cervical plexus block, but phrenic nerve loss on that side must be expected and spread of agents to the brachial plexus is a distinct risk.

Subdural, extra-arachnoid injection of neurolytic agents under radiological control is often useful, giving a success rate in the order of 70 per cent with, in experienced hands, an extremely low risk of side-effects. The technique is well described by Mehta and Maher (1977).

Pain in the distribution of the lower division of the trigeminal nerve is reasonably amenable to nerve block. The maxillary and ophthalmic divisions are better approached by thermocoagulation using a radiofrequency lesion generator; an incorrect placement of local anaesthetic or neurolytic agent during an attempt to block the upper two-divisions can lead to a disastrous intracranial spread of the agent injected.

Thoracic region

Thoracic vertebral pain will often respond to bilateral paravertebral block or to radiofrequency thermocoagulation of the dorsal spinal root, while rib pain responds well to intercostal or paravertebral injection. Thoracic visceral pain is a rare problem, but a paravertebral block may be of value. Ideally, visceral pain should be treated by sympathetic ganglion blockade, but this really needs x-ray screening, while a simple paravertebral block does not. In experienced hands, the incidence of pneumothorax from a paravertebral block is extremely small.

Abdomen and pelvis

If abdominal wall pain is arising from a surgical scar, local infiltration with steroid and local anaesthetic into the most tender points is the treatment of choice. Pain arising from rib or vertebral secondaries should be treated as a thoracic pain.

Pain from the abdominal viscera usually responds well to coeliac plexus blockade, with a success rate of over 90 per cent obtainable in gastric and pancreatic neoplasms. Hypotension is a normal side effect of this procedure but rarely requires therapy. In severe hypotension, intravenous colloid or vasoconstrictor will be needed, so an indwelling intravenous cannula is a wise precaution. It is extremely rare for postural hypotension to persist for more than 48-72 hours and most patients can be cautiously mobilized after 24 hours.

Pelvic visceral pain is often relieved by lumbar sympathetic or coeliac blockade, while perianal or perineal pain responds best to intrathecal block, although anococcygeal blocks may suffice.

Bilateral lumbar sympathetic block and, more rarely, coeliac block can produce failure of ejaculation, although impotence is virtually unknown.

Large ovarian masses can produce a dragging lower abdominal pain which is often responsive to a thoracic paravertebral block of the affected side. This can avoid the need for a coeliac block and is a much more minor procedure.

Other procedures

Radiofrequency thermocoagulation

This is an extremely useful procedure for selected cases, but radiological control is needed. The technique is used to destroy selected dorsal sensory roots, divisions of the trigeminal nerve, or to perform percutaneous spinothalamic tractotomy, which is most useful for unilateral pain as there is a definite incidence of respiratory tract damage. A bilateral procedure is not normally undertaken in one session, but is acceptable with a delay of a few days between the two sides.

Radiofrequency generators, with their accessories, are expensive items and require considerable expertise for safe use.

Transcutaneous nerve stimulation (TNS)

This technique releases enkephalin at spinal cord level by stimulating the fibres from the low threshold mechanoreceptors. Although useful for milder pain, it is uncommon for this technique to give useful results in severe pain. It is, however, extremely simple and safe, with the advantage of allowing the patient to take an active part in management by experimenting with electrode positions and the stimulator output settings. Patients with scar pain, post-herpetic neuralgia or benign musculoskeletal pains will often experience considerable benefit.

Acupuncture

In general terms, acupuncture is seldom sufficient for severe malignant pain, though it can be a useful adjunct to other therapy. It is particularly useful for musculoskeletal non-malignant pain, and treatment provides a useful relaxed euphoria. Like TNS, the technique releases enkephalin and the effects of both can be reversed by naloxone.

Various intensities of acupuncture treatment may be used, from passive needle insertion to electrical stimulation.

Cryotherapy

Repeated freeze-thaw cycles cause cellular disruption, and if a cryotherapy probe is placed so that a nerve is included in the iceball at the probe tip, sensory blockage is obtained. The duration of the blockade is variable, but a median of two weeks to five months has been reported in various series. Like neurolytic block, loss of all nerve function is obtained and this may limit the application. The usual probe is 15 gauge and incorporates a nerve stimulator, but a finer probe is available for use via the sacral hiatus in the treatment of perineal pain and coccydinia.

Less fibrous reaction is produced by cryotherapy than by neurolytic injection, and it is possible that repeated treatments are easier with cryotherapy.

Pituitary ablation

Hypophysectomy has been used for many years to control advanced carcinoma of the breast. A transnasal approach to the gland and application of a cryoprobe or injection of a small volume of alcohol offer the same benefits in pain control with a reduced morbidity compared to the conventional surgical approaches. The mechanism of analgesia is unclear, and it is surprising that even non-hormone-dependent tumour secondaries may show a marked reduction in pain. Best results seem to be obtained in carcinoma of the breast or prostate.

Psychological modification

Hypnosis, relaxation training, biofeedback methods and behaviour modification techniques are all being used in the treatment of chronic pain. Hypnotic techniques usually aim to teach patients to modify their perception of pain by interpreting the pain sensation as warmth, tingling or some other relatively pleasant sensation.

An alternative hypnotic approach is that of time distortion, allowing the patient to shorten the perceived duration of painful periods and lengthen the apparent duration of relatively pain-free ones. Hypnosis has been widely used in some units specializing in chronic pain with considerable success. There is a risk of releasing suppressed memories of traumatic experiences, with which a patient under stress from pain or imminent death may not be able to cope. These techniques should, therefore, be reserved for the experienced therapist.

The other psychological techniques mentioned above have all been used with success in various pain-relief units, but they have not gained very wide use. This may be because they all make extensive demands on the therapist's time.

Hypertonic saline

Intrathecal hypertonic saline instillation is an alternative to neurolytic procedures for some patients. Significant morbidity, usually in the form of paraesthesias, occurs in only 1 per cent of patients, and those at risk appear to be patients with myocardial disease or evidence of a compromised blood supply to the cauda equina. The technique may be particularly valuable for the younger ambulatory patient with pelvic bony secondaries, or with secondaries in the lumbar spine. There is no convincing evidence that cold saline is of greater value than isothermic, and addition of a low concentration of local anaethetic to the saline prevents any severe pain on injection. A solution containing 5 mg/ml (0.5%) lignocaine (lidocaine) and 60-80 mg/ml (6-8%) saline produces good results. Any analgesia lasting more than three to four hours would merit a repeat procedure, and several repeats may be necessary to obtain the best possible results.

Implanted stimulators

Implantation of cerebral electrodes can provide excellent pain relief in certain cases. The major disadvantages are that it is not easy to predict which patients will respond, the procedure is fairly major, and the electrodes have a tendency to displace.

An alternative approach is to insert a wire electrode into the epidural space and connect this to a stimulator. Analgesia over several spinal segments can be obtained and the electrode can easily be re-inserted if the analgesia distribution is not quite that required. If the electrode is tunnelled subcutaneously to the lateral or anterior aspect of the chest or abdomen, it can be left *in situ* for some time, attached to an external miniature stimulator. If longer-term analgesia is required, implanted stimulator systems can be used. These are, however, rather expensive. Although the epidural wire is usually inserted under local analgesia, it should be done under full sterile conditions and the electrode position checked with x-ray.

CNS opiates

Pain relief is readily obtainable by intrathecal or epidural injection of opiates. A considerable number of studies have been undertaken on this technique, and a low but definite incidence of late-onset respiratory depression has been reported with a number of different opiates. It seems likely that a strongly lipophilic opiate which would bind readily and rapidly in the spinal cord is needed to avoid this problem, and evaluation studies are continuing.

If one of the more promising agents is found to be suitable, the technique offers useful prospects for long-term epidural cannulation and regular opiate instillation, either by intermittent bolus injection or by continuous infusion from a miniaturized syringe driver pump. Unlike epidural or intrathecal injection of local anaesthetic agents, the opiates do not produce hypotention or motor blockade.

Inhalation

Some relatively immobile patients are pain free at rest and only experience significant pain when they are turned. Prophylactic administration of an inhalational analgesic agent, such as an equal mixture of oxygen and nitrous oxide, can be quite satisfactory for these cases. Calibrated inhalers to deliver analgesic concentrations of methoxyflurane or trichloroethylene in air are available. This technique is also useful for painful dressing changes and is used in a number of intensive therapy units as an aid to physiotherapy in patients who have had thoracic or upper abdominal surgery.

An outline has been given of the procedures available for the control of pain in malignant disease. It is not possible in a work of this nature to give detailed instructions for the performance of these procedures, and references to specialist textbooks is recommended for such information.

However, two other topics must be considered.

Non-malignant pain

Patients with cancer are as liable as any other population sample to suffer non-malignant pain. Ischaemia, scar pain, arthritis and post-herpetic neuralgia are the most common causes of chronic pain.

In many cases, the analgesia required for the cancer pain will control the non-malignant pain as well, but there is a wide range of specific therapies available for these problems.

Sympathetic blockade for ischaemia or herpes zoster, acupuncture or transcutaneous nerve stimulation for musculoskeletal problems and somatic nerve injections for scar pain or certain skeletal symptom patterns all have their place, and the advice of a pain-relief specialist may be very useful.

Domiciliary procedures

The introduction of the domiciliary care team in the management of cancer has produced improvements in patient care within the community comparable to those in hospital care that arose after publication of the early papers from the hospice movement.

One unforseen result of this has been the appearance of a group of patients who refuse to consider entering a hospital or hospice for treatment and who require one of the procedures discussed above. It is worth trying to find out why the patient has such strong objections to in-patient care. In some cases, the problem turns out to be a personality clash with hospital staff, and a change of ward or hospital will overcome the objections. If the patient's objections are insuperable, however, then consideration can be given to a domiciliary procedure.

Although no procedure requiring x-ray control can be undertaken in the patient's home, many others can be, provided that certain criteria can be met. A clean and well-lit room is essential, and facilities for resuscitation and treatment of side-effects must be provided. Adequate post-procedure nursing care must be available, either from the community nursing service or from the domiciliary care team. The nurse in attendance must be familiar with the problems liable to arise after nerve blocks and should be trained to carry out any necessary administration of fluids or other therapy, including vasoconstrictor drugs. An open channel of communication between the nurse and operator must be defined, and access to an in-patient bed in case of crisis is required.

Acutely life-threatening side-effects are extremely rare in neutral blockade. I have seen one cardiovascular collapse and two local anaesthetic convulsions in a ten-year experience encompassing some 5000 nerve blocks. Other side-effects have occurred, but not of a nature to produce an acute crisis. Of the three serious cases, two would not have been undertaken outside hospital, although both of these could well have been arranged for a day-case unit.

Although domiciliary procedures should not be condemned, they should only be undertaken with adequate assistance and on the clear understanding of both patient and relatives that there is an extra element of risk involved. It is prudent to obtain a signed statement from the patients and their relatives that they appreciate this fact, that the decision to undergo a domiciliary procedure is theirs, and that they have declined even day-case treatment in hospital. Criticisms and allegations of imprudence or even negligence may come from sources other than the patient's family should a crisis occur, and the operator should have documentation to protect both himself and his nurse from such allegations, should this prove necessary.

Reference and further reading

Mehta, M. and Maher, R. (1977). Injection into the extra-arachnoid, sub-dural space. *Anaesthesia* **32**, 760.

Anatomy

Dunhill, R.P.H., Colvin, M.P. and Crawley, B.E. (1979). *Clinical and Resuscitative Data*, 2nd edn. Blackwell Scientific, Oxford. (Contains dermatome and sclerotome charts, visceral innervations and useful drug and metabolic data.)

Medical Research Council Memorandum 45 (1976). *Aids to the Examination of the Peripheral Nervous System*. HMSO, London.

Procedures

Cousins, M.J. and Bridenbaugh, P.O. (eds.) (1980). *Neural Blockade in Clinical Anaesthesia and the Management of Pain*. Lippincott, Philadelphia and Toronto. (Probably the most comprehensive text, with the best list of references, available at present.)

7

Control of other symptoms

Mary J. Baines

'When you know why, you know how.'

'Feverishness is generally supposed to be a sysmptom of fever—in nine cases out of ten it is a symptom of bedding.'
   (Florence Nightingale)

Advanced malignant disease commonly affects many organs of the body, disturbs the biochemical balance and may be associated with ectopic hormone production. It is therefore not surprising that patients develop many symptoms in the last weeks or months of life. Good terminal care involves meticulous attention to each symptom, for without this foundation, the necessary emotional and spiritual support becomes impossible.

   As in general medicine, it is important to seek to diagnose the cause of each symptom and to base treatment on it; but such a diagnosis will depend more on a careful history and clinical examination than on investigations which may be impracticable in the very ill.

   Sometimes it is impossible to make an accurate diagnosis, and to let a distressing symptom continue in the hope of producing a clear picture can rarely, if ever, be justified. Symptomatic relief must be given, if necessary using several drugs at once; sometimes the response to such treatment makes the diagnosis clear.

Gastrointestinal symptoms

Dry or painful mouth

The following causes are commonly seen in the terminally ill patient:

Drugs, especially phenothiazines, tricyclic antidepressants, antispasmodics, antihistamines, diuretics and cytotoxics.
Dehydration.
Oral candidosis.
Ill-fitting dentures.
Aphthous ulceration.
Local radiotherapy.
Oral tumours.

Treatment
Good oral hygiene is most important and will prevent many problems. Regular mouth washes should be given, and some patients chew gum or suck pineapple chunks to increase the flow of saliva.

Artificial saliva, made with methylcellulose and lemon essence, is occasionally helpful.

Dehydration is probably fairly common in the last days of life. Fortunately the only symptom it causes is a dry mouth. At this stage, intravenous fluids are inappropriate and the dry mouth should be treated with frequent small drinks and crushed ice to suck.

Oral candidosis is very common and about 75 per cent of hospice patients have a heavy growth of yeasts on swabs taken from the oral mucosa, though some will be asymptomatic (Kirkham, 1983). It need not show the features of classical thrush, and several different clinical pictures may improve after topical antifungal therapy. These include a dry mouth with a furred tongue, a generally uncomfortable mouth and angular cheilitis, which is only rarely the result of riboflavine deficiency.

Nystatin suspension (100 000 units/ml) 1 ml four-hourly is given; dentures should be removed and treated.

Amphotericin (Fungilin) lozenges four-hourly can also be used, but they dissolve very slowly in the mouth.

Very resistant cases can be treated with ketoconazole (Nizoral) 200 mg daily, a systemic antifungal agent.

Aphthous ulceration is not common. It is treated with hydrocortizone lozenges 2.5 mg (Corlan) four times daily or a topical steroid such as adcortyl in Orabase.

Dysphagia

When a patient complains of difficulty in swallowing, it is important to identify which of the three stages is affected:

passing the bolus to the back of the throat,
initiating the swallowing reflex,
passage of the bolus down the oesophagus.

Questioning the patient will give some information, but more will often be gained by direct observation of swallowing. Such an approch, combined with a knowledge of the previous medical history, will usually elucidate the problem, although further investigations may sometimes be needed.

Certain causes of dysphagia are associated especially with the terminally ill, and merit discussion.

Candidosis
This may spread from the oral cavity to the pharynx and oesophagus and sometimes causes dysphagia when no oral lesions are apparent. It should be treated with nystatin suspension or, in very resistant cases, with the systemic antifungal agent ketoconazole (Nizoral) 200 mg daily for ten days.

Cricopharyngeal spasm
This may occur in motor neuron disease and other neuromuscular disorders that affect the pharynx. If tongue movements remain good, a cricopharyngeal myotomy should be considered.

Mediastinal tumours
Irradiation should be considered if the patient is fit enough (see Chapter 8). Glucocorticosteroids can cause a temporary improvement by shrinking mediastinal lymph glands either prior to radiotherapy or if this treatment is contra-indicated because the patient has already been fully irradiated or is too ill.

Carcinoma of the oesophagus
Increasing dysphagia due to progressive narrowing of the oesophagus by tumour is a most unpleasant mode of death, with the patient eventually unable to swallow even his own saliva. Palliative surgery with the insertion of an oeso-phageal tube (see Chapter 10) or palliative radiotherapy (see Chapter 8) should always be considered as medication has little to offer these patients.

'Dysphagia syndrome'
This may occur in patients with advanced carcinoma of the oropharynx and has been described by Carter *et al.* (1982). There is total or near-total dysphagia for solids and liquids which is usually attributed to mechanical obstruction by primary or metastatic tumour. However, autopsy shows minimal or absent narrowing of the lumen, but mechanical 'splinting' of one side of the pharynx by local fibrosis and tumour in the soft tissues of the neck and perineural spread into the ipsilateral vagal trunk. The cause of the dysphagia is complex and probably involves neuromuscular inco-ordination. It is important to recognize this, as temporary palliation can sometimes be achieved with corticosteroids.

Case history
Mr K.B. (aged 57) had a five-year history of carcinoma of the tongue (posterior third) with metastases in cervical lymph nodes. This had been treated with two courses of radiotherapy followed by combination chemotherapy, but the disease had recurred in the neck. He was readmitted to the referring hospital with severe facial pain and almost complete dysphagia, and treated with analgesics and the insertion of a nasogastric tube. A week after transfer to St Christopher's Hospice he was started on soluble prednisolone 60 mg daily given via the tube. Three days later he could manage soup, ice-cream and other fluids orally, though he continued with nasogastric feeding. He became much more cheerful and planned a home visit. The improvement in swallowing was maintained until his death two weeks later from a chest infection. Autopsy showed no mechanical block but tumour and fibrosis in the soft tissues of the neck.

General management
If specific treatment (as outlined above) is ineffective, there are three further considerations.

Feeding
This is a very individual matter and should be fully discussed with the patient.

With a partial oesophageal block, fluids and liquidized foods are usually toler-ated and the latter should be made as appetizing as possible. When the problem arises in the mouth or pharynx, semisolids may be swallowed better than liquids, for example ice-cream rather than a milk drink. Necessary medication can often be given in suppository form.

Nasogastric tube and gastrostomy
These are rarely indicated and should never be used without full discussion with the patients and their families. It is extremely difficult for them to have the tube removed once it has been inserted and its use sometimes appears simply to prolong the process of dying.

Most patients with severe dysphagia sooner or later develop an aspiration pneumonia. In most cases this should be treated symptomatically, with opiates, hyoscine and other sedatives if needed.

Anorexia

The cause of anorexia in advanced malignant disease is obscure; indeed it seems likely that just as pain and sickness have a number of different causative mech-anisms, there may be many causes of anorexia. Some of these causes can be identified and are amenable to specific treatment; these include nausea and vomiting, abdominal distension from ascites, constipation and depression. Taste changes may occur, with a common dislike of meat, and patients complain that 'everything tastes salty' or 'it has a metallic flavour'.

Treatment
Serve small portions of food, attractively prepared.

Find out what food the patient enjoys. Often stronger tasting food is preferred to the traditional bland invalid fare.

Alcohol before meals may improve appetite.

Corticosteroids are the only effective drug treatment for anorexia. Predniso-lone 15–30 mg daily or dexamethasone 2–4 mg daily is given; most patients report an improvement in appetite within a week, sometimes finding that their sense of taste returns first. In most terminally ill patients this dose can be continued without causing side-effects; if the disease goes into remission, the dose can be reduced slowly or even stopped. There are no absolute contra-indications but it is wise to prescribe cimetidine (Tagamet) in a patient with a history of peptic ulceration and monitor diabetic patients closely.

Cyproheptadine (Periactin) has not been found effective in this group of patients.

Nausea and vomiting

These are caused by stimulation of the vomiting centres in the medulla oblon-gata in one or more of many ways (Fig. 7.1).

The antiemetic drugs act at different sites and are therefore effective in different causes of vomiting. Clinical experience has been borne out by studies localizing high levels of neurotransmitter receptors in certain areas of the brain. Thus the ability of dopamine antagonists such as phenothiazines to relieve

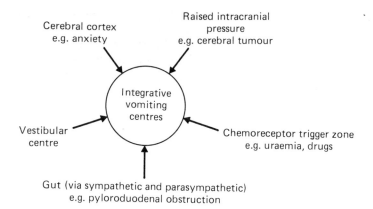

Fig. 7.1   Mechanism of vomiting.

vomiting due to biochemical changes presumably relates to the high density of dopamine receptors in the area postrema, which contains the chemoreceptor trigger zone (Peroutka and Snyder, 1982).

During the act of vomiting the glottis closes, the soft palate rises and the abdominal muscles contract, thus expelling the stomach contents. During the sensation of nausea the stomach relaxes and there is reverse peristalsis in the duodenum.

Table 7.1 shows the commonly used antiemetic drugs.

Some diseases cause vomiting through more than one mechanism, and com-

Table 7.1   Antiemetic drugs

Group	Examples	Dose (mg)/24 hours	Site of action
Phenothiazines	Chlorpromazine (Largactil)	50–150	
	Prochlorperazine (Stemetil)	15–50	Chemoreceptor trigger zone
	Methotrimeprazine (Veractil or Nozinan)	50–150	
Butyrophenones	Haloperidol (Serenace)	1.5–5	Chemoreceptor trigger zone
Antihistamines	Cyclizine (Valoid)	100–150	Integrative vomiting centre
	Promethazine (Phenergan)	30–75	
Anticholinergics	Hyoscine (Scopolamine)	0.4–0.6 single dose	Integrative vomiting centre
	Atropine	0.3–0.5 single dose	
Other	Metoclopramide (Maxolon)	30–60	1. Upper gut, increasing gastric peristalsis and relaxing pyloric antrum
	Domperidone (Motilium)	30–60	2. Chemoreceptor trigger zone
	Pyridoxine (vitamin B_6)	60–150	Not known. Vitamin B_6 may be depleted in some radiotherapy patients

binations of antiemetic drugs acting at different sites may prove more effective than a single agent.

Bearing in mind the mechanism of vomiting and the antiemetic drugs available, the causes of vomiting in the terminally ill patient are discussed below with suggested treatment (Table 7.2). (The management of cough, constipation and anxiety is covered elsewhere in this chapter.)

Table 7.2 Causes of vomiting

1. Chemical causes
   Drugs
   Uraemia
   Hypercalcaemia
   Irradiation
2. Gastric causes
   Local irritation from drugs, blood etc.
   External pressure
   Carcinoma of stomach
   Pyloroduodenal obstruction
3. Intestinal obstruction
4. Constipation
5. Raised intracranial pressure
6. Vestibular disturbance
7. Cough-induced vomiting
8. Psychogenic, especially anxiety

Drug-induced vomiting
Drugs can cause vomiting in three ways.

1. By direct effect on the chemoreceptor trigger zone—opiates, oestrogens, digoxin, chemotherapy. The drug should be stopped if possible, otherwise an antiemetic such as prochlorperazine or haloperidol is usually effective.

2. By causing gastric stasis—morphine. Treatment is with metoclopramide which increases peristalsis in the upper gut.

3. By causing local gastric irritation—aspirin and other non-steroidal anti-inflammatory drugs. Medication should be given with food or by suppository, or a similar drug substituted which has fewer gastrointestinal side-effects. Cimetidine (Tagamet) has occasionally been found to give symptomatic relief.

Uraemia
This is a common terminal event in patients with advanced pelvic malignancy. The resulting nausea and vomiting can usually be controlled by antiemetics acting on the chemoreceptor trigger zone, sometimes cyclizine is needed in addition.

Hypercalcaemia
The primary tumours associated with hypercalcaemia are shown in Table 7.3.

The symptoms of hypercalcaemia are usually described as weakness, anorexia, nausea and vomiting, leading to drowsiness, confusion and coma. However, in practice this progression is not often seen; the severity of symptoms does not correlate well with the corrected calcium level and may depend more on its

Table 7.3 Types of hypercalcaemia in malignant disease

Bone involvement	Primary sites	Probable mechanism	Alkaline phosphatase
With skeletal metastases	Breast Bronchus Kidney	Prostaglandins	Usually raised
	Myeloma Lymphoma	Osteoclast-activating factor	Normal unless pathological fracture
Without skeletal metastases	Squamous cell tumours especially bronchus, kidney	Ectopic parathyroid hormone	Usually normal

rate of change. Increased bone pain has been reported in hypercalcaemia, but in a series of patients with bony metastases at St Christopher's Hospice, it was found that the analgesic requirements were lower in the hypercalcaemic than the normocalcaemic.

Hypercalcaemia should be suspected in two clinical situations.

1. Persistent nausea and vomiting in a patient with widespread skeletal metastases, usually from a carcinoma of breast or bronchus.

2. Drowsiness and confusion in a patient with a squamous cell carcinoma, carcinoma of kidney or myeloma. This is often not preceded by vomiting and it may easily be confused with cerebral metastases.

Treatment
Severe hypercalcaemia (greater than 3 mmol/l).
This is a life-threatening condition so the decision whether to treat or not should be made carefully and be based on the patient's general condition, including cardiac and renal function and the extent of malignant disease.

Active treatment involves rehydration with 3 litres of saline intravenously in 24 hours, together with a loop diuretic such as frusemide 80 mg. These alone may be adequate, but other measures available are mithramycin 25 mg/kg intravenously on alternate days and oral phosphate 1–3 g/day (Phosphate-Sandoz effervescent tablets) (Hosking, 1983). The action of corticosteroids is slow as they reduce gut absorption of calcium, thus they have little place in the acute management of severe hypercalcaemia.

Mild hypercalcaemia (less than 3 mmol/l)
This will usually respond to corticosteroids alone. If the patient is vomiting and unable to take oral medication, an injection of hydrocortisone 100 mg should be given, followed by oral prednisolone 30 mg daily, reducing the dose as improvement occurs. If steroids alone are ineffective or if they are contraindicated, oral phosphate 1–3 g daily should be given.

There is a group of patients who are clinically indistinguishable from those with metastatic hypercalcaemia from carcinoma of the breast. They have widespread bony metastases, nausea and vomiting, a raised alkaline phosphatase but with a normal serum calcium. They respond to the above steroid regime and one can only label this as 'steroid-responsive vomiting' and postulate that it is due to some biochemical abnormality other than hypercalcaemia or to a specific antiemetic effect of corticosteroids.

Gastric causes

1. Extrinsic pressure on the stomach from hepatomegaly causes the 'squashed stomach syndrome' described by Twycross (Twycross, 1982). Symptoms include early satiation, flatulence, hiccup and vomiting soon after food. Treatment is with metoclopramide 10 mg before meals, with a defoaming agent such as dimethicone (Asilone).

2. Intrinsic involvement of the stomach from carcinoma, including linitus plastica, often causes severe vomiting. Treatment is not very satisfactory, but metoclopramide or cyclizine may help. A coeliac axis block may reduce vomiting as well as pain due to interference with efferent impulses from the stomach. Glucocorticosteroids sometimes give temporary relief (see below).

3. Pyloroduodenal obstruction. This is caused by malignant involvement of the pylorus, duodenum or a previous gastroenterostomy by carcinoma of the stomach or pancreas. There may be large vomits, sometimes with undigested food eaten hours before.

If the patient is too ill for palliative surgery, there has been, until recently, very little to offer medically. Metoclopramide is usually ineffective, and a nasogastric tube with regular suction often more distressing than the vomiting it seeks to relieve. However, glucocorticosteroids have been shown to be of use in this situation. The assumption is that the 'obstruction' is caused not only by tumour, but by surrounding inflammatory oedema. In a small series, half the patients showed considerable benefit with a marked reduction in vomiting lasting for several weeks. Dexamethasone 6–8 mg/day is given, if necessary by injection at first. If effective the dose can be gradually reduced.

Case history
Mrs L.T. (aged 69) had a cholecystojejunostomy, jejuno-jejunostomy and gastroenterostomy for a carcinoma of the head of the pancreas with extensive local spread four months before admission to St Christopher's Hospice. She remained well for three months, but was then admitted to a local hospital suffering with severe vomiting. Barium meal showed a grossly dilated stomach with gastric outlet obstruction due to recurrent tumour. She was treated with intravenous fluids and nasogastric suction but this was discontinued the day before transfer to the hospice. Her vomiting immediately recurred and she was started on dexamethasone 8 mg daily, given by injection. The following day the vomiting stopped and remained controlled for five weeks while the dexamethasone was reduced to 4 mg daily and given orally. One week before her death she started to vomit again, but was only partially controlled with antiemetic drugs.

Intestinal obstruction

Incidence
Intestinal obstruction is probably a larger problem than previously recognized. Cases were monitored over a nine-month period at St Christopher's Hospice and it was found that 1 in 23 patients died with obstruction. Tunca *et al.* (1981), in a series of 518 patients with ovarian cancer, found that intestinal obstruction developed in 25 per cent.

Pathology

A series of eighteen patients showed a M:F ratio of 5:13, the difference being caused entirely by gynaecological malignancy, predominantly ovarian.

Obstruction in a patient with extensive abdominal or pelvic malignancy is rarely caused by a single total occlusion of the gut lumen. Most cases are due to partial (or subacute) obstruction combined with some functional deficit, as in chronic intestinal pseudo-obstruction (Schuffler *et al.*, 1981).

Pseudo-obstruction can be caused by tumour infiltrating gut muscle or tumour with retroperitoneal spread involving the autonomic nerve supply; in both cases peristalsis will be impaired.

Autopsies on obstructed patients usually show multiple sites involving both ileum and colon where the bowel is kinked and narrowed by tumour masses and malignant adhesions. Microscopy shows peritoneal deposits in most cases and, in about half, significant infiltration of gut muscle coats by tumour.

Treatment

There are three methods of treatment to consider:

1. surgery,
2. intravenous fluids and nasogastric suction,
3. symptom control.

Surgery   Every patient who develops intestinal obstruction should be considered for surgery, and the decision as to whether this is the right treatment is not easy. Attention must be given to the patient's medical history—especially previous surgery—to his present condition and to his wishes. Straight abdominal x-rays may help.

The surgeon who advises the hospice on obstructed patients gave as his criterion for surgery: 'Good evidence of a single block in a relatively fit patient' (Howard, 1982).

Unfortunately, the results of palliative surgery are not good, measured both by mean survival time and symptom control. In this series seven patients had already had palliative procedures, four continued to have obstructive symptoms, the remaining three re-obstructed in one to four months; mean survival time was four months.

A study of 73 patients with small-bowel obstruction from metastatic tumour showed a 35 per cent surgical mortality, mean survival of six months in the remainder, but 10 per cent developed faecal fistulae (Aranha *et al.*, 1981).

Intravenous fluids and nasogastric suction   This is the traditional surgical management of a patient admitted with obstruction. Its value in decompressing the bowel and correcting electrolyte imbalance prior to surgery is not disputed. However, what is far from clear is the role of this treatment alone in treating malignant obstruction. Two papers have shown a 1 per cent and 15 per cent sustained response to conservative treatment (Glass and LeDuc, 1973; Aranha *et al.*, 1981), but the interpretation of this is made more difficult by the fact that obstructive symptoms are often intermittent, especially at first.

At St Christopher's Hospice no obstructed patient is treated with intravenous fluids and nasogastric suction. Symptoms are controlled with medication and this enables the patient to move about with ease or be cared for at home.

Symptom control   The main symptoms such patients exhibit are vomiting, intestinal colic, other visceral pain, diarrhoea and constipation. The last three are covered elsewhere, but vomiting and colic will be discussed.

The vomiting from intestinal obstruction is probably due to a combination of reverse peristalsis and toxic absorption. Its severity depends on the level of obstruction, and it may at first be intermittent. The vomiting is accompanied by considerable nausea and may finally become faeculent. Vomiting is present in the great majority of obstructed patients and is difficult to control fully. The most that can usually be offered is some improvement, a considerable lessening of nausea (which patients find worse than vomiting) and a diminution of vomits to once or twice a day.

The phenothiazines are probably the most useful group of drugs; three are listed here in ascending order of sedative effect:

prochlorperazine (Stemetil) 5–10 mg three times daily
chlorpromazine (Largactil) 25–100 mg three times daily
methotrimeprazine (Nozinan or Veractil) 25–100 mg three times daily.

These can all be given by mouth or injection; the first two also by suppository.

Methotrimeprazine is a sedating phenothiazine with strong antiemetic and analgesic properties. Some obstructed patients have terminal vomiting only controlled with this drug. It is the most suitable phenothiazine for use in the syringe driver for continuous subcutaneous infusion as it causes little skin reaction.

Haloperidol (0.5–1.5 mg 8-hourly) can be used instead of a phenothiazine; cyclizine 50 mg eight-hourly is sometimes given in addition as it has a different site of action. Both are suitable for use in the syringe driver. Metoclopramide has not been found effective and it may increase colic.

Colic is present in the majority of obstructed patients; it is usually intermittent. Persistent colic responds to loperamide (Imodium) 2 mg or diphenoxylate with atropine (Lomotil) given four times a day. Rapid relief of occasional colic can be obtained from sublingual hyoscine 0.3–0.6 mg (available as Kwells). Hyoscine 0.8–2 mg or propantheline (Probanthine) 60–90 mg can be given over the 24-hour period in the syringe driver for the control of colic in a patient unable to take oral medication. If high doses of anticholinergic drugs are required, there will be blurred vision with loss of accommodation; this may be helped with appropriate reading glasses.

A coeliac axis block may also prove effective (see Chapter 6).

The role of steroids in intestinal obstruction is not yet clear and needs further study. Occasionally there is a dramatic and lasting improvement in symptoms, and this appears to be in cases where a later autopsy shows extensive gut muscle infiltration rather than luminal occlusion. At this stage a trial of steroids using dexamethasone 8 mg daily for a week is justified if other measures fail.

Case history
Mr A.H. (aged 37). Fifteen months before admission to St Christophers Hospice this patient had a right hemicolectomy for a carcinoma of the hepatic flexure of the colon. He remained well for ten months but then developed obstructive symptoms: colicky abdominal pain, distension and vomiting. He was readmitted to a general hospital; abdominal x-rays showed fluid levels in the small intestine

but, at laparotomy, no procedure was possible as there were multiple malignant adhesions.

During the next four months he had three further admissions for obstruction. He was treated on each occasion with intravenous fluids and nasogastric suction but the obstructive symptoms persisted.

Prior to transfer to the hospice the intravenous fluids had been discontinued, and on admission Mr A.H. was started on suppositories using oxycodone pectinate 60 mg and chlorpromazine 50 mg, both given eight-hourly. He improved temporarily on this regime but after eight days his vomiting recurred and became faeculent. The syringe driver was therefore started and this continued for 23 days until his death. Both colic and generalized abdominal pain were minor problems, requiring hyoscine 0.6 mg/24 hours and diamorphine 50–60 mg/24 hours respectively for good control. Vomiting proved more difficult, but an increasing dose of methotrimeprazine from 50 to 150 mg/24 hours was well tolerated, and during the final two weeks he vomited about every second day, continued to eat small amounts with enjoyment and remained alert until about three days before death.

Post mortem showed multiple levels of obstruction due to widespread malignant adhesions involving a right-sided abdominal mass, the anterior abdominal wall and loops of bowel. The large and small intestines were grossly dilated and distended with liquid faeculent material.

Raised intracranial pressure

This is an unusual cause of vomiting, and many patients with large primary cerebral tumours or multiple metastases causing extensive brain damage never vomit, even if they show symptoms and signs of raised intracranial pressure such as headache, blurred vision and papilloedema.

The decision to use steroids should be made after considerable thought and taking into account the age and general condition of the patient (see p. 125). If steroids are not used, vomiting can usually be well controlled with an antiemetic such as cyclizine.

Hiccup

This may occur in uraemia, in diseases affecting the stomach or diaphragm, and occasionally with cerebral tumours.

Rebreathing into a paper bag may give relief but many patients are too ill to attempt this. The two most effective drugs are metoclopramide (Maxolon) 10 mg and chlorpromazine (Largactil) 25 mg. They can be given when required for occasional bouts of hiccup or three times a day if the symptom persists. A severe and distressing episode may respond to chlorpromazine 25 mg intravenously.

Constipation

The majority of patients complain of constipation, and for many of them there is more anxiety provoked by this symptom than any other. There are many causes of constipation; these include inactivity, a diet low in roughage, and the use of analgesic and other constipating drugs. Unfortunatly these factors are difficult to alter: bran is sometimes tried but is usually unacceptable to the very ill; mobilization may not be possible and analgesics continue to be required. In practice, therefore, the management of constipation involves the correct use of laxatives and rectal measures.

If a patient presents with a rectum loaded with hard faeces, evacuation from below is required. Bisacodyl (Dulcolax) and glycerine suppositories, or alternatively a phosphate enema, are often adequate but occasionally a manual removel or an oil-retention enema given at night may be necessary. The traditional soap and water enema is very rarely required.

Laxatives should be used after such rectal measures or if the patient presents with a rectum which is empty or contains only soft faeces or routinely after commencing opiate analgesia.

There are two main types of aperient.

1. Faecal softeners. These include methyl cellulose (Celevac) and magnesium sulphate (Epsom salts) which take up water and thus increase the volume of intestinal contents, docusate sodium (Dioctyl) and poloxamer (in Dorbanex) which are wetting agents increasing water penetration of the faeces, and liquid paraffin (in Milpar) which is minimally absorbed and thus softens and lubricates.

2. Stimulant purgatives. These increase peristalsis in the colon. They include bisacodyl (Dulcolax), danthron (in Dorbanex and Normax), senna (Senokot) and phenolphthalein.

Most terminally ill patients are best managed with a combination of both types of aperient. This will avoid either painful colic or a bowel loaded with soft faeces—problems which can arise if a stimulant or softening aperient is given alone. Dorbanex (danthron and poloxamer) and Normax (danthron and dioctyl) are convenient combined preparations. Milpar and Senokot have a similar effect. The dose should be gradually increased until a regular soft bowel action is obtained.

Occasionally, in spite of regular aperients, the bowels do not open regularly and a good general rule is for a rectal examination to be performed on the third day, inserting suppositories if the rectum is loaded. Such a regime will avoid the physical and mental distress of patients who are constipated for a week or more.

Intestinal obstruction is an occasional cause of constipation. If it is suspected, stimulant purgatives must be avoided and a faecal softener such as Milpar or dioctyl prescribed. These can be given while the obstruction is partial; when it appears complete they should be stopped.

Diarrhoea

The following causes are found in the terminally ill:

Malabsorption

This is usually due to a lack of pancreatic enzymes which occurs in patients with a carcinoma of the head of the pancreas. The diarrhoea is characteristic, the stool being bulky, pale and greasy, flushing away only with difficulty. There may also be complaints of wind and abdominal distension. Treatment is with pancreatic replacements, e.g. Tabs Pancrex V Forte two to three with each meal and snack.

The malabsorption in jaundiced patients, due to lack of bile salts to break down fat globules, is usually less severe and rarely needs treating.

Incomplete (or subacute) obstruction
About 40 per cent in a series of obstructed patients complained of diarrhoea at some stage, and untreated this can be very unpleasant with a constant fear of incontinence. It should be treated with an anti-diarrhoeal drug such as loperamide (Imodium). The dose should be adequate to lessen diarrhoea but not cause constipation which would increase obstructive symptoms.

Faecal impaction
This may cause spurious diarrhoea. It should be treated as for constipation.

Colorectal carcinoma
This may cause severe diarrhoea with associated rectal discharge and tenesmus (see below). A palliative colostomy or local radiotherapy should be considered if the patient is well enough. Constipating drugs cannot be given for fear of causing impaction, but occasionally glucocorticosteroids, locally or systemically, will help.

Neurological causes
Lack of rectal sensation and of anal tone occurs in paraplegic patients and results in constant soiling. This should be treated with a constipating drug such as codeine phosphate so that suppositories or a manual removal can be performed on alternate days.

Ileal disease or resection
The resulting failure to reabsorb bile salts can cause diarrhoea. The treatment is with cholestyramine.

Rectal discharge

This is a considerable problem for patients with colorectal carcinoma when only a palliative colostomy has been performed. A course of local palliative radiotherapy should be considered if the patient is well enough. Local application of steroids, a hydrocortisone foam enema (Colifoam) once or twice a day or prednisolone (Predsol) suppositories may help.

Tenesmus

This is fairly common in pelvic malignancies; it may occur after a palliative colostomy or even after the rectum has been removed. Not surprisingly, patients find it an embarrassing problem, one that they are reluctant to admit to unless directly questioned. The only effective drug treatment is with glucocorticosteroids, dexamethasone 4–6 mg daily to reduce peri-tumour inflammatory oedema. Some patients are helped by a coeliac axis block (see Chapter 6).

Ascites

This can often be improved with diuretics, using a combination of frusemide (Lasix) 40–80 mg daily and spironolactone (Aldactone) 50–100 mg daily.

If the symptoms persist, it is usually better to do a limited paracentesis, removing perhaps 5 litres of ascitic fluid, taken off slowly over 24 hours. This will increase comfort but without the risk of shock which may occur in debilitated patients following the drainage of a large quantity. If frequent paracenteses are required, a chemotherapeutic agent such as bleomycin or thiotepa can be instilled to seek to prevent or delay the recurrence of fluid.

Respiratory symptoms

Dyspnoea (Section written by Louis Heyse-Moore.)

Dyspnoea is an abnormally distressing difficulty in breathing. There are two components, the first subjective and the second the physical response to this distress, which is usually tachypnoea (fast breathing) and hyperpnoea (increased depth of respiration). These responses do not always occur, so it is possible to be dyspnoeic and breathing normally, and conversely to have an increased ventilation and yet not be dyspnoeic (as with metabolic acidosis).

Incidence

Patients admitted to St Josephs Hospice, April 1979–April 1980.

	Male	Female	Both
Total patients	168	213	381
Dyspnoeic patients	96 (57%)	83 (39%)	179 (48%)

Of these patients, 153 (40 per cent) had lung tumours either previously proven, or clinically. Of the patients with lung tumours, 69 per cent were dyspnoeic.

Mechanism

Respiration is controlled by neural and chemical signals to the respiratory centre in the brainstem. Two types of sensory nerve endings in the lung may be important in dyspnoea: the juxtapulmonary capillary (J) receptors, which are stimulated by stretching from pulmonary oedema, and lung irritant receptors.

Chemical signals are from a raised $P\text{CO}_2$, a lowered $P\text{O}_2$ or a raised H^+. All these signals feed into the respiratory centre, which then regulates the motor effort of ventilation.

Campbell and Godfrey (1969) suggested that, if abnormal motor effort is needed to maintain normal blood gases, there is a misalignment between muscle spindle tension and muscle fibre length, which is perceived as an inadequate breath for the tension generated, or dyspnoea.

Causes

Increased ventilatory demand
This will not, of itself, cause dyspnoea, but may tip the balance in someone

with a decreased respiratory reserve. The cause is a raised metabolic rate, such as with fever, anxiety, exercise, or anaemia.

Decreased ventilatory capacity
In all the causes listed below, ventilation–perfusion mismatch may worsen the respiratory dysfunction.

1. Airways obstruction.
   (a) External pressure: such as cervical and mediastinal lymph node metastases.
   (b) Within the air-passage walls: such as from bronchial or laryngeal tumours, or asthma.
   (c) Intraluminal: this may be a transudate (such as with congestive cardiac failure) or an exudate (mucus or pus), or inhaled vomit, or blood.
2. Increased lung stiffness. This will increase the respiratory muscle work needed to achieve a normal Po_2.
   (a) Pulmonary oedema: such as congestive cardiac failure, or lymphangitis carcinomatosa. In addition, this oedema will cause stimulation of the J receptors.
   (b) Pulmonary fibrosis: from asbestosis or after irradiation.
   (c) Tumours: if very large, or multiple.
   (d) Asthma and chronic bronchitis.
3. Loss of elastic lung recoil. Emphysema will lead to both inspiratory *and* expiratory muscle effort.
4. Painful chest lesions preventing full inspiration. Examples are pleurisy or fractured ribs. Here the Po_2 may fall, which will cause increased muscle effort to compensate, but this is frustrated by pain.
5. Loss of functioning lung tissue. If there is only moderate loss, compensation may be possible and so dyspnoea does not always occur.
   (a) Collapsed lung: this may be from a pleural effusion, post-obstructive collapse, tumour compressing lung or a pneumothorax.
   (b) Abnormal lung: either from pneumonia or oedema.
   (c) Pulmonary embolus.
6. Respiratory muscle dysfunction. If the respiratory muscles are paralysed, the problem of length–tension inappropriateness in the muscles does not arise and dyspnoea does not result, even if there is hypoxia. However, if only the intercostal muscles are paralysed leaving the diaphragm intact, or vice versa, then dyspnoea might occur.
   (a) Paraplegia affecting intercostal muscles.
   (b) Phrenic nerve palsy.
   (c) Diaphragmatic pressure from ascites.

Neural stimulation
1. Peripheral. This is by stimulation of the J receptors in the lung, as with lymphangitis carcinomatosa.
2. Central. Here the respiratory centre is stimulated but this will only alter the rate and depth of breathing and not cause dyspnoea of itself.

(a) Metabolic: such as uraemia and diabetic ketoacidosis in which there is a raised P_{CO_2}.
(b) Intracranial: such as infections, raised pressure, a stroke or tumour compressing the respiratory centre.

Anxiety
This worsens dyspnoea by increasing ventilatory demand, by raising intercostal muscle tone, and by increasing cortical awareness of respiratory difficulty.

Clinical features
It is essential to ask the patient if he feels short of breath, for, like pain, dyspnoea is subjective. Patients will describe dyspnoea in many ways, such as 'tightness' or 'not being able to get enough air'. They may have difficulty in giving precise descriptions, and just as there are different types of pain, there may be different types of dyspnoea.

Important points in examination are hyperpnoea, tachypnoea and often intercostal and sternal notch recession. Also, because the patient may feel he will die of lack of air, there is often a restless anxiety. Cyanosis may occur. Tracheal compression causing stridor and often associated with superior vena caval obstruction is particularly distressing.

Investigations
A chest x-ray may demonstrate previously unsuspected lung metastases or an effusion. Measuring the haemoglobin will help in deciding if dyspnoea from anaemia would benefit from a transfusion.

Treatment
For many causes of dyspnoea, such as heart failure, treatment is the same as in general medicine. However, sometimes a distinctive approach is needed.

Opiates
These affect respiration as follows.

1. Reduction of respiratory centre sensitivity to hypercapnoea or hypoxia.
2. Decreased anxiety.
3. Reduced subjective distress of dyspnoea.
4. Stopping pain associated with ventilation.
5. Improving heart failure.

Clinically, there is a reduced rate and depth of respiration with lessened anxiety. Thus opiates are very effective for dyspnoea from terminal cancer and may be used as one of the first treatments. Dosage of morphine is similar to that for pain control (see Chapter 5), except that high doses are rarely needed. However, in ordinary hospital practice, morphine is little used to control dyspnoea, for fear of causing respiratory depression and hence respiratory failure or pneumonia. Provided dosage is carefully monitored, this belief has not been found valid in hospice care for a number of reasons.

1. It is a clinical impression in hospice work that dyspnoeic patients on morphine do not necessarily die in a short time. Indeed, some improve so much

that they become mobile again and so avoid the risks of pneumonia and pulmonary emboli associated with being bedbound.

2. Walsh (1984) found that of 20 patients on regular high-dose morphine, 12 of whom also had chronic bronchitis, only 1 had a raised P_{CO_2}.

3. It is possible to be dyspnoeic and yet have normal blood gases. In lymphangitis, for example, ventilatory effort may be set too high. In this case morphine may reset the effort at a more normal level, not depress respiration.

4. Restlessness from dyspnoea will cause high energy consumption and hence further lack of oxygen in a vicious circle. Morphine will reduce agitation and hence break this pattern.

Sedatives and tranquillizers

Diazepam may reduce dyspnoea partly by an anxiolytic effect and partly by reducing the increased tone in the respiratory muscles. Clinical observation at St Christopher's Hospice suggests that diazepam 2 mg t.d.s. may markedly improve shortness of breath in patients with lung tumours. In acute dyspnoea, as with tracheal compression, diazepam 2–10 mg i.v. given slowly, titrating dose with effect, is very useful.

As with morphine, diazepam does not, if properly used, shorten life. Phenothiazines such as prochlorperazine may help by reducing anxiety, especially as adjuvants to morphine.

Glucocorticosteroids

These may help dyspnoea in various ways.

1. Relief of bronchospasm.
2. Reduction of tumour oedema in lung or mediastinal neoplasms and hence relief of tracheal or bronchial compression.
3. Reduction of lymphangitis carcinomatosa.

Dexamethasone 8 mg/24 hours is used to reduce tumour oedema, though probably the optimum dose varies with individuals.

Atropinic drugs

Hyoscine (Scopolamine) has the following actions.

1. It dries up secretions of all exocrine glands.
2. It relaxes smooth muscle.
3. It is markedly sedative, though rarely it may cause confusion and agitation in the elderly.

Hyoscine is used to abolish the so-called 'death rattle'. This is caused by accumulation of bronchial secretions from pneumonia and heart failure in a patient too weak to cough effectively, and can be very distressing to a watching family or others on the ward, though probably not to the patient himself, who may be semiconscious. Hyoscine will also relieve bronchospasm. The dose is 0.4–0.6 mg four- to eight-hourly i.m., but tachyphylaxis may occur. Diamorphine 2.5–10 mg i.m. four-hourly is usually added to reduce dyspnoea and prevent the rare agitation from hyoscine.

Antibiotics
There are many different opinions on the treatment of chest infections in the terminally ill. It is not so much a question of whether to treat a chest infection, but rather to ask what the appropriate treatment is in a patient with pneumonia; in some patients it is antibiotics, in others it is symptomatic treatment. There are several guidelines in making this decision.

1. What is the patient's physical state? A markedly reduced respiratory capacity, inability to cough effectively, being bedbound or with reduced immunity, will all make it less likely that antibiotics will help. A patient who is already dyspnoeic from lung disease and who recovers from pneumonia may be left even more short of breath.

2. What does the patient want? It is important to respect the wishes of the terminally ill patient with regard to further active treatment such as antibiotics. Many, however, will be too ill to decide, and guidance from the family may help. Finally, however, the doctor must make a responsible decision in the light of the points just mentioned.

3. Will the patient and his family benefit from more time to heal rifts in their relationships or to settle business affairs? Similarly, further time to discuss emotional or spiritual problems may be valuable.

The best antibiotic is chloramphenicol 250–500 mg six-hourly for seven to ten days, since bacterial resistance is uncommon and the minimal risk of blood dyscrasias (1:30 000 cases) can be disregarded. Chest physiotherapy may also help.

Cytotoxics and hormones
These may be used to reduce lung metastases or effusions, and hence decrease dyspnoea (see Chapter 9).

Bupivacaine inhalations
If there is stimulation of the lung J receptors, inhalation of bupivacaine may relieve dyspnoea (Taylor, 1979). This has been found helpful in some cases, especially with lymphangitis, but is sometimes unacceptable to the patient.

Bupivacaine 0.25% solution to a maximum dose of 30 ml/24 hours nebulized by ultrasound (Pulma-Sonic nebulizer) will give a particle size of 2 Å, which will reach the alveoli. A Bird nebulizer gives particle sizes of 2–10 Å, and these will tend to fall out in the larger bronchi and hence be more helpful in suppressing cough (Lunt *et al.*, 1981). Anaesthesia of the mouth or pharynx does not occur due to a laminar flow effect.

Oxygen
This may help in acute dyspnoea, but in longer term use, the benefit gained is outweighed by the distress to the dying patient and his family of the presence of an oxygen mask and cylinder. The treatments already mentioned will be more effective. Some patients use oxygen more to relieve anxiety than a low Po_2.

Radiotherapy

This may reduce the size of lung tumours or mediastinal lymph node metastases and hence reduce dyspnoea, and may help haemoptysis, or stridor. While waiting for the radiotherapy to take effect, dexamethasone 8 mg/24 hours will provide quick relief of symptoms and will also prevent transient oedema and worsening of symptoms from radiotherapy.

Transfusions

Many patients with advanced malignant disease are anaemic. The causes are multiple, and several factors may contribute to the anaemia of an individual patient. It is only rarely that there is a single curable cause such as iron deficiency. Anaemia will probably not cause severe symptoms, unless marked, as with a haemoglobin of less than 7 g/dl. Dyspnoea may be one of these symptoms but is usually not severe.

Transfusion rarely improves symptoms significantly. It may occasionally be helpful prior to further active treatment such as chemotherapy, or before an important family event such as a wedding.

Procedures

Tapping a pleural effusion may relieve dyspnoea. It is indicated if the effusion is the main cause of breathlessness, if a previous tap has helped, or as part of further active treatment. However, this procedure is rarely carried out for the following reasons: effusions do not usually cause much dyspnoea; the fluid often reaccumulates in a few days, even if a chemotherapeutic agent is instilled; and the procedure can be distressing to an ill patient. Paracentesis will relieve pressure on the diaphragm and hence dyspnoea.

The physiotherapist can help the patient to cough up bronchial secretions and can show him breathing exercises, and also relaxation techniques.

Counselling

Fear of choking and not having enough air is very common, and counselling techniques such as behaviour therapy may be very helpful in exploring these fears, refuting myths, and finding ways of dealing with anxiety. It is important, however, to be sure that the patient has enough time left to find solutions to problems uncovered through counselling before beginning such an approach.

Cough

A dry cough is usually caused by pressure on a bronchus by primary or metastatic tumour. It is also found in the mucosal inflammation stage of acute bronchitis and is exacerbated by the inhalation of irritants such as smoke.

A productive cough results in the expectoration of mucus which may or may not be infected. It is caused by chronic bronchitis, pneumonia, lung abscess or tumour with secondary infection. Pulmonary oedema due to heart failure causes white, frothy sputum.

The cause should be identified, if possible, and appropriate treatment offered; for example antibiotics for a chest infection and palliative radiotherapy for a tumour. However, in many cases such treatment is not possible and only symptomatic relief can be given. In general terms it is reasonable to suppress a dry cough, but a productive cough should be allowed to continue unless it is very exhausting and disturbs sleep.

Treatment

Antitussives act at two sites: on the respiratory mucosa and on the cough centre in the medulla.

Peripheral action

1. On inspired air. It is not often possible, or kind, to stop a patient smoking, but the inspiration of warm moist air will often relieve a hacking cough. This may be achieved with a steam kettle or humidifier or the use of benzoin inhalation B.P.C.

2. Mucolytics. Bromhexine (Bisolvon) and carbocisteine (Mucodyne) are claimed to reduce the viscosity of of bronchial secretions and thus aid expectoration. Many patients find then effective.

3. Bupivacaine inhaler. Bupivacaine 0.25% administered in a Bird nebulizer which gives 10 Å particle size is very effective in intractable cough. The maximum dose is 30 ml/24 hours. Unfortunately it is often not acceptable.

Central action

1. Codeine and pholcodine. These should be tried first in adequate dosage.

2. Morphine, diamorphine or methadone. One of these will often be required for patients with bronchogenic carcinoma. The dose should be titrated against the symptom and increased as necessary, as for pain. The regular use of methadone may cause sedation due to accumulation of the drug, which has a very long half-life (see Chapter 5).

Haemoptysis

Although a significant haemoptysis is usually due to bleeding from a bronchial carcinoma, there are a number of other causes which require appropriate treatment. The bleeding may come from the upper respiratory tract or from a pulmonary infarct or metastasis, and sputum stained with blood occurs in chest infections and pulmonary oedema.

Radiotherapy is the treatment of choice if the haemoptysis is caused by a carcinoma of the bronchus and if the patient is well enough and has not been fully irradiated (see Chapter 8). Occasionally bleeding is brought on by a secondary infection and will subside when this is treated with antibiotics.

The value of aminocaproic acid (Epsikapron) to prevent excessive fibrinolysis, and ethamsylate (Dicynene) to reduce capillary bleeding is quite unproven in this situation. They are occasionally prescribed, but perhaps their greatest value is for the anxious patient who feels that something is being done for a frightening symptom.

A major haemoptysis may cause sudden death, but if the patient remains conscious and distressed, his dyspnoea and fear should be treated with an immediate injection of diamorphine 5–10 mg with hyoscine 0.4 mg.

Urinary symptoms

Frequency and incontinence

These symptoms are often found in patients with advanced malignant disease and can cause great distress: 'I don't mind what happens to me as long as I don't become incontinent' expresses a sentiment that is commonly felt.

It is important to diagnose the cause of frequency or incontinence as specific treatments are available for some conditions.

1. Urinary infections. The urine should be cultured and a full course of an appropriate antibiotic given. Often, however, the infection is associated with a structural abnormality of the urinary tract and recurs after treatment.

2. Incipient paraplegia or a cauda equina lesion from metastatic tumour. Dexamethasone 30 mg daily should be commenced and the patient referred for urgent radiotherapy of decompression laminectomy (see p. 127).

3. Polyuria caused by diabetes mellitus or diabetes insipidus.

Unfortunately, many of the causes are not amenable to specific treatment, but the following can be considered.

1. Emepronium bromide (Cetiprin) 200 mg three times a day or 200–400 mg at night. This is useful in urinary frequency because it increases the volume of the bladder at which the first desire to micturate is experienced.

2. Urinary condom. This is useful for nocturnal incontinence, but is not often tolerated throughout the 24 hours for long periods.

3. Catheter. This is usually the best way of treating severe frequency or incontinence as the usual risks associate with long-term catheterization do not apply there. The procedure should normally be discussed with the patient a few days beforehand as there will be a few who will prefer to use a condom, a permanent urinal or incontinence padding.

A self-retaining catheter should be passed under full aseptic conditions; in most patients this is quite painless. For difficult catheterization—for example in patients with large vulval carcinomas or who are especially anxious—it may be helpful to give intravenous diazepam (Valium) a few minutes beforehand.

It is impossible to maintain a sterile urine in a patient with an indwelling catheter, and long-term antibiotics have no place as resistance occurs. Only symptomatic infections are treated with a short course of an appropriate antibiotic; if these occur frequently, a urinary antiseptic such as hexamine hippurate (Hiprex) 1 g twice daily will often prevent them.

Bladder washouts with chlorhexidine gluconate (Hibitane) 1 in 5000 are useful if there is a lot of sediment. Noxytiolin (Noxyflex) bladder instillations twice daily for two days are also used.

Urinary retention

The commonest cause of retention is constipation. It can also be caused by bladder neck or urethral obstructions, neurological problems and by certain drugs, especially anticholinergic drugs and tricyclic antidepressants.

Bethanechol (Myotonine) 10 mg twice daily can be used if there is no outflow obstruction, otherwise catheterization is required, occasionally suprapubically.

Bladder pain

This is usually caused by infection and treated with antibiotics. Occasionally bladder spasm occurs, mainly associated with catheterization; it is treated with emepronium bromide (Cetiprin). Phenazopyridine (Pyridium) 100 mg eight-hourly is both a urinary antiseptic and analgesic, it colours the urine a bright yellow.

Haematuria

This may occur with infection, but more profuse haematuria is normally associated with malignancy involving the urinary tract. Radiotherapy should be considered if the patient is well enough (see Chapter 8).

Clot retention or catheter blockage should be treated with citrate bladder washouts, if necessary using a three-way catheter.

In persistent haematuria, ethamsylate (Dicynene) 500 mg four times a day and aminocaproic acid (Epsikapron) 3 g four times a day sometimes prove effective.

Fistulae

A considerable proportion of patients with pelvic malignancies develop fistulae. These rarely occur unless irradiation has been given at some stage in the illness, and the risk of fistula formation will often deter the radiotherapist from treating or re-treating this area (see Chapter 8).

Vesicovaginal fistula
This can often be managed satisfactorily with a large-size indwelling catheter with or without vaginal tampons.

Rectovesical or colovesical fistulae
The presence of faecal material in the bladder and urethra causes a great deal of pain, not easily relieved by antibiotics or analgesics. An indwelling catheter may help, though it usually blocks with debris. A palliative colostomy should be considered.

Rectovaginal fistula
A palliative colostomy is the only satisfactory treatment.

Skin problems

Fungating tumours

Breast carcinoma is the commonest malignancy to cause fungation, but open lesions can also occur with other tumours. Such an obvious manifestation of disease is always distressing to the patient. It may also be painful and have an offensive smell.

The following methods of treatment have been found effective.

1. Radiotherapy, chemotherapy and hormone manipulation if appropriate (see Chapters 8 and 9).

2. Regular cleansing of the area is essential, usually twice a day.

3. Many local applications are tried; their purpose is to reduce local infection and the resulting odour, to soothe discomfort and to prevent the new dressing from sticking. An emulsion of 4% povidone-iodine solution (Betadine) with liquid paraffin in a ratio of 1:4 has been found most effective; it is used to clean the wound, then gauze soaked in it is applied as a dressing.

4. If there is persistent capillary bleeding from the tumour, a non-adhesive dressing should be applied and covered with gauze soaked in 1 in 1000 adrenaline.

5. Vulval lesions should be treated with frequent washdowns with 1 in 2000 chlorhexidine (Hibitane) solution.

Sometimes, in spite of such measure, there is a persistent problem with smell, embarrassing to the patient and his family. This is usually due to secondary anaerobic infection and should be treated with metronidazole (Flagyl) 400 mg orally three times a day or 1 g suppositories b.d. An alternative is chloramphenicol 250 mg four times a day. It is effective against anaerobes and is better tolerated in the very ill.

Some dressings incorporate a deodorant and there are many available for use either locally or in the room.

Bedsores

Cachectic and immobile patients run a great risk of developing pressure sores, and prevention is much better than cure. Regular turning, special mattresses and gentle massage of the areas at risk are important.

The large number of local applications available reflect the fact that there is little to choose between them, and the success of each depends considerably on the enthusiasm of the nurse and the time she is able to give.

Sometimes the development of slough delays healing, and desloughing agents such as Aserbine can be used with benefit. If there is considerable secondary infection leading to surrounding cellulitis or an offensive smell, then a course of systemic antibiotics should be given.

Skin sinuses and fistulae

Many types of these may occur and each presents considerable problems in management. A colostomy bag should be fitted if possible to prevent excoriation of the surrounding skin; otherwise a barrier cream such as Kerodex may help. An offensive odour can usually be prevented using local applications and antibiotics.

Itch

Many patients complain of a mild skin irritation, probably due to their dry skin. This can be helped by stopping the use of soap and using an emulsifying ointment in the bath. If the irritation persists, it may be eased by the use of crotamiton (Eurax) cream t.d.s., or the prescribing of an antihistamine such as chlorpheniramine (Piriton); the benefit of the latter is probably due to the mild sedation it causes.

In patients with jaundice there is an accumulation of bile acids in the plasma which may cause intense irritation. This can be relieved by cholestyramine (Questran) 4–8 g daily (1–2 sachets). This binds bile acids in the bowel and prevents their resorption. Unfortunately, Questran sachets are rather unpalatable for the very ill and are only effective if biliary obstruction is incomplete.

Neurological symptoms

Confusion

The differential diagnosis and management of confusion in a terminally ill patient are two of the most difficult problems that a doctor concerned with the dying has to face. The family will be distressed, wanting to know what has happened and what can be done to help. It is important to have in mind the common causes.

1. Drugs, especially psychotropic drugs, analgesics and alcohol.
2. Biochemical causes. Uraemia, hypercalcaemia, hypoglycaemia.
3. Anoxia.
4. Toxins, from infections usually in the chest or urinary tract.
5. Postepileptic.
6. Cerebral tumours, primary or secondary.
7. Other causes of brain damage, cerebral arteriosclerosis, cerebrovascular accidents.
8. Psychogenic, from depression or, in the elderly, an altered environment.

Often confusion is multifactorial and more than one of these causes is implicated.

From such a list, which is not exhaustive, it is apparent that specific treatment can be attempted in a proportion of cases: chest infections treated, excess sedation decreased, the dose of insulin or oral hypoglycaemic drugs reduced to match the patient's diminished food intake.

Even if the underlying cause cannot be treated, it is a great help to the family to be able to identify it and explain it to them. They are often greatly relieved to know, for example, that the confusion is due to kidney failure caused by cervical cancer rather than 'her losing her mind'.

Psychotropic drugs have only a minor place in the treatment of a confused patient; they cannot restore mental function deranged by disease, but only make a restless and aggressive patient easier to manage.

Haloperidol (Serenace) 5–10 mg by injection is useful in an emergency, to be followed by 5–10 mg daily by mouth in divided doses.

Thioridazine (Melleril) 25 mg three times daily is suitable for the elderly since it does not cause much sedation. Chlorpromazine (Largactil) 50–100 mg, immediately followed by 25–50 mg three times daily is useful if extra sedation is required.

Cerebral tumours

The terminal care of patients with cerebral tumours, primary or secondary, requires more detailed discussion.

Tumours cause symptoms in two ways.

1. Local effect of tumour depends on the site of brain affected. Hemiplegia, dysphasia, personality change or epilepsy may result.

2. General effect of tumour results in raised intracranial pressure which may cause headache, nausea and vomiting. Later there may be visual disturbances and finally drowsiness progressing to coma. Death usually results from transtentorial herniation (coning), with resultant pressure on the midbrain; terminally, there may be herniation through the foramen magnum with medullary compression and cardiorespiratory arrest.

Symptoms and signs of the cerebral tumour

These are due to the effect of the tumour together with accompanying oedema. The precise pathogenesis of cerebral oedema remains unclear; however, on the whole, the greater the rate of the growth of the tumour, the more the tendency for oedema to occur, and sometimes the extent of the oedema may be larger than the tumour that is producing it.

Treatment of cerebral tumours

Surgical removal.

Reduction in tumour size by radiotherapy, chemotherapy or, in certain cases, by hormonal manipulation (sse Chapter 8).

Glucocorticosteroid drugs to reduce cerebral oedema.

Symptomatic management.

The use of steroid drugs

1. Steroids should not invariably be used. If the patient is very old or frail, has widespread and distressing metastatic disease and/or death seems imminent, it will be wisest to give only symptomatic treatment.

2. Before starting steroids, the medical and nursing staff should get to know the patient and his family. Sometimes in conversation clues are given which will guide in treatment decisions: 'We were so looking forward to our golden wedding next month', or 'He often said that he hoped things wouldn't be too drawn out'. The decision to start steroid treatment must be a medical one, although full account should be taken of the the family situation. It can never be right to ask the family to make such a decision, with the inevitable heart searching and guilt that this could cause.

3. Before steroid treatment is started, the family and the patient, if possible, should be told that this treatment may cause a temporary remission; perhaps some explanation of cerebral oedema can be given. This should avoid the common distress of relatives who feel that the patient has been cured—only to be disillusioned later.

4. The action of steroids in cerebral oedema is not fully understood, but the effect is not simply proportional to the dose given. In each case there seems to be a critical level below which oedema increases.

5. Dexamethasone 16 mg daily is the traditional starting dose, this was the

dose originally used by Galicich *et al.* (1961). The great majority of patients who will respond to steroid therapy do so at this dose. (The occasional patient who would require up to 40 mg daily would need to be maintained at this level and unacceptable side-effects would quickly occur.)

6. If there is no response to steroids after a week, the dose should be rapidly reduced and stopped.

7. If a response occurs, the dose should be maintained at 16 mg daily for two weeks. Unless the prognosis is very short, an attempt should be made to reduce the dose to the lowest compatible with symptom control: the suggested rate is to cut the daily dose by 2 mg each week, working towards a maintenance dose of 4-6 mg daily.

8. If symptoms recur, the dose should be immediately increased to the previous level.

9. The purpose of keeping steroid doses as low as possible is to reduce the risk of severe Cushingoid side-effects developing.

10. Dexamethasone is only effective in suppressing cerebral oedema and has no effect on the tumour itself, which continues to grow causing further neurological symptoms. Thus the problems reversed by steroids will gradually return, and the doctor will be faced with the extremely difficult decision about the quality of life he is prolonging. The time will come, for example, if the patient is paralysed and confused, when no good purpose is served by continuing treatment and the steroids should be discontinued during the next week or so.

Symptomatic treatment

1. Headache. This is rarely severe and usually responds to simple analgesics such as paracetamol.

Sometimes oral morphine is required, it should be given regularly and in adequate dosage (see Chapter 5).

2. Nausea and vomiting, incontinence, bedsores and confusion are all covered earlier in this chapter.

3. Epileptic fits. These should be treated with anticonvulsants in the usual way. Sodium valproate (Epilim) 200 mg t.d.s. is given, increasing if necessary until fits are controlled or a satisfactory plasma level obtained. Phenytoin (Epanutin) 100 mg t.d.s. can be used similarly but is less suitable in terminal care as it interacts with other drugs which may be needed.

When a patient is unable to take oral anticonvulsants he should be changed to phenobarbitone injection 60-90 mg twice a day. The depressing effect of the drug is no longer relevant and it is a convenient small injection. Status epilepticus is rare; it should be treated with intravenous diazepam (Valium).

Paralysis

The loss of normal use of an arm or leg is one of the most distressing symptoms of the dying. It is usually of great significance to the patient and his family, who may feel that it implies that death is very near.

Advanced malignant disease can cause paralysis in a number of ways. For some of these there is treatment available which may arrest or reverse the condition. However, any treatment is dependent on a correct diagnosis and this will involve a careful history and clinical examination and sometimes further investigations.

Cancer causes paralysis in three main ways:

1. intracranial disease, primary or metastatic,
2. spinal cord compression,
3. involvement of nerve roots, plexuses and peripheral nerves.

Non-metastatic manifestations of malignant disease causing paralysis are not common. They are usually associated with bronchial carcinoma and include peripheral neuropathy and polymyositis—the latter may respond to corticosteroids (Posner 1978).

The three common causes of paralysis will be examined in more detail.

Intracranial tumours
Paralysis is caused by tumour involving the motor cortex or corticospinal tracts. The tumour may be a glioma or a metastasis, most commonly from breast or bronchus.

Clinical features
Limb weakness is usually associated with weakness of the other limb on that side, and sometimes of the face. There is no pain and only rarely any sensory loss. Examination shows an upper motoneuron lesion with spasticity, increased reflexes and an extensor plantar response.

Treatment
1. If paralysis develops in a patient with a previously treated cerebral tumour, primary or secondary, it is reasonable to assume that it is caused by extension of the disease and the only possible treatment is with corticosteroids (see p. 125).

2. If paralysis develops in a patient not known to have cerebral disease, the treatment will depend on the general condition of the patient and the accessibility of further investigations. If the prognosis is long, it is ideal to have a CT scan to confirm the diagnosis prior to treatment with surgery, radiotherapy or corticosteroids. In patients with a very limited prognosis it is reasonable to do a monitored trial of corticosteroids for a week. A physiotherapist should be involved to assess the degree of paralysis so that an objective response is not confused with a subjective feeling of wellbeing.

Spinal cord compression
This is a relatively common complication in patients with malignant disease. Untreated, it will cause irreversible paraplegia or quadriplegia, but with early diagnosis and correct treatment paralysis can often be avoided or reversed. It is therefore one of the emergencies in terminal care.

The common primary tumours to cause cord compression are those of the breast, bronchus, prostate and lymphoma. Less common are kidney, myeloma and melanoma. In 85 per cent of cases the tumour has spread to the vertebral body or pedicle; in the remainder there is spread from paravertebral nodes through the intervertebral foramina or an intramedullary metastasis. Compression can occur at all levels, but is most common in the thoracic area (below L1 the cauda equina is involved).

Clinical features
In over 90 per cent of patients the first symptom is pain, felt locally and/or referred, i.e. girdle pain with thoracic metastases. This precedes the diagnosis by a very variable time interval—one day to two years. By the time the diagnosis is made, 76 per cent will have developed motor loss, 57 per cent sphincter problems, and 51 per cent sensory loss (Gilbert *et al.*, 1978). On examination, the motor weakness is bilateral and relatively symmetrical; the majority have sensory loss involving all modalities and abnormal reflexes. With cauda equina lesions there is typically 'saddle' anaesthesia, sphincter disturbance and weakness of foot and calf muscles.

Treatment
Active treatment is contraindicated in a proportion of patients. In addition to those who are too ill, there are two groups in whom results of treatment are poor: those who are already paraplegic, and those whose symptoms have progressed very rapidly (in less than 48 hours). Corticosteroids alone are sometimes tried in this group, but probably have little effect.

There are a number of studies comparing radiotherapy and surgical decompression, both with adjuvant steroids. Results show that radiotherapy and steroids give better overall response with considerably less morbidity and mortality. Surgery remains the treatment of choice if the diagnosis of malignancy is in doubt, with radioresistant tumours such as chondrosarcoma, in previously fully irradiated patients, or if symptoms progress while radiotherapy is in progress.

If active treatment seems to be indicated, a bolus intravenous injection of dexamethasone 30 mg should be given while arrangements are made for urgent radiotherapy or, occasionally, for surgery. Investigations will depend on the clinical situation and the facilities: spinal x-rays are positive in 80 per cent, but a myelogram will be required prior to surgery and sometimes to confirm the diagnosis and if there are multiple bone deposits. Sterioids should be continued during radiotherapy and then gradually tapered off.

Results of treatment depend to a great extent on the degree of paralysis before treatment is started. If the patient is paraplegic, the chance or recovering the power to walk is only 3 per cent; if he was still walking, he has an 80 per cent chance of remaining so.

Metastatic involvement of peripheral nerves
Both cranial and peripheral nerves can be involved by tumour at any site along their lengths, thus there is a great variety of possible symptoms and signs. These will depend on the nerves involved and also whether they are affected as nerve roots, plexuses or distally.

Clinical features
Muscle weakness due to peripheral nerve lesions is usually preceded by pain, which is often severe and accompanied by sensory loss or paraesthesiae. On examination there will be signs of a lower motoneuron lesion with flaccidity, loss of tendon reflexes and muscle wasting.

There are two common clinical problems.

1. The weak arm. This is usually caused by neoplastic involvement of the brachial plexus (Pancoast syndrome) due to a carcinoma at the apex of the lung, and also in carcinoma of the breast and lymphoma. The lower cords of the plexus (C7, C8, T1) are involved first, leading to severe pain in the shoulder and elbow with weakness of the small hand muscles and forearm. A similar picture can be caused by vertebral metastases (C6–T1), but pain is also felt over the vertebrae radiating into both shoulders and associated with bony tenderness. Radiation injury involves the upper roots of the plexus (C5, C6, C7).

2. The weak leg. This can be caused by involvement of the lumbosacral plexus in the pelvis from carcinoma of the cervix, rectum and bladder or by lumbosacral spinal metastases associated with carcinoma of the breast, bronchus or prostate. The localization of pain and weakness depends on the actual nerves involved, but there is usually local tenderness with spinal deposits.

Treatment

Unfortunately, the paralysis caused by malignant infiltration of the brachial or lumbosacral plexus very rarely responds to any treatment and steadily increases in severity. However, when paralysis is secondary to bony lesions it can often be arrested by local radiotherapy.

Symptomatic treatment of the paralysed patient

Good nursing care is needed to prevent pressure sores.

Physiotherapy. Regular movement of paralysed limbs is important to prevent stiff joints, deformity and pain.

Support. Many patients will benefit from wearing a sling or a light splint, such as a toe-raise splint for foot-drop.

Spasticity may be improved by baclofen (Lioresal) or dantrolene (Dantrium).

Pain often occurs in paralysed limbs and needs appropriate treatment (see Chapter 5).

Emotional needs. The loss of use of a limb is a most psychologically distressing event and patients require a great deal of sympathetic help.

Psychological symptoms

Anxiety and depression

These are discussed fully in Chapter 4 and therefore only a summary of some important aspects of treatment is given here.

Meticulous attention to symptom control. This involves not only the management of major symptoms such as pain and dyspnoea, but the willingness to syringe ears, arrange chiropody, use dental fixatives etc.

Honest discussion about the future. This involves a willingness to talk not only about the final fatal outcome of the illness, but to discuss specific questions: 'Will I be in pain?' 'Will I become a cabbage?' 'How will I die and how will you know I'm really dead?' 'How long have I got?' The ability of a patient to voice these questions to nurses or doctors, without embarrassment, knowing that he will get an honest answer, does much to allay anxiety.

Full involvement of the family. They should be encouraged to meet staff regularly and be included in discussions about the future (see Chapter 11).

Avoiding boredom. The increasing physical weakness of the dying, associated sometimes with a slowing of mental processes, means that familiar pursuits may become impossible. Nursing and occupational therapy staff need all their skills to encourage alternative satisfying occupations.

Dealing with social and financial problems.

Spiritual help. Many patients suffer a sense of guilt over past failures, a feeling of purposelessness, an anxiety about what happens after death. All staff need to be aware of spiritual needs, if possible able to contribute support themselves, and willing to seek the Chaplain's help if appropriate.

Psychotropic drugs may be given in addition to these measures and not as a substitute.

The two useful groups of anxiolytic drugs are the benzodiazepines and phenothiazines. Individual patients seem to do better on one than the other. Diazepam (Valium) 2–5 mg three times a day or 10 mg at night, or chlorpromazine (Largactil) 10–25 mg three times a day can be used.

Some patients, especially those with protracted illnesses, seem to benefit from antidepressant drugs. The starting dose should be low: amitriptyline (Tryptizol) 10–25 mg at night increasing slowly to 75 mg, or mianserin (Bolvidon) 10–30 mg at night increasing to 60 mg.

Insomnia

Many patients with terminal illness suffer with insomnia due to unrelieved physical or mental symptoms such as pain, anxiety or nocturnal frequency. Insomnia improves as these are relieved.

Night sweats are an occasional cause of sleeplessness; they often respond to an indomethacin suppository 100 mg given at night or Indocid R, 75 mg, a sustained release oral preparation.

If hypnotics are required, the following are used.

1. Temazepam (Normison, Euhypnos) 10–30 mg at night. This is a short-acting benzodiazepine with little risk of cumulative sedation.

2. Nitrazepam (Mogadon) and diazepan (Valium) 5–10 mg at night can be used in anxious patients when some daytime sedation is required.

3. Chlormethiazole (Heminevrin) is a good hypnotic for the elderly as it is most unlikely to precipitate or increase confusion. The usual dose is two capsules (or 10 ml) at night, but a further capsule can be given with benefit in the early evening or if the patient is restless in the night.

Alcohol remains an excellent hypnotic, especially for the elderly. Antidepressant drugs given at night to depressed patients will improve their sleep pattern. The occasional person who has taken barbiturates for years should be allowed to continue.

Other symptoms

Weakness

Many doctors working in terminal care feel that the complaint of weakness is heard much more frequently now than some years ago. This is probably because other symptoms, such as pain, vomiting and dyspnoea, are better controlled, so that the patient becomes more aware of his lack of strength. Also the expectation of many nurses, families and patients has quite rightly risen, making it more difficult for them to accept that there are some symptoms which cannot be controlled.

The complaint of weakness seems often poorly related to any measurable loss of strength. Thus some patients struggle on when they can barely stand, insisting that they feel well. Others take to their beds, say that they are too weak even to wash and feed themselves, when they can, with encouragement, walk to the bathroom. It is apparent that 'weakness' as a symptom has both physical and psychological causes.

There are a few specific treatments available which will help a proportion of patients.

Glucocorticosteroids
Prednisolone 15–30 mg/day will usually lead to an improvement in appetite and general sense of wellbeing. This may be adequate to make the patient feel stronger, though continued steroids, expecially in high dosage, often lead to a proximal myopathy which will cause or exacerbate leg weakness.

Blood transfusion
This may help if lethargy is associated with other symptoms of anaemia such as dyspnoea and ankle oedema. It is disappointing for the treatment of weakness alone, probably because this symptom has so many causes.

Antidepressants
Clinical depression or, far more frequently, the natural sadness of the dying is often expressed in a complaint of weakness. This is dealt with fully in Chapter 4. The most effective treatment is the staff's support to the patient and his family, with attention to physical, emotional and spiritual needs. Antidepressant drugs may occasionally help.

Physiotherapy
To most people **exercise** seems the natural antidote to **weakness,** and faces light up when the suggestion of physiotherapy is made. It requires very special physiotherapy skills to prescribe suitable bed or chair exercises for the very frail, to mobilize when possible using the various aids available, and then to help the patient accept the almost inevitable decline in strength as illness progresses. Nevertheless, this is one of the most satisfactory ways of combating the helpless feeling of weakness.

For most dying patients, the only satisfactory way of coping with weakness is by acceptance and adjustment: acceptance that it is inevitable, and an adjustment of daily living to use limited strength wisely, to cultivate suitable pursuits rather than yearn for the impossible. The company of family and friends, the short outing, the game of cards, the good television programme can all bring great pleasure.

Terminal restlessness

This may be due to unrelieved pain or a distended bladder or rectum, but frequently no treatable cause is found and the restlessness may be due to cerebral anoxia, fever or some biochemical disturbance.

It is extremely important to treat restlessness actively because of the distress it causes to family and staff, if not to the patient himself. Those who visit the bereaved will be only too aware how the last hours become imprinted on the memory with unanswerable questions: 'I wonder if she was trying to say something to me?' 'Do you think he was in pain?'

Adequate medication must, of course, be given for pain, either by injection or suppository (see Chapter 5). Probably the best sedating drug is methotrimeprazine (Veractil or Nozinan). It is a phenothiazine with strong analgesic and antiemetic properties; 25-50 mg should be given by injection; it can be repeated four-hourly if necessary (Lamerton, 1979). If this drug is not available, chlorpromazine (Largactil) 50-100 mg four- to eight-hourly can be substituted.

Diazepam (Valium) 5-10 mg by injection or suppository is used in the last day or so to control muscle twitching, and it can be combined with methotrimeprazine and diamorphine (though not in the same syringe) when restlessness is not controlled by these two drugs alone.

Hyoscine 0.4-0.6 mg by injection will dry up excessive secretions which accumulate when a patient is dying, so causing the 'death rattle'. The dose can be repeated four- to eight-hourly if required, and is a most effective sedative in an emergency.

Medication, although important, is not the only way of managing the restless dying patient. Staff often notice that the presence of the family sitting by the bedside, holding the hand or speaking quietly to an apparently unconscious patient has a remarkable calming effect. As with every symptom, the successful management of restlessness involves the combined use of pharmacology and psychology: medication and loving care.

References

Aranha, G., Folk, F. and Greenlee, H. (1981). Surgical palliation of small bowel obstruction due to metastatic carcinoma. *American Surgeon* **47**, 99.

Campbell, E.J.M. and Godfrey, S. (1969). The role of afferent impulses from the lung and chest wall in respiratory control and sensation. In *Breathing: Hering-Breuer Centenary Symposium*, p. 219. Ed. by R. Porter. J. & A. Churchill, Edinburgh.

Carter, R.L., Pittam, M.R. and Tanner, N.S.R. (1982). Pain and dysphagia in patients with squamous carcinomas of the head and neck—the role of perineural spread. *Journal of the Royal Society of Medicine* **75**, 598.

Galicich, J.H., French, L.A. and Melloy, J.C. (1961). Use of dexamethasone in the treatment of cerebral oedema associated with brain tumours. *Lancet* **81**, 46.

Gilbert, R.W., Kim, J.H. and Posner, J.B. (1978). Epidural spinal cord compression from metastatic tumour: diagnosis and treatment. *Annals of Neurology* **3**, 40.

Glass, R.L. and LeDuc, R.J. (1973). Small intestinal obstruction from peritoneal carcinomatosis. *American Journal of Surgery* **125**, 316.

Hosking, D.J. (1983). Disequilibrium hypercalcaemia. *British Medical Journal* **286**, 326.

Howard, E.R. (1982). Personal communication.

Kirkham, S. (1983). Personal communication.

Lamerton, R.C. (1979). *The Practitioner* **223**, 813.

Lunt, M.J., Taylor, J. and Meldrum, S.J. (1981). A system of producing particles of controlled size from a nebulizer. *Journal of Medical Engineering and Technology* **5** (3), 138.

Peroutka, S.J. and Snyder, S.H. (1982). Antiemetics: neurotransmitter receptor binding predicts therapeutic actions. *Lancet* **i**, 658.

Posner, J.B. (1978). Non-metastatic effects of cancer on the nervous system. In *Cecil's Textbook of Medicine*. W.B. Saunders, Philadelphia.

Schuffler, M.D., Rohrmann, C.A., Chaffee, R.G., Brand, D.L., Delaney, J.H. and Young, J.H. (1981). Chronic intestinal pseudo-obstruction. *Journal of Medicine* **60**, 3.

Taylor, J. (1979). Personal communication.

Tunca, J.C., Buchler, D.A., Mack, E.A., Ruzicka, F.F., Crowley, J.J. and Carr, W.F. (1981). The management of ovarian-cancer-caused bowel obstruction. *Gynecologic Oncology* **12**, 186.

Twycross, R.G. (1982). Symptom control in terminal cancer. Long term prescribing. In *Drug Management of Chronic Disease and Other Problems*, p.163. Ed. by Eric Wilkes. Faber & Faber, London.

Walsh, T.D. (1984). Opiates and respiratory function in advanced cancer: a preliminary report. In *Recent Results in Cancer Research*, Vol. 89. Springer-Verlag, Berlin and Heidelberg.

8

Radiotherapy in terminal care

Thelma D. Bates

The last few weeks of a patient's life are usually a time when active treatment has ceased and he is moving towards being allowed to die in comfort and dignity. However, radiotherapy can, on occasions, be helpful during this period provided it is applied skilfully. If misapplied, it can be harmful. The purpose of such palliative radiotherapy must be to relieve distressing symptoms quickly and thus improve the quality of the remaining life. Radiotherapy is not, at this atage, aimed at anticipating symptoms which may never arise, nor in prolonging life, though both may be secondary results of successful treatment. There are rare occasions when radiotherapy may be used to prevent an impending complication such as paraplegia from a collapsing vertebra.

General principles of palliative radiotherapy

These principles are dictated by the limited expectation of life and the need to avoid causing the patient additional discomfort. At no time is a good clinical judgement more important. The radiotherapist must be able to make a correct assessment of the situation with the minimum of time-consuming investigations. He must also know what he can hope to achieve with treatment and what is impossible.

If radiotherapy is indicated, it should be given without delay: there is no time to go on to a waiting list. Nor should time be spent on numerous visits to the radiotherapy department. Effective palliation can sometimes be achieved in a single treatment but more often involves the patient in a course of five or six treatments spread out over a period of two or three weeks. Daily treatments over a period of several weeks are never necessary. Palliative radiotherapy at this stage of the disease should have few or no side-effects, and the benefits of treatment must be carefully balanced against the price the patient has to pay in terms of the time and trouble involved.

There are occasions when radiotherapy can be actually harmful at this stage of the disease. This applies particularly when a tumour is infiltrating a neighbouring structure such as the bladder, bowel or bronchus, when there is a very real risk that radiotherapy, even at palliative dosage, may lead to fistula formation: the symptoms which follow will be even more distressing than those caused by the untreated tumour. On a similar basis, it may be unwise to irradiate the pelvis of a patient dying from uraemia associated with advanced pelvic cancer; the relief of ureteric obstruction may keep the patient alive long enough for her to develop much more distressing terminal symptoms such as severe pelvic pain and offensive discharge. Cerebral metastases may be better untreated in a patient with rapidly progressing, disseminated bronchial carcinoma.

It is not always easy for a radiotherapist to refuse treatment to a patient who is terminally ill. Very often he has known the patient for years and has helped him in the past, and both the patient and his relatives may beg him to help once again. In addition, a radiotherapist may be pressed to treat a patient by his medical colleagues, who themselves have nothing more to offer but who wish to give some positive help. On the other hand, a radiotherapist who feels he can help a patient may be faced by medical or (more often) nursing colleagues, who seek to protect the patient from further therapeutic interference. In all cases, a radiotherapist must be clear in his own mind what he can hope to achieve by his therapy. Although he will take psychological factors into consideration, he must be motivated by the possible physical benefit to his patient. Occasionally a radiotherapist may be asked to 'pretend to treat' a patient, but this deception is never justified.

Three factors influence the potential value of radiotherapy in terminal patients. They are the likely radiosensitivity of the tumour itself, the radiotolerance of the surrounding normal tissues, and the degree to which these tissues have been irradiated in the past. All tissues, both normal and malignant, vary in their response to irradiation and there is a limit to the total dose which tissues will tolerate, even over a period of months or years. Some tumours are very radiosensitive. These include malignant lymphomas, seminomas, nephroblastomas and the rare dysgerminoma of the ovary. On the other hand, some tumours are generally resistant to radiotherapy and are unlikely to respond to palliative dosage. These include most of the bone and soft tissue sarcomas, the cerebral gliomas and malignant melanoma. Squamous cell carcinomas are moderately radiosensitive and adenocarcinomas, particularly those of the gastrointestinal tract, rather less so.

Of the normal tissues, the gastrointestinal tract is one of the most radiosensitive. Large-volume irradiation of the abdomen can be expected to cause nausea and diarrhoea, and even small-volume, palliative radiotherapy, when delivered to the region of the epigastium or upper lumbar vertebrae, will often cause either nausea or vomiting. Most patients and many doctors believe that radiotherapy is invariably associated with distressing nausea and vomiting, but this is not so. Quite wide-field irradiation of either the chest, head or limbs is well tolerated and is likely to be associated with no more than a sense of tiredness for a few hours after each treatment.

Relief of pain

Palliative radiotherapy has an important part to play in the relief of pain from bone metastases, most commonly those from a primary breast or bronchial carcinoma. A single treatment delivering 10 Gy to a painful metastasis in a limb bone or rib is often sufficient to relieve pain within 7-14 days. In a well-run department, this can be given on the same day that the patient is seen. Painful metastases in the bony pelvis or in a vertebra will, however, necessitate a fractionated course of treatment in order to keep side-effects to a minimum. Usually a maximum tumour dose of 20-25 Gy can be delivered in a course of four or five treatments spread out over two weeks. When metastases in the region of the upper lumbar vertebrae are irradiated, an intramuscular injection of prochlorperazine (12.5 mg) given at approximately 20 minutes before treatment will help to prevent nausea and vomiting. Irradiation of a collapsing cervical or dorsal vertebra is worth considering, even if it is not causing pain, as a prophylactic measure against possible incontinence and paralysis.

For patients with pain in several areas due to multiple bone metastases, a single dose of 8 Gy to either the upper or lower half of the body will often give rapid relief of pain within 24 hours. After an interval of four to six weeks, a second dose can be given to the unirradiated half of the body. This treatment is not without side-effects. Most patients will have nausea, vomiting and diarrhoea for up to two days, and if higher doses are used, there is a risk of radiation pneumonitis and haematological toxicity.

The bone and joint pain of both adults and children in the late stages of leukaemia often responds to irradiation. During their periods of hospitalization, doses of a few Grays can be given to the painful zones on a day-to-day basis as necessary.

Palliative irradiation can sometimes be given to achieve an indirect effect. The painful joints of a patient suffering from hypertrophic pulmonary osteoarthropathy can occasionally be relieved by irradiating a previously untreated primary bronchial carcinoma. In the same way, itching due to jaundice can be relieved by low-dose irradiation of hepatic metastases provided they are from a radiosensitive tumour.

Nerve root pain due to vertebral collapse, and the severe pain of nerve plexus involvement due to advanced breast, gynaecological or colorectal carcinoma are much more difficult to control by radiotherapy. Irradiation for pain resulting from rib erosion by bronchial carcinoma is also often unrewarding. Analgesic drugs and nerve-blocking procedures play a much more important role in these situations.

Control of bleeding

The presence of severe bleeding can be very disturbing to a patient, and a short course of radiotherapy to the chest or pelvis can be used to relieve haemoptysis, haematuria or vaginal bleeding, at least temporarily. A simple technique of opposed fields of suitable size can deliver a maximum tumour dose of 25 Gy in five or six treatments at the rate of two treatments per week. As an alternative, bleeding from a vaginal vault recurrence may be controlled by a single insertion of a radioactive isotope (usually Cobalt-60 or Caesium-137). This necessitates admission to the ward for a day or two but does not usually require a general anaesthetic. In a radiotherapy department with a Cathetron or other afterloading machine capable of delivering high-intensity irradiation in a matter of minutes rather than hours, this treatment can be given on an out-patient basis.

Control of fungation

One of the problems of radiotherapy is to deliver an adequate dose to the tumour without irreparably damaging the adjacent normal tissues, and it is therefore less of a problem to treat tumours of the surface of the body. Patients are not infrequently seen with disseminated carcinomatosis associated with a primary breast tumour which is either fungating or about to fungate. When time permits, a previously unirradiated tumour, even if quite large, can often be controlled (with healing of ulceration) by a few doses of irradiation. However, if a fungating breast tumour has been irradiated previously, other forms of treatment such as hormone therapy or chemotherapy may be more appropriate.

Using opposed fields of supervoltage radiotherapy aimed tangentially across the breast, a maximum tumour dose of 35 Gy delivered in six treatments at the rate of two treatments per week will control such a tumour just as well as any more protracted technique of daily treatments. In elderly, frail or very sick patients, a similar arrangement of fields can be used to deliver a single treatment of 8 Gy. If the patient is well enough, this treatment can be repeated a week later and again for a third and final time after a further fortnight. Either of the dosage schemes will restrain fungation and reduce discharge, and if the full dose can be given, the ulceration will usually heal. As the fields of irradiation are aimed tangentially and do not penetrate the body, treatment will not be associated with general systemic symptoms. The only disturbance to the patient will be that with full dosage the skin of the breast will become mildly erythematous and the nipple temporarily tender.

Other tumours fungating on to the surface of the body may warrant irradiation in an attempt to reduce a profuse discharge. A very elderly lady at St Christopher's Hospice had a huge fungating tumour on the anterior abdominal wall from a primary carcinoma of the gall bladder. This tumour was expected to be of only moderate radiosensitivity and, as it had been previously irradiated, further treatment was associated with a risk of producing a fistula. But as she had no distant metastases and as the only symptom which was keeping her in hospital was a profuse discharge (such that she was unable to stand without soaking her clothing), it seemed justifiable to risk retreatment. A maximum surface dose to the tumour of 15 Gy in three doses was sufficient to control the discharge and allow her to return home, and treatment was safely repeated on two occasions within six months before she died.

Patients with advanced rectal carcinoma whose obstructive symptoms have been relieved by a palliative colostomy sometimes may live many months with distressing residual symptoms. Severe perineal pain or profuse rectal discharge of mucus from an unremoved primary tumour is difficult to control, but a short course of palliative irradiation aimed at the tumour is worth considering as these patients have often had no previous radiotherapy (see Chapter 7). Computerized tomography can be useful in defining the extent of a recurrent rectal tumour so that the volume to be irradiated can be kept as small as possible.

Control of cough and dyspnoea

Cough and dyspnoea from an advanced primary bronchial carcinoma can often be relieved or improved by a course of palliative radiotherapy. A history of a previous course of palliative irradiation, especially if it has been temporarily successful, does not prelude a second course. Using a simple technique involving a pair of parallel opposed fields, a maximum tumour dose of 25 Gy can be delivered to the primary tumour and mediastinal nodes in six treatments over a period of three weeks. When time is short, similar results can be obtained with 20 Gy delivered in five consecutive daily treatments.

Palliative irradiation of lung metastases should not be considered unless the metastases are from highly radiosensitive tumours such as lymphomas, seminomas or nephroblastomas. In these instances, part or all of both lungs can be irradiated. It is, however, unwise to exceed a maximum dose to both lungs of 15 Gy in six treatments over three weeks because of the risk of producing an acute radiation pneumonitis. The irradiation of less radiosensitive tumours is unlikely to be of value.

Radiation of large lymph-node masses

Enlarged metastatic nodes in the mediastinum from a primary bronchial carcinoma or from a malignant lymphoma may cause the syndrome of superior vena caval obstruction. The resultant dyspnoea and congestion are particularly distressing. Occasionally these symptoms can be relieved by therapy with corticosteroids, but not infrequently a course of concurrent radiotherapy similar to that recommenced for the relief of cough and dyspnoea will be of greater value. It is usually wise to irradiate these patients as in-patients rather than by out-patient visits. Very occasionally, the first treatment may be associated with an exacerbation of the symptoms, although this appears to be less common than reported in the literature.

It may also be of value to irradiate radiosensitive tumours or nodal metastases if they are causing obstructive symptoms such as dysphagia in the last few weeks of life. A primary carcinoma of the oesophagus is not a particularly radiosensitive tumour, but an anaplastic carcinoma of the thyroid causing dysphagia often responds.

Intra-abdominal metastases from a seminoma of the testis or dysgerminoma of the ovary are very radiosensitive and, even if large, are worth irradiating.

Symptoms unlikely to be helped by radiotherapy

In general, the irradiation of extensive intra-abdominal carcinomatosis from a carcinoma of the gut or ovary is unrewarding. Even at palliative dosage, such a course of treatment is often associated with distressing nausea, vomiting and diarrhoea. In these circumstances, well-chosen chemotherapy may be preferable or it may be a time to withhold active treatment.

Radiotherapy is rarely, if ever, helpful in the control of pleural effusion or ascites. In the past, the instillation of radioactive gold was used, but more recently the instillation of a cytotoxic chemotherapy agent, such as thiotepa or bleomycin, has been found equally effective and much safer to use.

Side-effects of radiotherapy

The aim of palliative radiotherapy is to relieve symptoms with the lowest possible dose in the fewest possible treatments. Side-effects at the level of dosage described in this chapter are unlikely to be severe, except for the inevitable nausea produced by fields directed at the epigastrium.

Irradiation of fungating tumours on the surface of the body where a maximum dose falls on the skin may be associated with a temporarily uncomfortable erythema. This can be kept to a minimum by keeping the irradiated skin dry and avoiding the application of lotions, ointments or adhesives containing metal salts, such as zinc. Fungating tumours have to be kept clean and free from infection (see Chapter 7) but unnecessary washing should be avoided when possible. However, when irradiating the perineum, the benefits of brief bathing far outweigh those of the avoidance of washing.

Mucosal reactions in the mouth and oesophagus are unusual at palliative dosage, but as irradiation predisposes to mucosal infection with *Monilia*, it is wise to accompany irradiation with a prophylactic course of an antimonilial drug such as amphoteracin lozenges (10 mg four times daily). Irradiation of the mouth reduces the secretion of saliva and tends to dry the mouth. If food collects in the sulcus and the lips become dry and cracked, advice on oral hygiene can prevent a great deal of suffering.

Temporary diarrhoea may follow palliative irradiation of the pelvis, but it should only be moderate at the doses recommended. Kaolin and morphine mixture (10 ml three to six times daily) and codeine phosphate tablets (15–30 mg three times daily) are the most commonly prescribed remedies and, with an adequate fluid replacement, should control this side-effect. The mucosa of the bladder is more resistant to irritation and a course of palliative radiotherapy aimed at controlling haematuria is unlikely to cause troublesome bladder symptoms. Persistent dysuria and frequency are more likely to be due to the effects of the tumour itself.

Prochlorperazine (5–10 mg three times daily) is probably the most useful drug to control radiation-induced nausea and vomiting, and a liberal intake of glucose fluids also helps.

It must, however, be stressed that it is unusual to see side-effects from the type of palliative irradiation that has been described for use in the last few months of life. These patients are already ill and it is important not to confuse the progressive symptoms of disease with the symptoms produced by radiotherapy. However, on occasion, patients may be comforted by the erroneous belief that their symptoms are due to a recent course of radiotherapy, and this need not disturb a radiotherapist. What matters is the result of good care.

The care of a patient who is terminally ill, and of his family, is at its best when a team of experts works together. It is possible for the surgeon, the radiotherapist and the chemotherapist to deprive a patient of his final dignity, but it is also possible that working skilfully together they can contribute to his comfort.

9

Palliation by cytotoxic chemotherapy and hormone therapy

Thelma D. Bates and Thérèse Vanier

The use of cytotoxic chemotherapy and hormone therapy, though rarely curative, belongs primarily in the active phase of treatment of malignant disease. Because most of the cytotoxic drugs and some of the hormones have unpleasant side-effects, and as a response to treatment may be delayed for several weeks, their use in the terminal stages of malignant disease is very limited. However, although the palliative value of such treatment is not as predictable as that of radiotherapy, a successful response to these drugs is more likely to be associated with a prolongation of life. As with all other modalities of treatment, it is the quality of this life which is important.

At the moment, there are approximately 40 clinically useful cytotoxic drugs. None of them specifically damages malignant cells, and most act by interfering with cell division and cause a variable degree of damage to normal as well as to malignant cells. This leads to unwanted side-effects such as bone marrow depression and gastrointestinal disturbances, thus limiting their use.

Each of the cytotoxic drugs is of value in the treatment of several different tumours, and a higher response rate may often be obtained if several drugs are combined. The most successful combinations in use comprise three or four drugs which are individually effective against the tumour, each having a different mode of action and toxic side-effects which do not overlap. Cytotoxic drugs are also best given intermittently rather than continuously. This helps to avoid the development of drug resistance and immunosuppression which may be important if the expectation of life is to be increased.

Cytotoxic chemotherapy has to be modified and simplified for use in the terminally ill, when the emphasis is on symptom control. Unpleasant side-effects, which may be acceptable in the earlier phases of the disease, are no longer justified at this stage. Whenever possible, the drugs used should be effective by mouth, should require the minimum of specialist supervision and monitoring, and should have minimal, controllable side-effects. The drugs chlorambucil and cyclophosphamide satisfy these criteria. Both can be given by mouth and are effective against several solid tumours, including carcinomas of the ovary and breast, as well as lymphomas. When drugs have to be given intravenously, regimens should be simple and the frequency of injections kept to a minimum. Dosage also may have to be modified in order to balance the likely benefit to the patient against the side-effects.

Carcinomas of the breast, endometrium and prostate may respond to sex hormone therapy. By the time these patients reach the terminal stages of their disease, most will have exhausted this form of therapy, but if not, hormone therapy can be considered. Hormones have several advantages over cytotoxic drugs. They have fewer side-effects, can usually be given by mouth, and need less specialist supervision and monitoring. The main disadvantage of both sex hormones and cytotoxic agents in terminal cancer is that a response to treatment often takes four to six weeks to become apparent.

Prednisone and dexamethasone play an important role in terminal care as they act quickly and help to relieve a variety of symptoms (see Chapters 5 and 7). When given with cytotoxic drugs, they are alleged to give some marrow protection and to reduce nausea.

In general, a pre-existing course of cytotoxic drugs or hormones is stopped in these patients when the disease process shows no sign of control despite adequate duration and level of dosage. There may, however, be a place for continuing low dosage of these agents, (even when there is little chance of affecting the disease process) if the patient believes they are beneficial. It is not always easy to know whether the drug is responsible for an apparently static condition. Drugs may be inappropriate at one moment but if the patient's general condition improves and a longer prognosis is evident, they should be considered.

Experience at St Christopher's Hospice over a two-year period is shown in Tables 9.1 and 9.2. In the case of most patients referred to this specialist unit for terminal care, a decision will already have been reached that cytotoxic or hormone treatment is no longer appropriate. In a small number of cases, referral is made primarily for pain or other symptom control but with the option of continuing more aggressive treatment if this is considered appropriate. Stopping what is looked upon as active therapy will be much less traumatic if symptom control has been seen by patient and doctor as of major importance throughout treatment. The figures given for continuing or starting hormone treatment (6 per cent of total admissions) and cytotoxic treatment (1.6 per cent of total admissions) reflect the general principles underlying the use of these drugs at the present time, as does the breakdown of figures relating to primary sites. We submit that survival figures from St Christopher's Hospice reflect not so much the effect of these drugs as the stage at which patients are transferred to its care.

Breast carcinoma

Patients with breast carcinoma often respond to cytotoxic drugs or to hormones. The choice of treatment will be dictated by the patient's previous response to treatment, her general condition and the estimated possible survival. Cytotoxic drugs may show their earliest effects within two or three weeks, but with hormones one usually has to wait for four to six weeks. There is often a place for giving both together.

Single cytotoxic agents

Although single agents are not as effective as multiple drug regimens, they have an important role in the terminally ill because they are often less toxic and simpler to administer. Probably the most useful is cyclophosphamide which can be expected to cause a temporary but worthwhile response in one-third of cases. It can be given by mouth at a dose of 100 mg daily. Nausea, bone marrow

Table 9.1 Analysis of patients receiving cytotoxic drugs at St Christopher's Hospice during the period 1.1.80–31.12.81.

Primary site of tumour	Number	Percentage total admissions	Number given cytotoxic drugs	Percentage for tumours at this site	Continued	Started
Breast	225	16.6	2	1	2	0
Gastrointestinal	356	26.3	2	0.5	0	2
Ovary	40	3.0	1	3	1	0
Vulva	8	0.6	1	12	1	0
Bladder	55	4.1	1	2	1	0
Prostate	45	3.3	1	2	1	0
Myelomatosis	10*	0.7	3	30	1	2
Retroperitoneal	1	0.1	1	100	1	0
Other	612	45.3	0	0	0	0
Total	1352	100	12	1.6	8	4

Survival in days	Mean	Median
Treated with cytotoxics	61	44
Drug(s) started	117	74
Drug(s) continued	40	33
All admissions	24	13

Alive at the end of the study: 1 with myelomatosis (336 days).

* One with myelomatosis who received no cytotoxic drugs (89 days).

Table 9.2 Analysis of patients receiving sex hormones at St Christopher's Hospice during the period 1.1.80–31.12.81.

Primary site of tumour	Number	Percentage total admissions	Number given sex hormones	Percentage for tumours at this site	Continued	Started
Breast	225	17	56	25	52	4
Ovary	40	3	1	2.5	1	0
Prostate	45	3	20	44	19	1
Cervix	32	2	1	3.1	1	0
Kidney	18	1.5	6	33	6	0
Uterus	19	1.5	3	15	3	0
Other	973	72	0	0	0	0
Total	1352	100	87	6	82	5

	Survival in days	
	Mean	Median
Treated with hormones	66	32
Drug(s) started	107	60
Drug(s) continued	63	31
All admissions	24	13

Alive at end of study: 1 with carcinoma breast (350 days); 2 with carcinoma prostate (640, 551 days).

depression and alopecia at this dosage are rare and, if the drug is taken in the morning with plenty of fluids throughout the day, bladder irritation can be avoided. Although intravenous adriamycin is the most effective single agent for breast cancer, a high incidence of alopecia makes it unsuitable for these patients. Intravenous 5-fluorouracil 500 mg at weekly intervals is a well-tolerated alternative to oral cyclophosphamide.

Mrs S., aged 76, was admitted mainly for social reasons, with a local recurrence and multiple skin deposits. During the year she lived at St Christopher's she received three courses of oral cyclophosphamide (100 mg daily for six, nine and four weeks). The first two courses were followed by complete disappearance of the lesions. Despite deterioration in her general condition, she was sufficiently troubled by the local recurrence on the chest wall to justify a trial of 5-fluorouracil after the third course of cyclophosphamide was ineffective. She received three weekly injections of 500 mg but the drug was of no avail and she died three weeks later.

Mrs P., aged 65, was referred for terminal care with local recurrence, involvement of the opposite breast and secondaries in bone, liver, skin and lymph nodes. Her general condition was remarkably good and she was up and dressed for most of the day shortly after admission. She was started on a combination of cyclophosphamide 100 mg daily and tamoxifen 20 mg b.d. which caused rapid regression of node and skin secondaries. The remission lasted for eight months, during which time she was at home, leading a fairly active life. When relapse occurred she was re-admitted for consideration of multiple cytotoxic treatment, but she died suddenly before it was commenced.

Multiple cytotoxic agents

More aggressive cytotoxic therapy may occasionally be justified in patients with gross fungating tumours, especially those who have presented late in the course of the disease. The following intravenous quadruple regime can be given to out-patients.

Day 1	Cyclophosphamide	500 mg	*Day 8*	Cyclophosphamide	500 mg
	Vincristine	1 mg		Vincristine	1 mg
	5-Fluorouracil	750 mg		Methotrexate	50 mg

Each drug is injected singly into a butterfly needle and washed through with saline. Injections are given on two days a week apart, and repeated after three clear weeks. Patients usually complain of nausea on the day of injection and approximately half will develop alopecia. Full peripheral blood counts must be done before each course of injections. A worthwhile response lasting several months can be expected in 50-60 per cent of patients, and improvement is usually apparent in the responders within a month.

Mrs R., aged 67, had been given oestrogen therapy for four months before referral but without any benefit. Her general condition was remarkably good despite a gross fungating lesion and leucoerythroblastic anaemia. As these were causing her dominant symptoms, she was transfused with 2 pints of blood and treated for 15 months with a quadruple chemotherapy regime (cyclophosphamide 300 mg, vincristine 1 mg, 5-fluorouracil 500 mg on day 1 and cyclophosphamide 300 mg, vincristine 1 mg and methotrexate 50 mg on day 8 together with 10 mg metoclopramide (Maxolon) i.v. on each occasion) which produced no significant side-effects. The primary lesion dried up and shrank considerably and the post-transfusion haemoglobin level of 8 g per cent rose spontaneously to 12 g per cent. When she relapsed, tamoxifen 20 mg twice daily was substituted, and she had another remission which lasted five months, during which time she was at home. She was re-admitted because of progressive disease and died three months later.

Hormone therapy

The most useful hormone for the terminally ill is tamoxifen. This anti-oestrogen may benefit both pre- and post-menopausal patients and also those patients who have failed to respond to other hormones. It is given by mouth at a dose of 10–20 mg b.d. and is remarkably non-toxic. This is the best sex hormone to combine with cytotoxic therapy and is recommended for use with oral cyclophosphamide.

Premarin, a natural oestrogen, is less likely to cause nausea than stilboestrol. A dose of 1.25 mg is equivalent to stilboestrol 5 mg and may be of value in elderly patients with a longer prognosis even if they have failed to respond to other hormones. An appropriate dose is 1.25 mg three times daily.

Of the androgens, Decadurabolin is the least virilizing preparation. A dose of 50 mg intramuscularly every three weeks can be given to both pre- and post-menopausal patients, especially those with skeletal metastases.

Aminoglutethimide inhibits steroid biosynthesis in the adrenal cortex and induces a medical adrenalectomy. This is particularly useful for post-menopausal patients with painful bone metastases. Unwanted side-effects are more common in the elderly and include dizziness, lethargy, occasional nausea and, more rarely, a transient drug rash. Treatment should start with 250 mg twice daily and, in the absence of unwanted side-effects, the dose can be increased to three or four times daily. Tabs. hydrocortisone (20 mg twice daily) must be given at the same time as a replacement therapy.

Miss W., aged 63, presented for terminal care with bilateral breast involvement and pleural effusion. She failed to respond to quadruple chemotherapy but responded to tamoxifen 10 mg twice daily. The remission lasted 18 months. Relapse was treated with oral cyclophosphamide 100 mg daily and palliative radiotherapy which produced another remission lasting 14 months. Tamoxifen was then restarted but skin lesions worsened and she was given Premarin for four months. The disease remained static after this for eight months when a further transient improvement occurred on giving tamoxifen once more. She died some six years after the start of treatment and the quality of her life was good until the last 18 months.

Mrs P., aged 50, was admitted with a three-year history of breast carcinoma and bone metastases. She had been previously treated with androgens and recently had sustained pathological fractures of both femoral necks—one of which had been pinned. She was thought to be terminally ill and in need of pain control. After this was achieved it became evident that she was well enough to return home, albeit in a wheelchair. Tamoxifen 20 mg b.d. was started in the hope of holding up the progress of the disease and, if possible, preventing further pathological fractures. She was able to spend six months at home, during which time the dose of diamorphine required for pain control was reduced from 40 mg orally four-hourly to 30 mg. She died suddenly at home.

Ovarian carcinoma

This tumour does not respond to hormone therapy and, in most patients seen in the terminal stage, cytotoxic drugs will already have been used. If not, they should be considered, especially when recurrent ascites requires frequent tapping. The most useful and least toxic drug for these patients is chlorambucil given in an initial dose of 5 mg b.d. reducing to 5 mg o.d. Full blood counts will be necessary at monthly intervals, but at this dose level this drug has few side-effects. Less effective alternatives are tabs. cyclophosphamide 100 mg daily, caps. treosulphan 250 mg t.d.s. or the intraperitoneal instillation of thiotepa 60 mg or bleomycin 60 mg.

Cis platinum is probably the most effective agent for ovarian carcinoma, but it can only be given under specialist supervision. It causes severe nausea and must be given with intravenous hydration to prevent renal toxicity.

Miss M., aged 70, had refused laparotomy after presenting with severe ascites. Cytology of the ascitic fluid had been unhelpful but there was a large mass arising from the pelvis, and disseminating ovarian carcinoma was considered the most likely diagnosis. At first, tapping of 10–15 litres was required monthly to keep her comfortable. Chlorambucil and cyclophosphamide were then used sequentially (chlorambucil 5 mg o.d. for two months, then alternating two-week periods on 10 mg o.d. for five months; cyclophosphamide 100 mg daily for three months and then 50 mg daily for ten months), and only one further paracentesis was required over the following 18 months despite a gradual increase in the size of the abdominal mass.

Mrs P., aged 68, was found at laparotomy to have an ovarian carcinoma with pelvic and peritoneal spread. Radiotherapy had been started at the referring hospital but was discontinued because of a deterioration in her general condition. She improved to such an extent following admission for terminal care that chlorambucil 10 mg o.d. was started. She was discharged under the care of her general practitioner and lived a comparatively normal life for 13 months before dying at home.

Endometrial carcinoma

This tumour occasionally responds to progestogens but rarely to cytotoxic drugs. When progestogens have not been used previously, they can be tried in the terminally ill; none of these agents has unpleasant side-effects. The most useful drug is medroxyprogesterone acetate (Provera) which can be given by mouth at a dose of 100 mg b.d. An alternative is a weekly intramuscular injection of gestronol hexanoate (Depostat) 200 mg.

Cervical carcinoma

The rare adenocarcinomas of the cervix may respond to progestogens in a similar way to endometrial adenocarcinoma, but the common squamous cell carcinoma of the cervix does not respond to hormones. The most useful cytotoxic agents are adriamycin and methotrexate, but as both are highly toxic drugs they cannot be recommended for the terminally ill. If the expectation of life is somewhat greater, intravenous adriamycin 50 mg and methotrexate 20 mg on day 1 and methotrexate 20 mg on day 8 may temporarily relieve pelvic pain and bleeding.

Gastrointestinal carcinoma

The long-term results of cytotoxic therapy in this form of cancer are not encouraging. Less than 10 per cent of admissions to St Christopher's Hospice with this type of primary will have been given such treatment.

Patients with pelvic spread due to carcinoma of the rectum may live a long time and pain control may be particularly difficult. Radiotherapy remains the best palliative adjuvant to analgesics, but 5-fluorouracil may be useful if radiotherapy is contraindicated.

> Mrs R, aged 41, presented with gross pelvic invasion, including involvement of the vaginal vault. Pain was controlled with oral diamorphine but troublesome vaginal bleeding and discharge persisted when an effective pain-control regime allowed her to return home to care for a young family. Intravenous 5-fluorouracil was given, 500 mg weekly and then fortnightly over a period of three months, and these symptoms cleared during this time. Subsequently, increase in pain, liver involvement and general deterioration necessitated readmission and she died three weeks later.

> Mrs Y., aged 53, was referred because of gross pelvic spread, severe pain, vaginal discharge and bleeding. Two courses of quadruple chemotherapy at the referring hospital had made her feel very ill. When pain had been relieved with oral diamorphine, intravenous 5-fluorouracil 500 mg weekly and later fortnightly controlled the vaginal symptoms for several months. This allowed her to be at home for 7 out of the 11 months she lived after referral for terminal care.

Not surprisingly 5-fluorouracil is largely ineffective in controlling pain when used by itself in gastrointestinal cancer, but on rare occasions has proved helpful for pain due to carcinoma of the head of the pancreas.

Prostatic carcinoma

Most patients with prostatic carcinoma will be receiving hormone treatment, commonly stilboestrol (5-25 mg three times daily). This is usually continued into the terminal phase but the dosage may be reduced if the patient is vomiting or nauseated, or shows signs of fluid retention. A decision to start hormone treatment at this time is rare (see Table 9.2).

Bronchial carcinoma

Because of the poor response to cytotoxic drugs, no more than 5 per cent of lung cancer patients referred to St Christopher's have been treated in this way, except for small cell anaplastic ('oat cell') carcinomas. It is important to establish the exact histology since single agents such as cyclophosphamide may produce a remission of symptoms, even if this is short lived.

In the main, symptoms due to bronchial carcinoma are better controlled by radiotherapy or nerve block in conjunction with appropriate medication. In our opinion, tapping pleural effusion in the terminal stages either for fluid removal or instillation of a cytotoxic is rarely helpful as re-accumulation to the previous level is rapid. Dyspnoea is best controlled by small doses of morphine or diamorphine (see Chapter 7).

Head and neck carcinoma

Occasionally, patients with severe pain due to advanced squamous cell carcinoma in the head and neck can be helped temporarily by a course of intramuscular bleomycin. A dose of 15 mg twice weekly for three to four weeks is recommended for patients who have not had this cytotoxic drug previously. Side-effects will include nausea and fever; pulmonary fibrosis can be avoided if the total dose from all courses does not exceed 300 mg.

Lymphoproliferative disorders and leukaemias

Patients with these malignancies come into a special category in relation to cytotoxic agents. They will all have been treated with such drugs and also usually with blood and blood products. By the time they are terminally ill such treatment has become a way of life. This may make the decision to stop such treatment more difficult, but the change in emphasis will be easier if attention to symptom control is given prominence as the disease progresses.

Summary

When patients enter what is thought to be the terminal stages of malignant disease, the emphasis in treatment is on the control of distressing symptoms. On rare occasions, cytotoxic drugs and hormones can be used to relieve these symptoms and in doing so they may sometimes prolong life. As long as accurate prognosis remains difficult, these agents will continue to be useful.

10

The place of surgery in terminal care

Michael R. Williams

While there is still a prospect of cure or long-term control of disease, one can reasonably demand a great deal of patients in terms of pain, discomfort and time. Extensive ablations of tumour masses, amputations of limbs, the cosmetic disfigurement of major dissections of the head and neck—combined if necessary with exacting courses of radiotherapy and cytotoxic drugs—are all worth their while. But once the progress of the disease makes it clear that cure is no longer possible, the emphasis of treatment must be changed to secure the maximum quality of life for the period that remains at the cost of the minimum morbidity. Morbidity includes not only pain and discomfort but also loss of independence and dignity, clouding of consciousness and time spent in hospital. For those who have a home to go to, every day spent in even the best hospital is a day wasted which can be ill-afforded when life is limited.

There are some symptoms which no patient should suffer for long:

   intestinal colic;
   protracted vomiting;
   inability to swallow one's own saliva.
To which I would add:
   the stench of secondarily infected fungating lesions;
   the intractable itch of unrelieved obstructive jaundice;
   faecal or urinary incontinence;
   the throbbing pain of pus under tension.

When these symptoms arise they must be controlled. On occasion, radio-therapy and cytotoxic drugs may make a considerable contribution to palliation of the patient's symptoms (see Chapters 8 and 9). Failing that, control can almost always be achieved by adequate drug therapy which (if necessary) can be justifiably pushed to the point of shortening life; even without doing this, the dosage necessary to secure control may depress the level of awareness and deprive the patient of his independence and ability to exist outside an institu-tion.

It may be possible, however, to provide relief by surgery at the cost of a lesser morbidity, in which case it is essential to count the cost. Apart from minor procedures such as draining abscesses which are justifiable in the last days, my own rule of thumb is that one week spent in a surgical ward is justifiable if there is a prospect of three months useful life at home, two weeks for six months respite, while three weeks in hospital is justified for a year of worthwhile survival.

When presented with a patient with incurable malignant disease one should assess the present symptoms and signs and, in the light of the likely natural history of the disease, attempt to predict symptoms which may occur as the condition progresses and which are likely to prove troublesome and unacceptable. One then tries to devise some programme which will relieve the former and obviate the latter. The essence of effective terminal care is long-term planning so that the problems in the last days are manageable. Such planning implies working out an individual programme for each problem, using a common set of principles.

Take, for example, a patient with carcinoma of the rectum. The associated symptoms may be considered in two main groups: those due to the presence of the tumour itself, and those due to the narrowing of the lumen of the bowel. The tumour will cause by its presence increased mucus secretion, rectal bleeding and tenesmus. Fungating lesions are likely to become infected, with development of local abscesses and fistulae. The tumour may spread locally and involve adjacent tissues such as other pelvic viscera, the sacral plexus or anal skin, and it may cause venous obstruction with oedema of the legs. If the tumour obstructs the lumen of the bowel, the patient will develop colic, frequent and uncontrollable diarrhoea or incontinence and, finally, as the obstruction progresses, abdominal distension and vomiting.

A colostomy will relieve only the obstructive symptoms. Whenever possible, it is more satisfactory to remove the primary lesion and at least reduce the chances of local recurrence during the likely period of survival. If a patient at laparotomy is found to have a moderate amount of metastatic disease in his liver and he is likely to live a year or more, he will be best served by an abdominoperineal resection: this procedure will remove his primary tumour and reduce the risk of local recurrence at the cost of three weeks or a little less in hospital. With extensive hepatic metastases and a shorter prognosis of only six months or so, this approach would be inappropriate. It may, however, be possible to mobilize the tumour sufficiently to resect it and close the stump of the rectum below (Hartmann's operation), bringing out a terminal colostomy which must be carefully sutured to the skin with silk sutures to secure primary mucocutaneous healing. The patient can then begin to care for his colostomy without delay and, with no perineal wound to heal, he can be home in ten days.

If the primary tumour cannot be removed, a colostomy should be performed only if the patient has obstructive symptoms. In their absence, a colostomy is only an added burden. With a simple laparotomy and closure, the patient will be able to return to his family in a few days. If he develops colic later, a colostomy is a simple matter; but it may never prove necessary and a colostomy as such will do nothing to prevent the symptoms produced by the tumour itself.

If the patient has obstructive symptoms and a colostomy is performed, the bowel should always be divided and the proximal end carefully sutured to the skin with interrupted silk stitches to secure primary mucocutaneous healing with minimal reaction. The patient can then start to care for his own colostomy as soon as it works. There is no place in palliative surgery for the cumbersome loop colostomy which requires the assistance of nurses until it shrinks down. The distal end is best closed and dropped back into the abdomen. It never seems to give trouble, and by not bringing it out on the abdominal wall, one reduces the risk of a local metastatic deposit in the skin. The colostomy should be sited so that the patient can reach it easily himself even though the abdomen may subsequently become distended with a large liver or ascites. Continuing independence is more important than cosmetic appearance.

Using the same principles and lines of thought, a suitable plan can be produced for the management of incurable malignant disease at any site using surgery, radiotherapy, cytotoxic drugs and simple medicaments as indicated. Each programme must be planned on an individual basis, treating the patient in the context of his disease rather than the disease itself.

In general, removal of the primary tumour wherever possible is desirable in any lesion which is likely to fungate either on the surface of the skin or in the lumen of the bowel. This is particularly important with carcinoma of the breast, where an offensive ulcerated mass can readily be removed and primary healing at least temporarily secured by some form of local mastectomy; this may well be accompanied by hormonal therapy in suitable cases, either by drugs or by ablative surgery.

The surgeon should resist the temptation to refer such patients for radiotherapy merely as a method of disposal. Radiotherapy should be advised only after careful discussion with the other colleagues in the team, taking into account the possible advantages and disadvantages for that particular patient.

Even in the last stages, it is often worthwhile to excise particularly troublesome skin metastases, which can often be done under local anaesthesia.

To revert to the gastrointestinal tract. Patients with intestinocutaneous fistulae may have pain from inadequate drainage and secondary abscesses which are frequently subcutaneous, lying superficial to the muscles. Laying the fistulae widely open and saucerizing the abscesses will relieve the pain instantly and make the lesions easier to dress by the district nurse at home.

If persistent colic is a problem, not controlled by danthron with poloxamer (Dorbanex) and enemas, and if there appear to be some months of useful life left, a fistula should be established proximal to the obstruction—either a colostomy or even an ileostomy. It is a mistake to think that the latter is particularly troublesome to the patient with modern appliances. Mucocutaneous suture should always be done and training in the management of the stoma must be begun at once.

If it is clear at laparotomy that there are multiple obstructed loops of bowel secondary to numerous peritoneal seedlings on the serosal surfaces (as is often the case in disseminating carcinomas of the ovary), no attempt should be made to separate these or perform several side-to-side anastomoses for fear of producing multiple fistulae. It is wiser to close the abdomen and control the symptoms with adequate analgesia. The same is true of obstruction in the last stages of the disease, when the patient is unlikely to have long enough to enjoy the relief he has earned through the discomforts and stress of the operation.

Each case must be considered on its merits, taking into account not only the disease and the stage it has reached but also the patient's particular problems and aspirations. A woman with two boys at boarding school was dying from recurrent carcinoma of the cervix causing colonic obstruction. The ureters were also involved and her blood urea was raised, but her principal problem was uncontrollable diarrhoea which kept her housebound. A terminal colostomy with mucocutaneous suture was performed in the third week of July and she was out of hospital in seven days looking after her own colostomy. She was able to accompany the boys on various expeditions, visiting the theatre twice and going to restaurants and museums throughout the summer holidays. She died of uraemia a few days after the beginning of term. In spite of the shortness of the respite, this was worth her while.

Fungating lymph-node metastases in the neck, axilla and groin present particular problems. In advanced cases it is rarely possible to achieve surgical clearance. Radiotherapy and cytotoxic drugs may help to control pain, but are unlikely to secure healing. Secondary infection of surrounding normal tissues can be controlled by courses of systemic antibiotics, but it is impossible to sterilize the fungating lesion. The local management of fungating tumours is dealt with in Chapter 7.

Death in such cases may well be from secondary haemorrhage (see Chapter 2). If haemorrhage occurs, there is no place for resuscitation and transfusion: narcotic drugs in adequate dosage, to which hyoscine 0.4 mg can usefully be added, must be instantly available. Normally there is a small warning bleed, before the final fatal haemorrhage. This is not an indication to isolate the patient behind screens, but instead he should be encouraged to pursue his normal activities. It is, however, kind to arrange for the traditional red blanket to be draped about him to lessen the distress of any onlookers if a large bleed ensues.

In inoperable carcinoma of the oesophagus and cardia, the great problem is that the patient will finally be unable to swallow his own saliva. Every effort must be made to enable him to do this and it is justifiable to incur very considerable risks to achieve it. I find a Mousseau–Barbin tube the best method, but it is essential to trim off the green rim before inserting it (if this is not done the orifice of the tube tends to crinkle up when it is in position and obstruct the lumen). If the tube becomes blocked with food, fizzy drinks or soda water will frequently clear it. On no account should a gastrostomy be established in these patients or they will be kept alive to die of drowning in their own spittle.

In obstructive jaundice, as opposed to the terminal jaundice due to intrahepatic metastases, patients are frequently depressed and much troubled by an intolerable itch, which can be dramatically relieved by free drainage of the bile.

The presence of dilated intra- and extrahepatic ducts can be reliably and non-invasively demonstrated by ultrasound and, if necessary, the actual site of obstruction and frequently its nature can be shown by a percutaneous cholangiogram, which is a relatively simple and unexacting manoeuvre under local anaesthesia, well tolerated by even the fairly grievously sick.

If the obstruction is fairly low in the common duct, as in incurable carcinoma of the head of the pancreas, a choledochoduodenostomy with a wide anastomosis is a satisfying procedure because it leaves so little dead space and consequently a low risk of cholangitis. Failing this, a cholecystojejunostomy or even an external fistula via a T tube will secure relief.

If the percutaneous cholangiorgram shows that the obstruction is higher up the biliary system, due either to a carcinoma of the bile duct or external pressure on this duct from enlarged lymph nodes in the porta hepatis, which would make surgery impossible or unduly hazardous, it is frequently possible to feed a guide wire through the needle into the dilated duct system and then guide it down through the obstruction into the duodenum. Over this a catheter with multiple holes can be fed, thus draining the bile into the duodenum with consequent relief of symptoms. The end of the catheter should be left on the surface after withdrawal of the needle, so that if the catheter becomes blocked with sludge it can be cleared by syringing with saline.

If the obstruction is due to a primary carcinoma of the bile duct, temporary palliation can sometimes be achieved by placing a radioactive wire in the catheter at the site of the obstruction.

If later the catheter becomes irretrievably blocked by sludge or extension of the tumour, it is worth attempting to resite the catheter by repeating the procedure if a further dilated duct can be tapped.

Apart from such specific considerations, there are various points which a surgeon as a member of the team caring for the incurable patient must continually bear in mind.

Urinary and faecal incontinence is very distressing to the patients and their attendants and may be kept hidden from the doctor unless specifically asked about. It is due to overflow, until proved otherwise. A urethral catheter, either intermittently released or with free drainage into a bag, can transform the situation. The catheter should be on the small side to prevent irritation of the urethra and, in the male, it is often more satisfactory to use a fine suprapubic catheter such as a Riches which can be inserted blind under local anaesthetic and does not require such frequent changing. The use of antibiotics in catheterized patients is discussed in Chapter 7.

Most analgesics are constipating, and faecal impaction is common. As well as uncontrolled diarrhoea, it may cause considerable perineal discomfort. Once faecal impaction has occurred, it is advisable to do a manual removal rather than attempt multiple enemas, which are often unrewarding and always exhausting. It is essential to examine the rectum daily for some days afterwards. Reimpaction may occur as further faeces come down from the rest of the colon.

Perineal abscesses, whether secondary to fistulae or arising *de novo*, are frequently overlooked and should be searched for when doing the routine rectal examination to exclude faecal impaction. In the terminally ill, abscesses can arise very insidiously and the site of new pain must always be examined carefully to make sure it is not due to an abscess rather than neural involvement by neoplastic disease. Such discomfort can be relieved by simple drainage of the abscess.

Pus may form under tension beneath a slough of dead tissue in a pressure sore on the buttocks, heels or elbows. Excision of the slough, which does not require an anaesthetic and is painless, will give relief.

Finally, it is a mistake to think of malignant disease as a steadily and relentlessly progressive process. Periods of stabilization between the host and the tumour may occur, either spontaneously or as a result of treatment; occasionally, regression to a dramatic extent may occur. One must be constantly on the lookout for such a fortunate, if unusual, event. The patient should then be reassessed and may well be put back in the category mentioned in the first paragraph of this chapter where more active therapy such as 'second looks' or active treatment of comparatively minor disabilities may well be appropriate.

To sum up: the surgeon has frequently been involved in the care of the patient in happier days. Once it is clear that the disease is incurable, careful planning and foresight will help to make the last months and weeks as comfortable and valuable to the patient as possible. Even during the last weeks the surgeon may well have something to contribute, and careful reassessment of the patient's problems to see what can be offered is well worthwhile. The surgeon's continuing interest will be a boost to the patient's morale.

11

In-patient management of advanced malignant disease

T. S. West

'My Rule is to receive you with hospitality and to let you go in peace.'
(*Sayings of the Desert Fathers*)

The need for admission

Some patients suffering from advanced malignant disease will need in-patient care. However competent the general practitioner, or however willing the family, situations may arise when full-time skilled nursing and medical care will become essential if the patient's symptoms are to be properly controlled (Saunders, 1973).

Admission from home may be precipitated for any of the following reasons.

1. Inability to control the symptoms of the disease, for example:
   pain,
   restlessness,
   confusion,
   nausea,
   breathlessness,
   incontinence,
   pressure sores.
2. When the family are in special need, due to:
   exhaustion,
   lack of sleep,
   concurrent illness,
   financial worries,
   overwhelming anxiety,
   inability to share the truth and support each other.
3. Lack of, or insufficient, appropriate services, for example:
   incontinence laundry,
   home adaptations or equipment,
   night sitters,
   home help.
4. The patient's wish to be no further burden to his family.

Admission can be postponed by:

1. ability of the general practitioner and his team to control the symptoms of the disease and the distress of the patient and the family;
2. a close and competent family and/or good neighbours;

3. the strength which can come from sharing the truth;

4. applying for the full range of benefits available from the local social security department;

5. applying for the full range of services available from the local social services department;

6. the security which comes from the knowledge that admission to a suitable bed can be arranged without delay should the need arise.

Temporary admission may give the time necessary for any of these factors to be sorted out.

Preparation to admit

Good management of advanced malignant disease will be achieved only if those concerned are trained:

1. to distinguish between what is appropriate and inappropriate treatment at each stage of the patient's illness;

2. to accept the change of direction from cure to care and to be alert to its possible reversal;

3. to learn the special medical, nursing and social work skills involved in competent terminal care;

4. to comprehend family relationships and friendships;

5. to ensure good lines of communication within the caring team and between its members, the patient and the family.

The phrase 'the doctor said there was nothing more he could do' may sometimes represent a patient or family's misunderstanding of a statement made in a limited context. Sometimes it really has been said, yet the combined skills of teams caring for people who are dying consistently refute this conclusion (Saunders, 1975).

Little imagination is needed to picture the usual course such patients will have followed before they are admitted for terminal care. A long series of hopes and disappointments, of various more or less successful treatments and of relating to a host of new medical, nursing and paramedical faces will have left the patient exhausted, often despairing and sometimes cynical.

By now, the patient and family may have become the responsibility of no one, and transfer to another and unfamiliar unit will increase this sense of helplessness, despair and lack of support. Therefore, if it is possible, patient and family should be given the opportunity to discuss future care and even to visit the new unit. This can convey an important message: the patient, his family and the professionals are to unite in one sharing, planning, decision-making team. This invests patient and family with a sense of responsibility and control over their situation. Decisions regarding terminal care can never be purely medical, and the family team needs to be united with the professional team in the pursuit of total care.

The first step must be for the staff in the new ward to be interested enough to make the patient feel wanted and welcome as himself rather than for his physical condition and also confident enough that they can deal with the factors which have precipitated his admission. The family must be welcomed, both to be cared for and to be members of the caring team.

Admission must be efficient, quick and warm. This is no time for a junior clerk to search for a patient's number or for the patient, trolley and family to be left in a cold corridor. A senior person representing the institution should welcome the patient and his family and see them quickly through to the ward where the nurse in charge, having welcomed them herself, should introduce the new arrival to the other patients, and their families, in the bay or ward.

Admission to a specialized unit

Should admission become necessary, the general practitioner may have no choice as to where he sends his patient. All the same, neither a geriatric unit nor the busy medical or surgical ward of a general hospital will be appropriate unless the staff of the ward concerned have time and enthusiasm for terminal care.

We would be very grateful if you could give us the following helpful information:
Is there any special reason for referral to St. Christopher's?

....

....

....

(A preliminary visit to St. Christopher's can be arranged through the Admissions Secretary)

Have you been having any community support?

Social Worker? Name...

Home Help?..

Meals on Wheels?...

District Nurse?...

Church? Which?...

Other? Please specify..

Are there any special factors within the family you would like to be taken into consideration?

....

....

....

....

Are there likely to be problems in visiting should the patient require admission at some stage?

....

....

....

....

Date:...

Our booklet gives details of visiting hours, facilities, what to bring, etc.

Fig. 11.1   Page 2 of the Application Form, to be completed, if possible, by patient or relative.

A specialized unit or hospice dealing mainly with terminal care may be available. Such a place might be thought to engender a death-house image, as indeed could the palliative care unit or the symptom control team—or the screened bed or single room at the end of the ward; but a reputation for good nursing care and efficient symptom control will keep ahead of this image and, in practice, has been shown to challenge the standard of pain control and terminal care in wards or other institutions that it borders (Melzack, 1976).

A specialized unit is directed towards care rather than cure, possesses a corpus of specialized knowledge, and can provide an appropriate setting for the patient and his family as they come to terms with the final stages of a life. Medical, nursing and social work staff who have the confidence of their own experience in controlling the pains and the losses of terminal disease, and who do not regard death as a final failure, can sit by a patient's bed and listen to him. With appropriate treatment and successful symptom control, barriers of silence and of chatter can be lowered (see Chapter 4). In such an atmosphere, the visits of children are very important; they should be encouraged to bring their toys, their games or their homework. It is important that they too come to trust the people who are looking after their sick relative.

Before admission from either home or hospital, a specialized unit will expect the patient's doctor to fill out an application form. Current medication needs to be accurately listed, e.g. if steroids have been used, indications for their use and doses prescribed must be stated. Some indication of the patient's and the family's awareness of both diagnosis and prognosis is useful. It is particularly helpful if the family fills in part of the application form themselves (Fig. 11.1).

Admission to the ward

Unless the patient is in pain, the first half-hour after admission should be unhurried. During this time the ward staff will begin to make their own observations of the patient and the family. They will inform the doctor if the patient is in pain or the relatives are in a hurry to leave.

If the patient arrives in pain, he should be seen by the doctor as quickly as possible. Sometimes he will not have been given analgesics that morning. Sometimes a long and uncomfortable ambulance journey will have exacerbated his pain and the drugs will have to be written up before the nursing staff are allowed to administer them.

It is sad to receive a desperately ill person who has been packed off in a sitting ambulance, without adequate drugs for the journey. This is particularly true for patients who have come not from home but from another institution and where an experienced member of the staff should have been able to make some better assessment of their suitability, that morning, for transfer. Having obtained information from the application forms, the doctor's note, the social worker's report and, most useful of all, the letter from the ward sister or district nurse and from the new ward staff, the doctor, in his turn, makes the patient welcome. He may then choose to interview the family or friends. Often the patient is ill and tired and it is the family who can best and most easily describe the events which have led up to admission. It may seem right to interview and examine the patient first and, perhaps more often than we realize, it is right to interview husband and wife together.

Admitting the family

Every effort should be made to meet the family and to give them time to talk. The day of admission for the patient is a crucial time for the family as well. The patient who is going to die has relatives who are going to be bereaved. This is a crisis situation that will affect everyone and, from the outset, thinking must be in family terms. Appropriate inclusion of all concerned enables the patient as well as relatives to cope with the illness better, and after death it enables relatives to look back and gain strength, comfort and confidence from their contribution to the patient's care and their own ability to survive. The drawing of a genogram (or 'family tree') in the notes enables staff to have a clear picture of the family who surround the patient and who will be bereaved. It may well highlight individuals who have already suffered losses in the past and indicates potential family support systems (Fig. 11.2a).

For the family, the preceding weeks may have been as hard or harder than for the patient. If he has come from another hospital, the chances are that he is already very ill or that the family, for whatever reason, were unable to have him home. If the patient has come from home, the recital of anxiety, pain, soiled linen and sleepless nights, so often told with a minimum of self-pity, can only impress one with the family's love and strength.

Often, however, the family will feel that they have failed the patient by not succeeding in keeping him at home until the end. Part of the doctor's duty is to tell the family that, having seen the patient and having read his GP's letter, it is obvious that they really have done everything humanly possible and that the patient now needs the full-time nursing care and skills which can be given only with admission. But they must be reassured that their involvement with the patient is by no means over.

If the patient has come from home, a lot of the necessary but simple facts can be obtained from the family: 'What can he keep down? Is there anything he specially fancies? Alcohol? When did he last get to the bathroom unaided? Is movement a trigger for pain? Is it pain that keeps him awake? Does he sleep during the day? Is he incontinent?'—and here assurance can be given that the nurses are used to these common problems, and that the patient will not be humiliated.

Although some indication of the rate of deterioration may be obtained from the family, in the experience of most doctors an accurate prognosis is impossible. 'Days rather than weeks' or 'weeks rather than months' are probably as far as one should go—with the statement that 'We may be able to tell a little more when we have watched him for a few days'. Sometimes the family are not really asking, 'How long?' but rather, 'What is the end going to be like?' An assurance that symptoms will be controlled and that dying itself will not be distressing— suffocating, choking, uncontrolled pain or isolation are the common fears—will help to reduce the dread of the unknown which may oppress the family as they sit round the patient's bed. Less factual knowledge can also be sought: insight, religious faith and the place truth holds within that family.

Permission to tell the patient 'the truth' as he *wants* and *needs* to know it can almost always be obtained from the family if it is carefully explained to them that this is likely to be a gradual process. The family who has perpetuated the concealment of truth from the patient will need to be assured that they will not

OFFICE USE ONLY:

1. Risk : High: _____   5.   Telephone Call: _____
2. Immediate Support: __✓_____   6.   Group: _____
3. Score: _36_____   7.   Others: _____ _____
4. Counsellor Assigned: 8a. Not referred: _____
    FAMILY'S OWN SOCIAL WORKER   8b. Referred elsewhere: __✓___

FAMILY PROFILE

This form to be completed in <u>black biro</u> by staff about the family at ward
meetings before and after the patient's death:

Patient's Name: _ANN MURRAY_____ Hospice No: _83/535_____
Date of Birth: _15.11.36_ Date of Admission: _3.10.83__ Date of Death: _9.11.83__
Out-Patient: YES: __✓_____   NO: _____   WARD: _____

PATIENT'S FAMILY TREE: (Include extended family or other person most
affected by loss)

Complete this section as soon as possible after the patient's admission:

ASK PATIENT/FAMILY: "Is there anyone in the family you're worried about?"
                         "What are the strengths and resources in your family?"

LIST persons who may be most affected by loss:

NAME	ADDRESS	TELEPHONE	AGE	RELATIONSHIP
STEVE PHILIPS	)		48	FRIEND
MARY MURRAY	) 15 BROMLEY CLOSE	460 1334	17	DAUGHTER
SUE MURRAY	) S.E. 26		15	DAUGHTER
JACK CARTER	35 STANLEY RD., S.E. 21	698 1545	79	FATHER

- -

WHAT SUPPORT DO THE FAMILY HAVE:

(1) EACH OTHER: (YES)   NO

(2) OTHERS: Name: _MRS. SMITH_____   Name: _REV. J.E. BROWN_
                  Designation: _SOCIAL WORKER_ Designation: _VICAR (JACK CARTER)_
                  Telephone: _460 3500___   Telephone: _460 1231___

Fig. 11.2a.

<u>COMPLETE AT WARD MEETINGS THROUGHOUT ADMISSION/AT DEATH</u>

INDIVIDUAL OR FAMILY RISK FACTORS

1.	Are there children or adolescents in the immediate family	(yes) no	??
2.	Are there dependant family members (handicapped, elderly, sick)	(yes) no	??
3.	Loss of primary care giver/constant companion/emotional support	(yes) no	??
4.	Loss of financial provision	(yes) no	??
5.	Loss of home, <u>feared or actual</u>	(yes) no	??
6.	Anxiety about making decisions	(yes) no	??
7.	Is a parent still alive	(yes) no	??
8.	Family unable to share feelings	yes (no)	??
9.	Reluctance to face facts of illness or death	yes (no)	??
10.	Did the family feel unprepared for the death	yes (no)	??
11.	Marital or family discord	(yes) no	??
12.	Communication difficulties in the family	yes (no)	??
13.	Was the care of the patient by the family unduly stressful	(yes) no	??
14.	Presence of concurrent life crisis (adolescent daughters,	(yes) no	??
15.	Difficulty in dealing with the previous losses (separation of parents) *father's illness)*	(yes) no	??
16.	Excessive or prolonged emotional reaction/mental illness/suicide risk	yes no	(??)
17.	Self-care difficulties	yes (no)	??
18.	Lack of Spiritual Support	yes (no)	??
19.	Lack of Community Support	(yes) no	??
20.	Distress over <u>changed body image</u> or personality	(yes) no	??

Comments by ward staff seeing family the day after the death:

(e.g. present at death? viewed in chapel? mood? expression of emotion?
      numb? any special worries? family/friends giving support?)

Mrs. Murray died suddenly during night. Family not present. All came today and were very tearful. The two girls and Steve wanted to spend time in the chapel with Mrs. Murray's body. This seemed to help them to take in what had happened and to say goodbye. Very supportive of one another; but otherwise without support of relatives or friends. Sue feeling particularly frightened about the future in case her father will come and "take them away". Steve seems numb and reluctant to take responsibility for the girls.

Mr Carter's vicar will bring him to the Hospice tomorrow to see his daughter, tho' may decide he would rather remember her as she was. Ward Sister

I.	Is the family or individual high risk?	(YES) NO
II.	Is there any need for immediate family support	(YES) NO

Revised August 1983
(being evaluated)

Fig. 11.2b.

31. 9. 82 Tension and anxiety in this family is making it difficult for them to give Mrs. Murray the care and support she is needing. The General Practice social worker reported that family relationships deteriorated after Mrs Murray's diagnosis was made. There is rivalry between the 2 girls which, although normal at their age, is distressing for Mrs Murray. Her father, Jack Carter also has cancer and is distressed about his daughter's illness and frightened about his own.

                                    A. E. SHORT (Domiciliary Sister)

3.10.83   Arranged with British Telecom for a telephone installation funded by N.S.C.R. grant.

                              Anne Otter (Social Work Assistant)

3.10.83 (day of admission) Arguments between family members on the ward. Mary & later Sue, seen by Hospice social worker. They have little understanding of their mother's illness – "Where is the cancer? – When will she die? – How do you die?" Dr. Jones called in to be with us while we discussed their questions. Suggested family meeting with doctor, ward sister & their own social worker, which they would like & they want to bring their grandfather.

                                          P. PEARCE
                                          (Ward sister).

5.10.83 Family Meeting Those present: Mrs. Murray, Mary, Sue, Steve Phillips, Jack Carter & family's dog. Dr. Jones, Ward Sister, Mrs. Smith (Social Workers G.P. Practice.)
Discussion covered the following areas:
(i) Ward sister welcomed the family to the ward and said she hoped they'd feel at home! discussed what they could do for Mrs. M. including taking her home for Sunday lunch or weekends when well enough.
(ii) The pain of the past year and the continuing anxiety of the family. Mrs. M. said she had no pain now but was frightened in case it came back. Dr. Jones described how we would control the pain.
(iii) Jack Carter: "I wish I could take my daughter's place. I'm worried about the girls without a mother." Mary, Sue & Steve now more reconciled and showing great affection for one another, and support for Mrs. M. and Jack Carter.
Arranged to meet again next week or sooner if family wished.

                                    Staff nurse Keen.

Fig. 11.2c.

now be let down, for it may well have been right for them to have carried the burden of knowledge to this point; the patient would have done the same for them. Now they may share—and they often do so.

Often it seems that patient and family when first told the diagnosis and prognosis are in a state of shocked denial. Denial may be a common reaction during a period of remission, but when the disease begins to progress the family, too often with the connivance of the doctors, continues to deny the patient the truth and let him walk the lonely path towards realization and dying by himself.

It is wrong and should be unnecessary to tell a patient direct lies. But neither is the whole truth and nothing but the truth the order of the day. Death from cancer is seldom a sudden catastrophe. If we are sensitive and are travelling with our patient, he will be the one who lets us see if and when he is ready to know more about his condition.

By this stage, patients who ask for the truth rarely give up when they receive it. Rather, they sum up all that their life has been and, having looked, with their family, at the fact of death, are then better able to live out the time which remains profitably and even happily.

Admitting the patient

The patient may be very ill and tired. His admission need not be long but must appear unhurried. The identification of his main complaints and a general physical examination, which may not have been carried out by a doctor since active treatment was stopped, are probably all that is necessary at this first interview.

The reassurances that we are glad to see him, have taken note of what he complains of and will do something about it and that the bed is his for as long as he needs it are astonishingly therapeutic. Unless it is essential, it is wise not to change medication for the first 24 hours. Previous medication given with new confidence may now become more effective and, in any case, the first night in a strange place is not the ideal situation in which to introduce new drugs.

Although the drugs the patient has been taking may no longer be controlling his symptoms, he must be given time to transfer his trust to the new team caring for him. Only then can he be expected to dispense with the old drug regimen on which he has been forced to rely as the only defence against unbearable pain. In practice, by taking the same analgesics the patient has been given 'on demand' and giving them to him regularly, *before* pain breaks through, previously unrelieved pain can often be controlled (Melzack, 1976). As one patient said: 'At St Christopher's you do not pursue the pain, you anticipate it.'

Telling

Quite often, when asked to tell us about their illness, patients will reveal that they are fully aware of their diagnosis; at this first meeting, truth can sometimes be brought into the family situation, often with dramatic results. Family members who may have spent weeks and months in lonely isolation protecting each other from the truth may now be able to look at one another, to grieve and face reality and life together.

More often, the questions and anxiety which point to a request for the truth come gradually and obliquely from the patient and are presented at different times to different members of staff. At St Christopher's Hospice, a special pink page is kept in the patient's notes for any member of staff to record conversations which could help us understand the patient and family better (Fig. 11.2c).

Who should tell how much and when is a matter for which there is no umbrella answer. The doctor should never tell a direct lie to a patient, if for no other reason than that the lie will almost certainly be discovered and confidence, not only in the doctor but also in his successors, will be undermined. However, the busy consultant on a teaching round is unlikely to have time to sit down and listen to a patient's hesitant questions. Some consultants make a point of returning alone. It seems reasonable to expect that those who cannot do so should make it clear that responsible members of the team have permission to listen to their patients' questioning and to answer as best they can. Most of us can sympathize with the consultant who said, 'I never tell my patients the truth. I did so once . . .', but that should not be the end of the story. Even when things go less than perfectly, the team members must be able to rely on each other's support. To tell a patient he is going 'for convalescence' when in fact he is going to a home for terminal care may get the sending hospital out of an awkward situation; it will almost certainly put the receiving team in a difficult one. Far better to say, 'We are sending you to a place where they have the staff, the skill and the time to give you the care you now need . . .'.

The family doctor would seem to be the obvious person to introduce the truth at the appropriate time. Slowness of communication between the hospital and the general practitioner and finally a letter containing a list of findings without any statement about what the family and the patient have been told do not make his task any easier.

The most important question is not 'What do you tell your patients?', but rather, '*How* do you tell them and what do you let them tell you?' This sounds simple, but in practice involves a sensitivity to the questions being asked and to the answers which, at each particular stage in his illness, the patient can accept (Abrams, 1974).

Staff communication

After admitting the patient and the family, the doctor reports back to the senior nurse and discusses with her his findings, defining the problems and listing proposals for care. Uncontrolled pain and inadequately shared insight are the two problems which most commonly head the list.

Effective management will depend not only on the skills and knowledge of the medical and nursing staff, but also on the speed and ease with which communication can take place between all members of the caring team—which should include the family itself.

Ward reports may be little more than a list of names, procedures, drugs and current bowel problems, but there should be a time when the ward sister and her team are able, without visitors or members of other disciplines present, to discuss the problems of particular patients in some depth. The nursing staff remain the front line; they are the only people constantly with the patient.

The doctor, doing his round, should first go through the list of patients on the ward with the ward sister, giving her a chance to report to him changes in a patient's condition or anxiety about him or his family. Changes in medication and arrangements, when appropriate, to meet with the family can be planned.

'The doctor's round' itself should normally be done alone. But a consultant and his registrar or houseman with a member of the nursing staff should sometimes go round together. This can be particularly useful, if they work well as a team, in helping patients and families who are still trying to manipulate the staff in the hope of altering the facts, or who are presenting complicated problems of management—often the physical and emotional are inextricably intertwined. Contrary to what is thought, this need not inhibit the patient, who often feels able to look to the nurse or junior doctor for support, and who is reassured rather than distressed by the presence of a concerned team. The doctor must give the patient time to talk. Only in this manner will the symptom control discussed in Chapters 5 and 7 be maintained; for 'pain' can be thought of as whatever the patient experiencing it says that it is—not what the doctor thinks that it ought to be, not what the nurses report that it is, not even what the family complain that it is. Very ill patients may take long pauses between perfectly lucid sentences as they look for words and estimate the real interest of their doctor. The doctor's ability to sit with a patient in an unhurried but attentive manner puts the time available to proper use. Such a careful round should take place at least twice a week; on other days, as long as the nursing staff are experienced, a visit to the patients with specific problems and a few words of greeting to the others in the bay may be all that is necessary. A doctor's visit to a dying person reassures him, the relatives, neighbouring patients and ward staff that 'everything possible is being done'. Routine investigations have no place but particular procedures may be indicated in individual patients (Mount, 1976).

Patients who are very ill should be protected from having to meet too many new people, but it seems useful if each patient is cared for by two doctors during the week. Some patients open up to one doctor along a wide but fixed frontier but choose to step over that particular frontier with another doctor with whom they have not developed quite so personal a relationship.

It is important that after each round the doctor reports back to the nurse in charge of the ward and records any problems or conversations that will be of use to the ward team in the total care of the patient and his family. The whole ward staff must make this journey with the patient and his family and must not stand aloof from his increasing weakness or their exhaustion. They are all involved with the problems of physical distress and may have to support a growing awareness of truth.

Good terminal care requires enough ward staff to sit with patients who are anxious or dying and to spend time with families who are under stress and, later, when they have been bereaved. In most cases, temperature, pulse and respiration charts and a number of investigations can usually be dispensed with and the time saved more profitably used. When families telephone to enquire about a relative the nursing staff should, if possible, ask the enquirer to wait while they go to see the patient and then report back. The phrase, 'As comfortable as can be expected', has little meaning.

Sometimes a patient or family member is seen to be under severe strain. A life-threatening illness arouses in everyone powerful emotions which may be evident in irrational behaviour, uncontrollable weeping, anger or withdrawal. Here the social worker with her particular skills in understanding psychological and emotional problems, and her experience of working with distressed individuals or with a family as a group, may provide not only therapeutic help for patient and family members but also sufficient understanding of the situation to enable others in the ward team to respond more appropriately to very distressed people.

Whenever possible, a social worker who is already working with a family before an admission should continue to do so throughout the terminal phase of the illness and on into bereavement. This provides continuity of emotional support, based in the community, which is where the family have to pick up the threads of living again. A social worker from the community can also help the team to gain helpful insights into a particular family's problems and resources.

But nothing removes the responsibility from the ward staff to notice stress and to find appropriate support.

The interdisciplinary meeting

Nurses' ward reports and doctors' rounds done in close liaison with the ward sister still leave room for a weekly ward meeting, an essential opportunity for the exchange of important information. Such a meeting, after the confidence of the staff has been gained, will bring to light anxieties, questions and unrecorded information from the most unlikely sources. This meeting should normally only include staff who work with the patients in that particular ward: doctors and nurses, social workers, physiotherapists, occupational therapists, chaplain and others. It must be constructed so that any person present, however junior, feels able to question or contribute. It is a comfort to find that everyone else is also finding a particular patient difficult or that others have noticed with anxiety the strain a particular family is enduring. And it is good to hear of a patient's courage or wit, or of the mutual support families and patients can give the staff as well as each other. The drug management of a patient is sometimes questioned and needs discussion. Although the prescription must finally be written by the doctor, it is the ward staff who will help him to decide what is appropriate treatment and what could be inappropriate and to balance dose levels to individual need.

When lines of communication are properly used, the assessment of a patient's pain, be it physical, mental, social or spiritual, concern for the family and signs of strain among the staff should not take too long in coming to light. A broader awareness of unsolved problems and unexpected successes than any individual member can recognize is gained as a team.

The caring team

The ward sister rather than the doctor heads the caring team in the ward, unravels the strands and calls in the 'experts'. The doctor, with his knowledge of appropriately applied pharmacology and his special role of talking with authority to patient and family about the disease process, about prognosis and about the physical and mental manifestations of grief, maintains his ultimate clinical responsibility and has no need to feel his *amour propre* insulted by queries and suggestions.

The social worker, aware of the problems that can enmesh a patient and his family, must search for the resources and strengths within each situation. By facilitating discussion of the present, and as far into the future as the family is willing to go, the social worker encourages people in crisis to take control of their destiny and to regain their self-respect. The sorting out of practical problems should be done in such a way as to enable family members to remain in control of their affairs. To discover ways of obtaining appropriate help from social service, housing or social security departments, albeit with the backing of a social worker, should be seen as a means of marshalling strengths in a family who will then enter a future without the patient with greater confidence and effectiveness (Earnshaw-Smith, 1982).

The chaplain or appropriate minister of religion may be needed to give spiritual support with the authority of the church or faith he represents, to listen to confession and to give reassurance of forgiveness. It is not unusual for patients and families to find a new understanding and help in sacrament and service. He also has a special importance as a listener, as has the social worker, just because he is a person on whom the patient is not physically dependent.

The physiotherapist has two goals: the maintenance or restoration of the patient's physical independence, and the prevention of deformities which will curtail this independence. To keep a patient mobile or to get him to walk again is to raise his morale and self-respect enormously. To need to ask for everything, even if it is no further away than the locker, is to lose a basic independence which many patients find almost unbearable. It is irrelevant that this independence may not be long lasting. The physiotherapist's work is also to prevent deformities; if they occur, unnecessary stress and discomfort and unnecessary difficulties in carrying out nursing procedures will make the last weeks of a patient's life a time of increasingly painful dependence. Part of the skill in controlling physical distress in advanced malignant disease is to use drugs in such a way that the patient is still mentally alert and that even if there is pain on movement, it is tolerable. If this is achieved, the physiotherapist can often continue her work until the last day or two of the patient's life. Massage and passive movement or instructions about relaxation can also be most helpful.

The occupational therapist, and sometimes the speech therapist, if they are people of enthusiasm and imagination, interested more in day-to-day progress than in long-term rehabilitation, will help to maintain the physical dimensions of a patient's life as long as possible (Weisman, 1977). It should never be forgotten that diversion may be the best pain reliever of all.

The basis of good terminal care is good nursing and its apex is a ward sister who is a skilful and sensitive leader. The nurses must have come to some sort of terms with dying and with death; they must also learn not to hurry. The rest of the caring team can only function well in such a context (Charles-Edwards, 1983).

Family meetings

It is usually the social worker's task to orchestrate family meetings with doctor, nurses, chaplain and other appropriate members of the team present.

When the family meets a caring, united ward team, they begin to feel that the patient's illness, with all the physical, emotional and social problems which arise from it, is more manageable and less frightening than they had imagined. Alarming fantasies can be shared and replaced by an understanding of the facts of the disease; the resources for its management can be openly discussed. Children, by their openness and ability to voice the fears which adults often hide, often facilitate these meetings, bringing into focus the conflicts and stresses that operate within the family.

The presence of a concerned, empathetic, interdisciplinary team of people who are prepared to acknowledge their own emotional vulnerability, can enable family members to reveal their feelings of helplessness and fear. Also, because of their differing skills and ability, as they work together as a team they model for a family a way of restructuring relationships and working together in a crisis. Within the bounds of confidentiality, it is important that the outcome, if not the content, of such family meetings is made known to members of the caring team who were not present.

Remission

Admission can be turned into welcome by courtesy. The pains of dying and death can be alleviated by care and knowledge. Sometimes, however, between admission and death an unexpectedly long period may elapse. It is here that more than technique is required. This time can be hard for the patient, for the family and for the staff. Each day has to be got through as best it can and it may seem that death would be a merciful release. But in retrospect this time of waiting often turns into a time of deepening relationships within the family and sometimes what can be called 'spiritual growth' in the patient. To have shortened such a patient's life, denying him and his family this time, would be a tragedy. Patients who survive longer than expected may become sources of irritation or they can become focal points in the ward to whom other patients and the ward staff can relate. They can take a place with the orderlies, the volunteers and the families as essential parts of the working ward team. When such patients die, the whole ward may be bereaved.

Care of the dying calls for great flexibility on the part of the caring team. Although the emphasis has shifted from cure to care, the condition of the patient must be constantly reviewed and reassessed. If symptoms are properly controlled or the disease process slows down or enters a stage of remission, the patient may well experience a new lease of life. If the family have had their confidence restored and have had a rest from constant nursing, they, in turn, may be able to look after the patient for another period at home. For some it may be possible and more appropriate to arrange a stay in a convalescent home with sufficient medical and nursing supervision. Occasionally even a holiday abroad can be contemplated.

Patients whose illness has been labelled 'terminal' must still be constantly assessed by all members of the caring team for potential improvement in their physical and mental well-being. Further active treatment may sometimes, and surprisingly, be indicated. Palliative radiotherapy, palliative cytotoxic therapy, antidepressant drugs or steroids may produce dramatic improvements in patients for whom no further active treatment had been considered appropriate. Such an improvement may well enable the patient to return home and enjoy valuable extra time with his family. The patient himself should be encouraged to treat the ward as if it were his second home, from which he can go out for the day or the weekend. Sometimes his symptoms will be sufficiently controlled for him to be discharged home. Such a discharge will work only with the cooperation of the patient's general practitioner and his staff, the involvement of a domicilary service (if there is one) and the assurance to the patient and to his family that should the home situation break down in any way, readmission can be arranged immediately. For the patient, there can be no waiting list.

This constant reassessment of the patient in the context of his family and the regular reviewing of the rate of progress of the disease itself calls for careful and regular clinical observations and consultation with all members of the ward team. It may also involve visits from or to a consultant in another discipline.

Management of dying and death

The moment of death is rarely unexpected and therefore the nurses will have had time to prepare the relatives. Young children are not usually present but teenagers should not be discouraged if they wish to be there. A nurse endeavours to join them at the time of death or to watch if for one reason or another the family cannot be there. It is she who draws the curtains and gently tells the relatives when death has occurred. This is a hard moment, as death to them is often not obvious. The relatives around the bed almost always accept the offer of the simple set prayers which in many hospices are then said by one of the nurses. For some families this offer is obviously unsuitable and it is not made without thought.

After death the relatives may well wish to be left alone behind the curtains. When the time is right the nurse takes them to a quiet room and gives them a hot drink and sympathy and sometimes just silence. Special customs or cultures will be respected.

The remaining patients in the bay are told of the death. As they will have witnessed the dying, it will not be too much of a shock to them, but again they must be given time to react and express their own grief or fears.

When the relatives are ready to leave, the ward staff will have checked on the home situation and the availability of friends and transport. At this moment a bereaved person should not have to return to an empty house. A bereavement visitor or volunteer may be available to accompany such a person home. The ward team will have made it clear that they can always be telephoned in times of particular anxiety or depression.

A time on the following day will have been arranged for the family to collect the death certificate and property. This is an important occasion. Reception should inform the ward staff that the relatives have arrived and the ward staff should be responsible for greeting them and taking them to the visitors' quiet room. Refreshment should be offered and after some conversation the death certificate is handed over and clear instructions given on how to get to the registrar's office and what will happen there. On this visit, funeral arrangements and any other immediate problems can be discussed. The doctor, the social worker, the chaplain and the funeral director should all be available if necessary. Should relatives wish to view the body, this should be made as easy as possible and a nurse they already know should accompany them.

Many relatives wish to go back and see the remaining patients in the bay. Indeed, they will sometimes continue to visit regularly, a fact which underlines some of the advantages of not hiding away the dying person. At St Christopher's Hospice, relatives will be invited to come back to the monthly 'Pilgrim Club'.

Here they can meet with members of staff and sometimes with patients whom they knew during the time they had been visiting the hospice. Once a patient has died, the form used during the admission is completed, enabling the social worker to assess the relatives' need for support. This might involve a telephone call after the funeral, a visit from a bereavement counsellor, or later on an invitation to join a small therapeutic group of bereaved relatives for a limited period of time. The bereaved must be helped to discover their own resources and help must not develop into dependency.

In-patient management in advanced malignant disease demands that the specialized knowledge of symptom control now available is used successfully. With symptoms controlled, the patient is freed, if he so wishes, to contemplate both living and dying; the family as a whole can come to terms with the truth; they can be grateful for all that has been good and say goodbye—not necessarily in words. Sadness will not be removed but bereavement may be lightened.

> 'Tranquil talk was better than any medicine;
> Gradually the feelings came back to my numb heart.'
> (Po Chu-I, 1946)

References

Abrams, R.D. (1974). *Not Alone with Cancer.* Charles C Thomas, Springfield, Illinois.

Charles-Edwards, Alison (1983). *The Nursing Care of the Dying Patient.* Beaconsfield Publishers, Beaconsfield.

Earnshaw-Smith, Elisabeth (1982). Emotional pain in dying patients and their families. *Nursing Times* **78**, (44), 1865.

Melzaok, R. (1976). The Drompton Mixture: effects on pain in cancer patients. *Canadian Medical Association Journal* **115**, 125.

Mount, B.M. (1976). The problem of caring for the dying in a general hospital; the palliative care unit as a possible solution. *Canadian Medical Association Journal* **115**, 119.

Po Chu-I (1946). *9th Century Chinese Poems.* George Allen & Unwin; London.

Saunders, C.M. (1973). The need for inpatient care for the patient with terminal cancer. *Middlesex Hospital Journal* **72**, 125.

Saunders, C.M. (1975). Terminal care. In *Medical Oncology*, pp. 563–76. Ed. by K.D. Bagshawe. Blackwell, Oxford.

Weisman, A.D. (1977). The psychiatrist and the inexorable. In *New Meanings of Death*, pp. 108–113. Ed. by H. Feifel. McGraw-Hill, New York and Maidenhead.

12

A specialist nurse in a district general hospital and in the community

Winifred Morris

'The secret of the care of the patient is in caring for the patient.'
(Peabody, 1927)

Until very recently, death has too often been seen as a failure by the medical and nursing professions, and the care of the dying has frequently been neglected in general hospitals. Now, despite the enormous scientific advances of the last decade, we again realize not only that death is not a failure but that it is part of life. With this 'discovery' has come the realization that we need to care more adequately for terminally ill patients.

The trend today is to discharge patients much earlier than a few years ago: appendicectomy patients are often discharged after four days instead of seven to ten days, hernia patients may only spend part of a day in hospital. Patients with inoperable cancer are also discharged home, to be cared for by their families. These early discharge schemes optimally utilize scarce nursing skills but do not give the opportunity for personal nurse–patient relationships to develop. Added to this, modern technology and advanced pharmacology are in danger of producing within our profession an academic rather than a practical nurse who finds it easier to relate to a progress graph and digital read-out than to the patient in the bed. Other aspects of professional behaviour, like the shorter working week and rotational shift system for nurses and UMTs (units of medical time) for junior doctors 'unsocial hours', have fragmented continuity of patient care to such an extent that often the patient does not know with whom to relate. This is particularly hard for the very ill and often frightened patient.

In our enthusiasm to provide better technical care for patients, we may have overlooked the needs of the terminally ill. Over the last 15 years this gap in our caring system has gradually been filled by the hospice movement, which has developed a number of foundations caring almost entirely for patients facing death. Many new hospices have opened and are operating very successfully in this country, but, as Ford and Pincherle state in their article in *Health Trends* (1978), a team of staff within a district general hospital with the necessary skill and expertise can achieve many of the objectives of hospice care, counselling, symptom control and help after bereavement.

Today's National Health Service is in dire financial straits and yet we talk of building and running more hospices which carry a capital cost of at least a quarter of a million pounds, with a similar sum needed on a recurring annual basis to meet the revenue implications. Paradoxically, while there is a demand for hospice accommodation, many district general hospitals have up to 30 per cent of their acute beds empty (Yates, 1982). Would it not, therefore, be sensible to utilize these facilities by providing the dying patient with a proper, adequate and caring service within the confines of an existing district general hospital rather than squandering hard-to-come-by capital money on more bricks and mortar?

It is the duty of every nurse and doctor to be able to care adequately for the dying patient in terms of the control of pain and other physical symptoms and in emotional and family support. Midwifery is now a very specialized subject, and not every doctor is trusted to do obstetrics, yet every nurse should be able to care for the dying patient. If we remove all the dying patients to hospices, we are going to make this important field of medicine and nursing extremely specialized and, in years to come, we will live in a society where only a few can care competently for a dying patient and his family.

In November 1978, a post was created within North Tees General Hospital at Nursing Officer Grade to care for the needs of the dying patient. It is a specialty that has aroused my interest for some years and which became more obvious some 10 years ago, when, as a ward sister, I nursed a young girl of 18 for four months before she died. During these four months I spent many hours with her and her parents and a close link was forged between Susan and me. However, in retrospect, as a ward sister, I was wrong, for I had 24 other patients in my care who, at times, I must have excluded by caring so totally for Susan. After her death, however, I knew that there was a great need for a person or persons who could devote skill, energy and, most importantly, time to care for the dying patient, and therefore in 1978 I accepted the post of Nursing Officer Special Care.

Because the post was the first of its kind, there were few guidelines as to how it should progress and build up. I am lucky, having worked in this health district since 1960, as a ward sister and nursing officer surgery, and am therefore well known by most consultants and ward staff as well as by general practitioners. Much time was spent with these people discussing my role and also trying to convince them that I was not meant to take over but to complement their role. I do not normally 'nurse' as such, for that is left to the ward sister and her team who are the experts. The main thing that I can offer which they often cannot is **'time'**.

I spoke to community nurses who also tended to see me as a threat to their patient care. I hope that now, some three years later, they realize that this is not so, but that my role is only possible as an addition to theirs. This aspect of relationships requires constant attention. Social workers were also interested in this new post and I had many discussions with this group.

The Anglican, Roman Catholic and Free Church Chaplains were involved at the onset. Liaison is essential because the two jobs, while different, are interrelated. Whilst the chaplain's remit in this context is to care for the spiritual well-being of the dying, mine is to deal with the physical and emotional health of these patients and their families. The roles of the nurse and the chaplain may overlap, particularly when the objective is to give emotional support to the relatives of dying patients. Between them they must decide how this support can best be given and by whom. Being a Christian is a help to me, but this particular job could be done as efficiently by a non-Christian. Indeed, in our present multiracial and tolerant society, an evangelizing Christian attitude to the care of the dying may well prove counterproductive.

Patients are referred to me by the consultant and ward sister. Whilst in theory this is a nurse-to-nurse referral, I feel that the support of the consultant medical staff is very necessary because the treatment of the patient in hospital is his responsibility and he alone has prescription rights. If, therefore, I have his support, I am able to discuss all aspects of patient care with him and can often tell him of apparently unimportant details which may have repercussions on the state of mind of the patient. These 'details' can only be gleaned by offering to the patient and his family that very scarce resource—**time**.

Patients are also referred by their general practitioners. This form of referral was slow to develop:

in 1978–79 there were 2 GP referrals
in 1979–80 there were 5 GP referrals
in 1980–81 there were 12 GP referrals
in 1981–82 there were 20 GP referrals

Since the beginning in 1978 to the time of writing, there have been 557 referrals to the special care service from every department except psychiatric and maternity services. Geriatric patients have been referred since June 1980 and, at the request of an obstetrician, the service is about to expand further to include counselling of mothers following neonatal death. Most of our patients have suffered from cancer, but we have been involved with patients with multiple sclerosis, motoneuron disease and Hallervorden Spatz syndrome. We attend ward rounds with consultants to see specific patients and also see the consultants on a one-to-one basis.

When a patient is referred (usually by a telephone call), I go along and introduce myself to the patient by saying that I am a nursing officer with more time to spare than most nurses, to talk, listen and answer questions if I can. At this first visit, I make a practice of staying only 10–15 minutes and, on leaving, I tell the patient that I will visit again the next day unless they feel the need to talk before that, in which case I can be easily contacted by asking the ward staff to 'bleep' me at any time within the 24 hours. Although officially my working hours are from 8.30 a.m. to 5.00 p.m., there is an official on-call service which covers the needs of the terminally ill patients for 24 hours a day.

Once a patient is referred to me, I see him daily in hospital and weekly at home. As the disease progresses I see him more frequently. The 24-hour call system operates from the first visit onwards. My average case load is 15–20 patients, at least half of whom are likely to be in their own homes. A second part-time sister has been added to the service.

There are many aspects of patient care covered by the special care nurse. One of the most important is pain control, and this can only be achieved by the full co-operation of all the nursing and medical ward staff in hospital and district nurses and general practitioners in the community. Time spent with the patient, in unhurried communication, not necessarily by speech but observing all the time, is the best way to discover whether the analgesic prescribed is adequate for the prescribed time. Often a patient will not admit to pain if a nurse can spare only a few minutes and appears busy, and here I can give help to the ward team. I also have time to remember that while not all terminally ill patients have pain, other symptoms may be more distressing and time may be needed to identify them. The patient who uses the time to reveal previously unrecognized symptoms will be discussed with the ward and nursing staff. The suggestions for treatment developed in hospices and discussed in Chapters 5 and 7 can be used wherever the patient may be. The drug charts are written up by the ward doctor or by the general practitioner who is caring for the patient.

Anxiety is always present in a patient who is dying and can only be alleviated by giving time to the patient to express, however haltingly, his thoughts and fears. It may then be possible to analyse the reasons for the anxiety and obtain help for the patient or his family from an appropriate source. Many problems arise from anxiety, and again time is almost the main factor which eventually helps to build up a mutual trust relationship between the patient and the special care nurse.

Once that trust has been established, fears and anxieties gradually unveil themselves. These are usually manifold and range from the fear of death (which may not previously have been mentioned) to financial strain incurred by prolonged illness, fear for the future of loved ones to be left, and in many cases fears of whether they will be a 'trouble' to the family at home.

A patient is usually referred to the special care nurse when it is felt that active treatment is no longer able to save or prolong life and when the patient can no longer lead an active, independent life. At this time the special care nurse *must* spend time listening—talking only if required to do so. Often questions will be asked which require no answer. In this way, the relationship of trust may be formed and hope is offered.

Even though the patient is dying, it is of paramount importance to him to go on hoping, although the way such hopes are expressed will change. Periods of time at home may be arranged, requiring the full support of consultant, ward staff, general practitioners and community nurses. Also social workers, voluntary workers and the hospital chaplain (who will commend the patient to the parish priest or vicar where applicable) are involved in the organization of the patient's discharge, and the special care nurse becomes the liaison person or facilitator during this procedure. About 40 per cent of the patients referred so far have been discharged, and approximately the same percentage have finally died in their own homes.

Patients are always asked if they would like me to visit them at home, and, if the answer is 'yes' (which it usually is), then the general practitioner is contacted by the consultant and his permission sought for a home visit. I, in turn, discuss the patient, his treatment and care with the community nurse. When and if the patient is discharged and later re-admitted, my service is mainly one of counselling and liaison between home and hospital. There are various ways in which I can provide special nursing care. Patients may prefer their own china cup and saucer, their own pillow and even their own sheets. This is a novel idea in a general hospital, but it is not wrong to help a patient to die in comfort and dignity. In past years we have not had the time to think about it because we have so often expended all our energies on the patients who will live.

Patients require a confidante because quite often they are unwilling or unable to communicate with their loved ones. It is a time for honesty, and I endeavour to offer them integrity and trust as I listen to their problems. Although I always seek medical advice and accede to the wishes of the individual doctor, if questioned about diagnosis or prognosis I also try to be honest, for to tell lies destroys any trust between the patient and myself. The patient soon realizes that his body is getting weaker and his pain or vomiting more prolonged, therefore if he has been told anything other than the truth in answer to his question 'Am I going to die?', he has no one in whom to trust or confide and must face the reality and fear of death in total isolation.

After the first visit to the patient, I make an appointment to see the relatives because I feel that part of my remit is to provide a supportive service for relatives as well as patients. I rarely need to say more than that I can offer time and perhaps some answers to questions they inevitably want and need to ask. Usually I need only to listen to them because I am seen once more as a confidante. Friction between relatives, financial strain, fear of whether they will be able to support the patient, and the very real fear of whether they will be able to go on living after the patient has died all slowly unveil themselves and need to be discussed with them and reassurance given.

I spend many hours with relatives in my office or in their homes away from the ward situation, until eventually they appear to treat me as a friend as well as a nurse. In most cases, for both patient and relative this is the ultimate aim. There is no more rewarding phrase than to hear a patient or relative say 'We feel safe as long as we know that you are around and we can get you.' Emotional cost is high to the special care nurse and care must be given that the counsellor is counselled when necessary.

It would be impossible to carry out my job alone. All the caring professions have a major role to play, and during the three years that I have been in post this has become more and more clear. I have been given co-operation, guidance and support from staff in almost all disciplines and they have always been most helpful. Catering staff have taken trouble to satisfy the whims of my patients by producing special diets on request—on one occasion tripe and onions! Staff in the supplies department have ordered special pillows, back rests and sheets. Laundry staff produce, as if by magic, sheepskin rugs etc. Social workers have given their support, not only in providing equipment at home, but also by helping with rehousing and obtaining 'attendance allowances'; without this support we could not have made patients at home so comfortable and relaxed during the final weeks of life. The local branch of the National Society for Cancer Relief must also be praised for the ready help given financially to those patients in financial need. Consultant medical staff, many general practitioners, ward staff, community staff and hospital chaplains of all denominations have helped me to make this a valuable and co-ordinated service. They have also involved me in teaching. I speak to all learners in an introductory block and to second-year learners. I lecture to the Joint Board of Clinical Nursing Studies (JBCNS) course in care of the elderly and to the stoma course and have attended many seminars outside the hospital.

I feel that the most important thing is that we are proving that in a busy 1000-bedded district general hospital we can and do allow the patient to make his needs known and to die as most of us wish to live—in dignity and peace.

References

Ford, G.R. and Pincherle, G. (1978). Arrangements for terminal care in the N.H.S. (especially those for cancer patients). *Health Trends* **10**, 76.

Peabody F.W. (1987). *Journal of the American Medical Association* **88**, 877.

Yates, J. (1982) *Hospital Beds. A problem for diagnosis and management.* Redwood Burn Ltd, Trowbridge, Wiltshire.

13

Domiciliary hospice care

Harriet Copperman

'When all the world is old, lad,
And all the trees are brown;
And all the sport is stale, lad,
And all the wheels run down;
Creep home, and take your place there,
The spent and maimed among:
God grant you find one face there,
You loved when all was young.'
  (Charles Kingsley, 1863)

Introduction

'The house of every one is to him as his castle and fortress.'
  (Sir Edward Coke, 1552–1634)

This statement is well recognized by most people. Even if only briefly considered, it is easy to realize how distressing it is for many seriously ill and dying patients if they have to leave that 'castle' for the last weeks or days of life.

Acknowledgement of this distress has resulted in a spectacular growth in specialist domiciliary services for these patients and their families. Less than ten years ago, there were only two or three fledgling specialist services in this country. Today there are nearly 100, each having evolved to meet the special needs of a particular area. Many are based in a hospice or continuing care unit, some in a district general or teaching hospital, and a others run entirely within existing community services.

These services have two central aims: (1) to care for and support the patient and his family, so that, where appropriate, the patient may die peacefully at home; and (2) to share and disseminate expert knowledge gained in recent years about death and dying among professional colleagues, particularly the primary care team of general practitioners and community nurses. Sadly, these two basic aims may conflict with each other. The difficulty lies in ensuring that the teaching element does not in any way diminish the level of specialist care given to the patient and his family.

Many dying patients are, of course, well cared for by the existing primary care team and no additional help is required. But other patients may have more intractable problems and require more time spent with them than can be afforded by the primary care team, and in such circumstances, additional help from a specialist domiciliary hospice service may be appropriate.

The rapid increase of knowledge in so many fields of medicine has resulted in a corresponding rise in specialization: health districts may employ nurses who specialize in the care of dying patients, as well as those expert in stoma care, diabetes, or psychiatry. It is essential that community nursing staff are able to utilize all these new resources and not, as in some instances, feel threatened by them. This utilization can, in some areas, result in approximately 70 per cent of patients (mainly with carcinomatosis) dying comfortably at home—a reversal of national statistics.

Requirements

A domiciliary hospice team must be multidisciplinary, each discipline contributing its particular knowledge for the benefit of the individual patient. Communication with community colleagues may be facilitated if it is between the respective professions, doctor to doctor, nurse to nurse. Better patient care results where harmony exists within the team and nobody's professionalism is threatened. For example, if during a doctor's visit to a patient there is an obvious need for suppositories to be given to treat constipation, it would be absurd to ask a nurse to visit, which may mean 10-20 miles of travelling, when the doctor is perfectly well able to perform this service. It is also likely to enhance his relationship with his patient! Thus the team may include doctors, nurses (generally with community training), social workers, clergy, clerical staff and perhaps a physiotherapist, each having a flexible role. Help from committed and trained volunteers is also invaluable in augmenting the service.

A 24-hour service is essential and is usually shared between the doctors and nurses of the team. Some general practitioners are available by day or night for their dying patients, but more use a deputizing service. However well-meaning the deputizing doctor may be, his prescribing is likely to be inappropriate as he does not know the patient's history or current diagnosis, seeing only the presenting symptom of perhaps a troublesome cough or a pain in the abdomen. A member of the domiciliary hospice team, if called, would know the patient and his problem, or have access to his notes and therefore be able to respond more aptly to the situation.

Such a team is aware of the need for frequent reappraisal of the service it offers; research projects which will not cause inconvenience to the patient may be undertaken and in-service training to keep abreast of current trends is another priority. New members to the team will acquire many of their skills by 'apprenticeship'. The founders of such teams have usually served one or more years with an established hospice.

The area and size of population served will tend to vary—a rural team may cover many more miles with a smaller population than a team working in an inner city area.

Ease of access to equipment and medication is necessary. Most teams seem to 'acquire' a supply of commodes, urinals, backrests and bedpans, etc., so that if a local authority is unable to meet the need—say on a Friday afternoon—the equipment can be supplied. Anticipation of the need for equipment or medication is desirable but not always possible. As the patient deteriorates, numerous changes of medication may be necessary. Repeated visits to collect prescriptions from the chemist can be exhausting and worrying for a spouse and it may be difficult to find a chemist who keeps a stock of a particular medication. Thus many domiciliary hospice teams have organized a method of supplying some medication which would otherwise be difficult to obtain.

An expression which some teams use to describe themselves is that of 'gap fillers'. Where there may be difficulties in providing some aspect of care, be it medical, nursing or social, the team will attempt to meet that need, either directly, or indirectly through co-ordination and advice. The amount of direct care given varies according to the needs. If, for example, a nurse (or doctor!) visits and the patient has been incontinent, she will obviously deal with the immediate situation. It is, however, not practicable to be involved with daily care on a regular or long-term basis.

Assessing the needs

In hospital the assessment is centred on the patient. In the community there is much more to evaluate. The use of the senses provides the key. Before entering the home, sight, sound and touch (e.g. broken glass underfoot) will inform about the patient's environment. On the threshold the senses will again indicate the outward condition and impression of the home—whether it is well cared for or neglected and whether perhaps the neglect is long-term or recent due to illness. What sounds are heard before the door is opened? Is the person opening the door anxious, tired, suspicious, relieved, welcoming—or a combination of all of these?

Initial impressions of the home and mode of living of the patient are important. Sight may reveal an orderly or disorderly home, sounds may be pleasing or disturbing, touch and smell will also reveal much. How does the patient look, sound, feel and smell? Much information can be gathered before anything other than greetings and introductions have been exchanged.

The first visit may take an hour or more and is crucial to the subsequent relationship. The trust of the patient and family has to be earned; it is not an automatic right conferred as soon as the home is entered. For this trust to develop, an open and approachable manner is essential, so that patient and family feel able to discuss some of the questions and fears that may not have been voiced previously.

A great deal of information has to be gathered concerning medical, nursing and social needs, preferably during the first meeting. Many people are only too pleased to have yet another opportunity to parade their illness and problems before an attentive audience, others find this a tedious experience. It is therefore a courtesy to warn the patient that there are a number of questions to be asked, although much can be gleaned during the course of simply conversing with the patient. Without precise information there is no useful baseline against which future changes of condition can be measured. For example, if a patient says his bowel habits are 'ok', what exactly does this mean? He may in fact be too embarassed to admit he has a problem, though the professional can guess constipation is likely because of the patient's recent need for more analgesia. The degree of symptoms and problems, as described in Chapters 5, 7 and 10, are assessed. There are many symptoms such as sweating or headache (particularly if mild) which will not be mentioned by the patient unless he is asked directly about them. The patient's religious views should also be established accurately. Many people will say they are 'C of E' although they do not practise their religion, and offering to arrange a visit from a minister once a patient has become very ill and weak may be inappropriate and cause needless distress. Knowing the patient's previous occupation can also be important as it may be possible to claim industrial disease benefit for an illness such as asbestosis.

Note should be taken of all previous and current medication. This is usually an excellent opportunity to help the family empty their bathroom cabinet of medication accumulated over the years! It may also provide an opportunity to go into another room with another member of the family and perhaps be given additional information.

A limited physical examination is carried out, taking care not to tire the patient in the process. If done by a nurse, it will necessarily be less precise, but she should be able to palpate the abdomen to estimate whether it contains an enlarged liver, a palpable bladder, ascites or constipated faeces. A rectal examination is performed if there is doubt about the diagnosis of constipation or the cause for spurious diarrhoea. The condition of the pressure areas is assessed at the same time. A nurse should be able to estimate the likelihood of chest infection from a description of any cough or sputum and the sound of the breathing. The mouth is inspected for signs of monilial infection.

Subsequent visits

It is normally not possible to predict or establish a regular pattern of visiting. At the conclusion of one visit agreement can be reached about the timing of the next one according to the current condition of the patient and family. A vague 'I'll see you next week sometime' is discourteous and leaves the family with an unnecessary degree of anxiety. Generally, patients require fairly frequent contact, perhaps daily, while relationships are being established and symptoms and problems are being resolved. After that, there tends to be a plateau of weeks or months when the situation is relatively stable and the patient may only need a weekly visit, augmented by a telephone call. When he begins to decline, the visits will increase again—perhaps to two or three a week—becoming daily or even more frequent in the last few days.

The family

The attitude and circumstances of the family can make the difference between a patient having to be admitted to hospital or not. An effective domiciliary hospice team is able to preclude most admissions for medical or nursing reasons. Admission may become necessary, however, where a spouse is elderly, physically frail, or is unable or unwilling to give up work to care for the patient, or if there is inadequate support from other family members.

Much can be done to support or assist family members. This can begin even before the first introduction is made to the patient, when the spouse often says, before entering the patient's room, 'Don't tell him what he's got, it would kill him'. Being able to reassure the spouse calls for some 'fancy footwork' if the nurse is not to be manoeuvred into the position of having to lie to the patient. As a guest in that house, the professional can be refused entry. A family in hospital is less likely to be assertive.

Many relatives believe that they will not be able to cope because they fear the whole situation. Many fears can be dispelled quite easily, but sufficient time must be allowed for these fears to be expressed. The fading of the fears gives way to a new-found confidence and determination and the frequently used words, spoken with amazement, 'I don't know where I got the strength from. I didn't know I had it in me.'

A very basic fear is of death itself. Nowadays, people frequently have no personal experience of death until an elderly relative or friend dies, their knowledge having been previously restricted to the violence and drama of the television or cinema screen. There is often a belief, perhaps subconscious, that cancer, particularly of the bronchus, is something that is alive and growing and creeping slowly around the body. Thus if a patient develops a recurrent laryngeal nerve palsy, both he and the family may fear that he is slowly being strangled to death. Another belief is of the body bursting open and leaking everywhere when the patient dies—a simple explanation about relaxation of the sphincters will banish this fear. The 'death rattle' conjures up terrifying images—until it is explained that the patient is simply too weak to cough up secretions. Families may have witnessed a painful and distressing death of another relative many years earlier, before skills available today were developed. They may be afraid that they will not recognize death when it occurs, or of what to do when it has. Before the death there will be fears about ability to cope with both the practical and emotional problems, hence the need to offer the reassurance of a 24-hour service. Fear of suffering is common, particularly when the patient is peacefully unconscious. It is important for onlookers to realize that it is they and not the patient who are suffering, otherwise their bereavement will be haunted by a picture of unmitigated suffering and agony. Fear of the future filled with loneliness will often be tinged with guilt at having such thoughts while the loved one is still alive.

Feelings of inadequacy may be reduced by emphasizing that a loving relative, often a wife, is the best nurse a patient can have, and teaching simple nursing techniques will improve her confidence. It is vital to emphasize that there is no need to rush any manoeuvre, such as repositioning the patient, and that each move should be planned before it is made, to avoid unnecessary movement and fatigue for the patient.

Adequate rest and recreation for the care-givers must be ensured; a continuous stream of well-meaning visitors can add extra strain sometimes, almost turning the house into a cafeteria. Grown-up children may want to help but be restricted by the commitment to their own families, or may use that as an excuse to hide their fear of the situation.

It can on occasion be very difficult to decide whether or not a patient should be admitted. The family may feel they can no longer cope but the professional knows that the patient will soon die and recognizes that the relatives will be pleased if he does in fact die at home. Usually, though, the indications for admission are clear, but the family may then need much reassurance that the decision is right if they are not to feel guilty. It is very helpful to be able to reassure a spouse that the ward staff will allow him or her to help care for the patient.

Children

Children are an integral part of the family. If shielded from the situation, they will grow up believing that death is a totally terrifying event. This may have to be explained to some parents, who will then usually understand the children's needs. After the death, they should be allowed to cry and grieve with the adults and be given the opportunity to go, accompanied, to the bedroom to say 'goodbye to grandma'. If they do not wish to do so, this should not, of course, be forced. Similarly, children should have the opportunity of attending the funeral if they wish. School teachers should be informed of the home situation, so that allowances can be made for any deterioration in work or absenteeism, particularly if children are preparing for examinations.

Pain and symptom control

Sometimes a doctor or nurse will say that they encounter few problems with their dying patients. It is very easy, when busy and short of time, not to appreciate the extent of the problems that a patient or family mentions, perhaps tentatively, and just attend to the immediate need such as a breast dressing or a chest infection. However, most problems, once acknowledged, can be treated at home. One of the main essentials is the provision for frequent change of prescription—particularly towards the end of the illness.

Patients are often confused by the profusion and timing of medication prescribed. This may result either in them taking it haphazardly or else consigning it to that notorious bathroom cabinet. There are several ways of improving patient compliance. Aiming, where possible, to prescribe twice-daily medication can be most helpful and there are now many preparations available for that purpose. Although perhaps more expensive, their use may be justified by making medicine time more tolerable and acceptable to the patient. The use of 12-hourly slow-release morphine tablets has in many instances reduced or eliminated the need for four-hourly mixtures. The tablets are small and easy to swallow. Steroids are given as a daily dose of dexamethasone rather than divided doses of prednisolone. If an anti-inflammatory agent is required, benorylate suspension (Benoral), or diflunisal (Dolobid) may be given 12-hourly. Antibiotics, particularly tetracyclines, are available as once- or twice-daily preparations, notably doxycycline hydrochloride (Vibramycin) and tetracycline hydrochloride (Tetrabid).

Another method of improving patient compliance is by using a drug card (Fig. 13.1). This is prepared clearly and meticulously after ascertaining convenient times for the patient to start and finish his medication—to fit in with the household routine. If it is written out hurriedly and illegibly, it would be better not to write it at all, because it will not be understood. When complete it should be handed to the patient or whoever is giving the medication to ensure it is understood. If many changes are made in successive days or weeks, the card is re-written before it becomes illegible.

In order to prevent unnecessary and tiring visits to hospital or hospice, abdominal paracentesis is easily performed at home, using a peritoneal dialysis cannula, a receptacle for drainage (usually a bucket), a little local anaesthetic and a suture. There does not appear to be a need for slow decompression.

NAME *Mr. N. O. PAYNE*   DATE *4.12.83*

TIME	NAME OF MEDICATION	DESCRIPTION OF MEDICATION	DOSE
7 am	MST	Purple tablet for pain	1 tablet
	DEXAMETHASONE	White tablet for appetite	1 tablet
	MODURETIC	Diamond-shaped water tablet	1 tablet
	PHYLLOCONTIN	Pale yellow tablet for breathing	1 tablet
7 pm	MST		1 tablet
	PHYLLOCONTIN		1 tablet
	DORBANEX FORTE	Orange medicine for bowels	1-2 tea-spoons

Fig. 13.1   Drug card.

Infection should not be a problem either. Chest aspiration can likewise be carried out at home if the patient obtains relief from the procedure. A local hospital would probably lend the equipment. For a few patients, a fast intravenous infusion containing chemotherapy may also be given at home. It is amazing what can be found to use as an i.v. stand! The chemotherapy is prescribed and monitored by an oncologist. Intermittent compression pumps for lymphoedematous limbs can also be lent to patients for home use. Some of the more simple nerve-blocking procedures, not requiring a special table or screening facilities, may be carried out either by an 'ordinary' doctor, or an anaesthetist from a pain clinic, depending on the nature of the block.

When the patient is unconscious, an eight-hourly regime of medication by suppository can be employed. For example, oxycodone, prochlorperazine (Stemetil), chlorpromazine (Largactil) and diazepam (Valium) are available in this form. Four-hourly morphine sulphate suppositories may be used instead of oxycodone where a higher or lower dose of analgesia is required. Often relatives can be taught to give suppositories, but careful and detailed instruction must be given if they are not to feel nervous about doing this.

Nursing care

Frequently, most of the physical care of the patient can be managed by a spouse until the patient begins to lose consciousness and is unable to move himself. Great skill and sensitivity are needed by the nurse so that the patient is comfortable and the family satisfied. Many patients, unless very dyspnoeic, look and feel more comfortable nursed from side to side and supported by a number of pillows. The patient's skin, which is likely to be poorly nourished, may easily be scratched by the nurse's finger-nails, or wristwatch if worn. Washing a sick patient so that he is not left damp, chilly, soapy and tired is a great skill. Excessive noise and movement are disturbing for most patients.

Pressure sores should be prevented. It is most distressing for relatives to have to witness black and bleeding areas. This can usually be avoided by teaching the family how and when to turn the patient and by the judicious use of such aides as a large-cell ripple mattress, or gentle massage around a sore area.

Care of bowel and bladder should receive high priority. If a patient requires rectal medication when he is unconscious, it is essential that the bowel is emptied just before he is too ill to get onto the commode. This will also prevent the distress and inconvenience to the family of faecal incontinence in the last few days.

Urinary incontinence should be anticipated and a plastic draw-mackintosh inserted under a drawsheet, *before* the patient is incontinent and a mattress ruined. Catheterization should be performed for the last few days if incontinence is a problem, following discussion with the relatives. These and other needs must be anticipated if the patient is to be peaceful and comfortable and the family spared unnecessary distress and anguish.

As death approaches, it is usually necessary to spend an increasing amount of time with the relatives during a visit. An opportunity for discussion should always be given, either in the kitchen or on the doorstep, if the relative wants to be out of earshot of the patient. Enough information is given so that the family is prepared for the deterioration as it occurs. Too much information will frighten them as much as too little. It is often useful to gather the whole family into the living-room and give them the opportunity to ask any questions or make any comments about the approaching death. Families will often ask about prognosis, perhaps because of various commitments elsewhere, or the need to inform relatives away from home, about the situation. A prognosis should never be given as it can increase the anxiety—so often patients live a shorter or longer time than anticipated. It is necessary to be very sympathetic and understanding with the relatives at this point, perhaps advising them whether or not to cancel a holiday or contact a relative to come home urgently.

Following the death, the body should be straightened as appropriate and dentures inserted. The jaw can be supported by a small object such as a cigarette box or a new bar of soap. With the sheet just covering the chin, the deceased person will look peaceful and at rest and the relatives can then be invited to see him if they wish. If relatives wish to assist in performing these last actions, they should be allowed to do so.

Some families, unsure of the next step, appreciate it if the nurse informs the doctor of the death and makes the initial contact with the funeral director. (The doctor should have seen the patient within the previous two weeks.) If someone from the team can attend the funeral, this is much appreciated by the family. Bereavement visits may be undertaken, but if there are long-term problems, referral to a social worker or other counsellor is necessary.

Other professionals and services

A social worker may initially earn the trust of the family by practical help such as expediting the installation of a telephone or unravelling financial tangles. She can then deal with the emotional problems which may be present or looming. Generally her input is required where there are existing social problems, or the likelihood of them, for instance where a young patient is dying, leaving a single parent to care for the children. Health visitors may also undertake this role, particularly where the children are under 5 years old. Most group practices will have such workers, but if not, they should be contacted through the local social services or in the hospital previously attended.

Spiritual needs should be met as appropriate. Some families will require help and advice about religious practices and contacting the minister concerned. Others will have the situation under control.

Physiotherapy and recreational therapy can be vital sources of help to a patient, perhaps confined to the boredom of four walls and a window without a view. Helping a patient not to feel a useless burden on his family can change the whole atmosphere in the home.

The home-help service is often invaluable, and meals-on-wheels may be particularly useful for an elderly spouse not used to cooking for himself. The incontinent laundry service is of limited use, as the incontinence, if any, usually occurs in the last few days.

The Marie Curie Memorial Foundation's assistance in providing a night sitter service can make the difference between a patient remaining at home or being whisked semiconscious into hospital at the last minute. The latter situation is always very distressing for the patient and family, as well as for the hospital staff and other patients in the ward.

The National Society for Cancer Relief also plays an important role in supplying financial assistance to families with a low income. It will, for example, give grants for purchasing bed linen, installing a telephone or help with an outstanding bill. It may also pay a weekly allowance to be used as desired by the patient and family. Only a few patients with advanced malignancies are likely to fulfil the six months qualifying period for Attendance Allowance. The Department of Health and Social Security has discretionary powers to give supplementary benefits and to make grants in exceptional cases.

Thus many people may be involved in caring for a patient in order that he may die comfortably and contentedly at home, and that the family be left with some feeling of peace and newfound strength as well as their sadness. For the 'outsiders', a strong sense of privilege can be experienced at having helped a patient and family during such a special time.

References

Kingsley, C. (1889) *The Water Babies*, p. 80. Macmillan and Co., London and New York. (First edition 1863).
Coke, Sir Edward (1644) *Third Institute*, Ch. 73.

A comment: the general practitioner and the dying patient

M.J.F. Courtenay

The inception of the National Health Service in 1948 split the previously integrated pattern of medical care, separating the hospital from community care, and, by implication, making the hospital the 'centre of gravity', in spite of the fact that general practitioners still looked after more than 90 per cent of illness.

The rapid advances in medical technology which were applied in the hospital context reinforced this division, and encouraged the public to think that all good medicine was practised within the hospital walls. A collusive pattern arose in which patients and their relatives came to feel that only hospital treatment could provide what was best in medical care, while the doctors came to feel that anything which could not be cured was not their responsibility. General practitioners now felt that they were excluded from the hospital facilities, but were still expected to receive patients discharged from hospital, frequently without warning or discussion and often in a condition for which the community sources were inadequate.

The revolution in the control of infective conditions produced by antibiotics altered the relative prevalence of other conditions such as cardiovascular disease and malignant disease. As terminal care for malignant disease assumed a greater importance in terms of total medical care, it challenged the altered functions of the hospital; though these patients were not curable (and therefore considered 'unsuitable'), they and their relatives felt that they would receive only proper care if they remained in hospital. General practitioners were faced with a feeling that they were expected to send their patients to the appropriate consultants and receive them back only if those specialists failed to cure and therefore discharged the patient. As general practitioners were trained in hospital, they mostly shared the current medical opinion that proper medicine was hospital medicine, and felt doubly denigrated by being clerks in the first instance and nursemaids in the second. The concept of the caring personal doctor nearly perished.

The situation was not helped by the fact that the district nurses were not working closely with the general practitioners on a day-to-day basis, although ever willing to do everything to help patients. Ironically, in the light of one comment by a nurse who felt that 'many (doctors) seem unaware of the patients' distress and are unwilling to prescribe adequate analgesia until the last moment', other district nurses felt that general practitioners were too ready to give large doses of potent analgesics. The scene was set for someone to review the alleviation of pain in advanced malignant disease, and this came eventually from outside the National Health Service.

Whatever the future of special units for the care of advanced malignant disease, it is certain that proper analgesic regimens might never have evolved without them. The pain-relief protocol of St Christopher's Hospice (as developed from St Luke's Hospital and St Joseph's Hospice) is now available for 'education of the profession'. The literature available which lists the various drugs which may be useful has shown that the medication must be arranged so that symptoms, including pain, should be prevented rather than just treated when they occur (see Chapters 5 and 7).

This does present difficulties in treating the patient at home, since someone other than the doctor must be relied upon to administer the medication in the correct way while the doctor monitors the dose and the procedure. In case of sudden emergencies, the limits of the delegated responsibility must be sharply drawn, and the methods of calling assistance set out in detail. The home-nursing service is the key to this kind of management, though the responsible person may have to be the spouse or other close relative. Fortunately, nursing resources in the community are usually good and when the nurse has dealt with special problems, there are other ancillary services to call on, such as night attendants, who may allow the relatives to get adequate sleep or prevent an isolated patient remaining alone. Even so, the help of good neighbours is often essential to adequate care.

Apart from this pioneering educative role, special units will probably always be needed in the foreseeable future. The demand for acute beds in a hospital service starved of adequate resources and the inappropriateness of keeping certain patients at home will leave a gap which can be properly filled only by a special unit. For the general practitioner there must always be a back-up in case domiciliary care breaks down because either the patient or the relatives reach breaking point. Increasing anxiety often renders a plan of symptom relief ineffective—what will work in a special unit or hospital does not always work when the patient is constantly worried that he is not in a 'safe place'.

The general practitioner has an important role to play in the management of terminal malignant disease, but only if he has absorbed the necessary information and developed the necessary skills. These are gradually becoming more available, largely through the GP trainee schemes which have been established over recent years.

The first fact for the GP to realize is that the number of patients in an average practice likely to need such care is very small, so that although it may involve extra time for each case, the total workload is not greatly affected. The second fact is that, once the GP has divested himself of the feeling that the whole exercise is one of failure, this kind of care can be immensely rewarding. The perennial anxieties over what to tell the patient and how to handle the relatives' wishes or how to conduct the management wither away, provided the doctor can allow them to talk out their anxieties, and can assure them that the control of pain will be maintained one way or another, even though this may eventually mean admission to a hospital or a special unit.

The more professionals involved in the care of one patient, the greater the problems of day-to-day communications. While ideally one doctor should be in charge, and may arrange a special system whereby nurses and relatives can get in touch with him while otherwise off duty (and here doctor-initiated phone calls can be immensely useful), it is probably adequate if the care is shared with one partner, so that they can share the daily decisions about management. The extra work is more than repaid by what the patient can teach about the last voyage of discovery. To be with another person by turns frightened, angry, fighting and denying reality is a training process in itself. The doctor needs to identify with the patient, and then stand back professionally to seek the best way to meet his needs. Paradoxically, the certainty of losing the battle allows the GP the greatest possible freedom in being the patient's personal doctor. While exercising the highest skills in symptom control, he is involved with the twin dreads of separation from loved ones and the fear of death itself, which are in some degree common to us all.

The rate of deterioration itself is an important factor in deciding how the patient is best to be served.

The question of morality itself must inevitably be faced by every GP who enters this type of relationship. It is not necessarily a question of religious or philosophical belief; it is more the conscious realization of one's own feelings about dying. It is not so much answers that are required, but the need to remember Donne's words that 'no man is an island entire of itself'.

14

Care of children dying from malignant disease

Janet Goodall

'O, little body, do not die.
You hold the soul that talks to me
Altho' our conversation be
As wordless as the windy sky.'
    (John Betjeman, 1980)

I shall go to him but
he shall not return to me.
    (King David, 2 Samuel 12:23)

Introduction

The official figures for 1975 (HMSO, 1977) show that deaths from malignancy form a relatively small proportion of all childhood deaths. In that year, about 9500 children died before their first birthday in England and Wales: the majority of these deaths were perinatal, but many were from acute infection or congenital handicap. In contrast, in the same year, a little under 700 of all children under 14 years of age died from neoplasms, including all childhood cancer and leukaemia as well as a few benign tumours.

The majority of childhood deaths are sudden, following acute infection or accident (Table 14.1), and this could well be the major reason why terminal care for children has lagged behind that for their elders. Doctors and others involved in child care are used to doing all that they can to save life at times of acute crisis. The average paediatric team, trained to assist at child birth and to encourage child health, finds it hard to participate in a child's death. For general practitioners and community nurses, such an event is rare and so even more abhorrent. The whole atmosphere can be one of promise unfulfilled and

Table 14.1 Major causes of death in childhood and teenage, England and Wales (from Court, 1976)

	<1 year	1–4 years	5–9 years	10–14 years	15–19 years
	Perinatal	Respiratory infection	Accidents	Accidents	Accidents
	Congenital anomaly	Accidents	Malignancy	Malignancy	
	Respiratory infection	Congenital anomaly	Respiratory infection Congenital anomaly		
Male:Female	4:3	7:6	7:5	3:2	9:4

hopes dashed, and the natural drive is to fend off the end for as long as possible. The advances of technology mean that so much more can be done and it seems almost improper to ask whether it should be done for each child. Because for so many children the action has to be swift and intensive, we need to be reminded that for some the pace must become slower. Instead of battling it out on the high seas we are heading for harbour: most hands are still on deck, but the hope now is to give parents and child a period of calm together before the journey ends. Such a change of tack requires sensitive timing and skill in its accomplishment, but unless we can so adjust our outlook and our expectations to consider our treatment in this light, we could ourselves provoke shipwreck. Those involved in the care of dying children must therefore be very clear about the diagnosis and likely prognosis for each patient. They should also be experienced enough to judge when the time has come to stop efforts at restoration and aim instead for relief. If prolonging effort is merely prolonging dying, and no longer enhancing the life that is left, then we must be prepared to consider cessation of such efforts, whilst never ceasing to relieve distress. The amount of intervention possible may be affected by a shortage of time or of resources, but where endless resources allow an indefinite playing for time, we need to be all the clearer about our priorities.

Paediatric practice and philosophy

Much of what has been written about the terminal care of adults applies in principle to children dying from malignant disorder. However, it is outdated to regard children as being merely mini-adults, or paediatrics as a minor offshoot of medicine. Both the practice and philosophy of child care vary in significant ways. In such vital areas as physiology, biochemistry, clinical pharmacology and psychology, even the different age groups within childhood itself have different norms. The distribution of disease and the progress and prognosis of different illnesses also alter greatly with age, so that not only are causes of death very different, but disorders bearing the same name may have very different behaviour and outlook as age advances. Applied to malignancy, both the organs affected and the course of the disease processes show wide variation. Thus, cancer of lung or stomach is rare in childhood: nephroblastoma occurs proportionately more frequently in children and also has a better prognosis in very young infants (although advances in medicine are affecting this bias).

On a broader footing, those caring for children must pay more assiduous attention to the child's basic needs. Adult patients can speak for themselves, but a child's messages are not always received unless care-givers are tuned in. It is traditional to separate nursing from medical needs and for a patient's need for love, food, warmth and comfort to be considered separately from the need for either medication or surgery. Paediatricians tend to regard this distinction as artificial, for comfort may depend on carefully selected drugs as well as on clean sheets, and even parental love may need to be educated by professional understanding if a child's anxiety is to be properly relieved. Comfort includes being understood, and the paediatric team should therefore be prepared to consider the needs of the whole child, which must include knowing something of intellectual and emotional growth as well as the ability to diagnose physical disorder and to institute appropriate therapy.

The importance of the parents, or the child's natural parent figures, must never be forgotten as they are vital members of the team. Particularly at times of crisis, it is all too easy to push them out, but their involvement can be both beneficial to the child and instructive to other members of the team. Not only may they act as interpreters between a young child and the doctor, but their familiar presence can of itself be one of the best anxiolytics in paediatric practice. In order to fulfil this role, however, the parents themselves must be supported, knowing their own anxieties to be understood and, where possible, met.

This attitude of attention to the child's basic needs is fundamental to paediatric care, whether children are curable or incurable. The child and parents (or other family supporters) are considered together at the centre of the circle of care, whether activity is still being directed towards saving life or whether the time has now come to ease into mainly supportive management. The importance of this concept cannot be overstated, yet still hospital staff can sometimes behave as though the child is theirs and the parents are intruders.

Guidelines for paediatric terminal care

Set goals.
Uphold parents.
Assess the child's understanding.
List symptoms and plan treatment.
Function as a team.

Setting goals

Whether the illness is acute or chronic, we need to keep checking which way it is moving and what we are aiming at (Fig. 14.1). For all sick children, our obvious hope is to restore as nearly as possible to normal, and as long as bearable treatment is producing reasonable results, this attempt will continue. When it becomes clear that there is no longer hope of cure and that intense

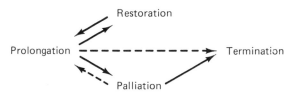

Fig. 14.1 Possible goals in the management of illness.

activity is merely prolonging suffering, it is important to avoid the trap of thinking that there is no more to be done. There will always be some symptoms left and our aim now is to relieve them. The change of direction into palliative care means that goals become immediate instead of very long term, although attempts to relieve symptoms will continue for the rest of the child's life. Occasionally, a child who is nearly dead from the onslaught of aggressive treatment has an unexpected lease of life when the focus is changed. In the management of malignancy, there will rarely be circumstances when it has to be decided to discontinue abruptly treatment which was life supporting. To switch off a ventilator is more likely to be necessary for an unresponsive neonate or accident victim than for a child dying from cancer. Such a mode of death should normally be considered inappropriate in malignancy (or in other inexorably advancing disorders of childhood). When this happens, it is usually because goals have not been appraised or altered. To lose a patient has been considered as a failure so that prolonged attempts at restoration have gone on, even when it is evident that the child is dying. The failure then is not the death itself, but that it was unseemly. We cannot save the lives of all our patients, but we can attend to a child's basic needs right through to the end. For many this should include consideration as to whether the last stages of illness could be catered for at home.

It is not always easy to know when to change direction, but this enhances rather than excuses the importance of vigilance. The sadness that we all feel at the thought of a child's death can lead us to rationalize our persistent efforts to avert it, but we must continually balance the rewards of treatment with the cost to be borne by the child in carrying it out. To embark on spinal surgery for metastatic vertebral collapse is likely to cause more distress than would the possible paresis. To treat septicaemia when the marrow is terminally aplastic may tie the child to an intravenous line in hospital and could also allow a more unpleasant death from haemorrhage a few days later. In such decisions, we are torn between giving up too soon and being aggressive for too long, between anger at being beaten and denial that the battle is being lost. To keep focus on the needs of the child, key members of the team must regularly review together what is the current aim of treatment, whether this aim is being met and, if not, whether it is the aim or the therapy which needs to change.

Upholding parents

Amongst other team members, the parents rank high. Their grief will be greatest for they are losing a part of themselves and may, at times, be distraught. Even so, they must never be given the sense of having been left out of all discussion and decision making, yet neither must they be given the added burden of feeling that vital decisions have been left to them. It is a natural reaction for those responsible for treatment to shrink from painful conversation with parents, but we must learn to respond rather than to react and to recognize them as people in pain who also need our help. As well as their child being our patient, the parents, too, need our care if they are to cope in their role as the child's chief supporters. At all stages of the illness, therefore, we must include, inform, prepare and stand by them.

The pattern of grief described in those facing death themselves (Ross 1970: Parkes, 1972) is also to be found in parents of dying children (and amongst the therapists as well), although it is probably better to consider the varied emotions as a cycle rather than a sequence (Fig. 14.2). This means that conversations with parents need to continue regularly throughout the illness. An apparent lack of co-operation during a time of denial may alter, even after a few hours, to the bargaining mood of 'If it's really the best thing for her, then we will agree to it'. Parents, too, are caught up in the moods likely to be there in other team members, swinging between false optimism and undue pessimism. Small changes in the child's condition, or alteration in treatment, or even the tension of waiting for a laboratory report, can cause a renewed whirl of emotion which might seem unjustified to junior medical and nursing staff for whom these things are part of the routine. It is the responsibility of senior staff to be aware of the atmosphere likely to be surrounding the child, and be ready to give time to earthing the tension. The involvement of a trained social worker can be invaluable, but there must also be considerable senior paediatric input for the sake of both parent and child.

Young and old children quickly sense disturbance in their parents: the less vocal the child, the more likely this awareness is to show itself as disturbed behaviour. Unless on the outlook for this, it would be all too easy to assume (and investigate) a physical explanation of the symptoms when a child's apathy, tearfulness, abdominal pain or sleep disturbance are all, in fact, on an emotional basis. Of course, grief cannot be completely dispelled, but parents can slowly be helped to come to terms with it and so to emanate a calmer feeling.

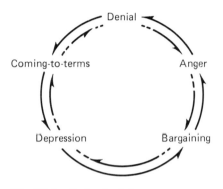

Fig. 14.2 Cycle of grief.

'Acceptance' is too final and optimistic a word to apply to actual or impending death, but many parents are enabled, in time, to take a steadier look at it and even help their child to do the same (Schiff, 1979). A potentially major obstacle about which it may be thought appropriate to warn parents is that each may move at a different pace through the grief process. Whereas not all people experience all of the cycle of possible emotions, it is an added sadness for partners to find that they are feeling and behaving differently at the very time when each might expect unprecedented support from the other. A father may steel himself against breaking down to the extent that his distraught wife feels that he does not care, either about the child or for her. Anger may break out between the parents themselves (as well as its being directed variously against the GP who missed the diagnosis, the consultant who made it, or the God who allowed it). It might be felt insensitive to draw for such parents a diagram of their likely behaviour reactions, yet it can still be a relief for them to be told that these emotions are normal. Encouraging a little forbearance with each other will go a long way to helping this added tension, but unrecognized or unexplained it could become a serious rift in the marriage.

Practical support can help to reduce other anxieties and funds are available to help patients with cancer.* Accommodation for parents to stay in is now standard in paediatric units and should be offered whatever the age of the dying child. If it is possible to conduct terminal care at home, good liaison between hospital and community teams should provide practical necessities such as bedpans, incontinence pads and sheepskin blankets, as well as close supervision of the child's dosage and continued availability of paediatric advice. Families must never feel abandoned to their own devices when a child goes home to die.

Not only should parents be included in the team and informed about their own reactions and the resources available to them, but they must also be prepared for the pattern that the illness is expected to follow. Many of them have never been so closely involved with death before and may be quite ignorant of what will happen before, at, or immediately after death. When invited to do so, different parents have expressed fears that the child's kidneys could break up and come away, that he might choke to death in his own blood, or that the body would start to decompose immediately after death. Unexpressed fears about such events may make them reluctant to take a child home, when an explanation of what can reasonably be expected, and assurance that they will always have help on hand, may encourage them to make the move. Unless warned, parents may also be unprepared for questions posed by the dying child or by their other children and may have little idea of the likely level of understanding to be expected of children of different ages. As this area can also be unknown territory to the child's professional attendants, it will be considered separately, but it is a most important area to be covered with parents. The pre-school child, unused to treating other adults as authorities, will naturally turn to a parent for answers to burning questions. A child old enough to sense that parents would find some questions intolerable is more likely to address them to the student nurse, the ward teacher, the ward maid, or (less often) to the paediatrician. It is therefore the child whom parents least suspect of having clear awareness of what is happening who may suddenly ask (as did a five-year-old) 'Am I going to die, mummy?'. Unprepared, the parent is utterly shocked and in response either speechless or dishonest. Children are implicitly trustful and it is important to keep their trust by tactful truthfulness, but many parents need to be forewarned if they are to achieve this. They also need to be sure to answer the question actually being asked. 'I wonder what you mean?' may be a wise beginning. To add further to their stress, parents may also have to deal with questions and criticisms from their own parents. In all this, they need to feel supported, and those caring for a dying child need to stand by the parents as well as the patient. We have to be ready to be the target for their varied emotions, to make repeated explanations and to anticipate events and possibilities. Bereavement counselling following the child's death will include attention to the needs of their other children, and thus act as preventive medicine. Thus, to uphold parents is not merely a humanitarian exercise, but a direct means of helping their children. Introduction to a parents' support group may, in time, be accepted and give long-term help.†

* The Malcolm Sargent Cancer Fund for Children, 6 Sydney Street, London SW3 6PP.
† The Society of Compassionate Friends, 5 Lower Clifton Hill, Bristol BS8 1BT.

Assessment of a child's understanding

This topic must perforce be dealt with sketchily here: the interested reader is referred elsewhere (Beard, 1969; Beadle, 1970; Pulaski, 1979), but some knowledge of this subject is essential if we are to meet the sick child or that child's siblings on a level appropriate to their needs. *A dying baby* is unlikely to register attempts at restoration in any other terms than being unpleasant attacks on the person, and this reaction is likely to hold until at least 2 years of age. Yet there is now good evidence to show that babies are born with a need for relationships and parents are the natural first comers for their establishment. A newborn infant chooses a face as the favoured object for regard even on the first day of life and, given contact with the mother, will indicate that she smells familiar to him, even by 5 days of age. Technologically minded professionals may think that because a child is so young, emotions and feelings can be discounted, but the converse is true: thought must be given to emotional needs, and the sensory pathways even of a dying baby should be fed by personal stimulation, which means parental involvement both during the period of active intervention and when the pace is slowing (Klaus and Kennell, 1976).

Up to 10 months of age a child has little conception that those out of sight are not also out of existence, so that the withdrawal of parents can be desolating. After this age, desolation can be even worse because it is recognized that they are alive, but have opted to be absent. In the infant's terms parental presence spells love (their touch and their voices and glances holding a different quality from even the most caring of professionals) and their absence spells loss of love (Bowlby, 1980).

Between 18 months and 3 years the child is slowly learning the thrill of power over the adult world. Still egocentric, he can recognize his own ability to cause pleasure or displeasure, but he interprets all parental reaction as being provoked by his own behaviour. The sequence of a heavy nose bleed, visiting the doctor and having more blood taken, followed by his mother bursting into tears and himself being sent to hospital, could be totally misinterpreted as his having caused so much mess that he is being sent out of the way. This misconception would only be relieved if his parents came to hospital, too, and showed that they still loved him.

Adults can also seriously misunderstood. Because a child screams and clings to her mother when threatened by separation, this is taken to mean that she will be uncontrollable and must be held down or sedated before any clinical procedures, when, in fact, the continued presence of the mother might have acted as the necessary reassurance. For a parent to go away leaving the child in strange surroundings for hours on end, may be to earn no recognition at all from the child on return. This does not indicate that she has 'settled down' to hospital life but that she was deeply wounded by the inexplicable abandonment and will, for a time, be mistrustful of parental overtures—sometimes to the point of active rejection. Conversely, a child may be abnormally gregarious with strangers in a pathetic attempt to hold on to the relationships that remain.

Up to 6 years or so the child continues to make face-value judgements and can regard injections and physical deterioration as being punishment for misdemeanours. Thus, a $3\frac{1}{2}$-year-old child thought that his operation was retribution for secretly tipping his small brother out of his perambulator, yet he could not articulate this reasoning for another three years. (After all, the grown-ups must have known about it as that was why they had gassed him and cut him.)

This age group, too, tends to think in very pragmatic terms about death. It is a familiar concept, playground wars and television films making their contribution: rural children often see death in the farmyard or in the fields. The implications of human death and its finality are not appreciated and it may even be thought of as a reversible process. The inner meaning of parables and proverbs is not understood, although because of the child's face-value approach, comparisons may be useful, such as likening death to a person's moving house or going on a journey. Concepts such as heaven may be bewildering because never experienced, although concepts to do with relationships may be better understood. 'Going to live with grandpa' or 'going to live with Jesus' can be comforting ideas if grandpa and Jesus are already recognized as comforters and have not until now been complete strangers. Even so, many children show a grasp of spiritual truths ahead of their intellectual age, and the simple faith of a child, either dying or bereaved, can be a great solace to grieving adults.

Between 6 and 10 years deductive reasoning develops, although two and two may be added up wrongly as double meanings are still not fully understood and the mental gymnastics needed to work out implications, or to engage in abstract thought, are still out of reach. Influenced by tele-viewing, therefore, a child may associate hospitals with inevitable surgery, so that his own admission promotes mounting anxiety, unrecognised and so unrelieved by medical staff—and, as he believes them to be in the know, the fear remains unexpressed. Experience accelerates understanding and a chronic illness may bring a conceptual maturity ahead of expectation. A leukaemic child will therefore quickly recognize that blood-test results can bring elation, gloom or another marrow aspiration: although repeating what adults say about bad and good cells, the concept of the disease itself may actually be very misty, even though its consequences are all too clear. If an acquaintance has died of the same disease, even a very young child, as well as older patients, may assume that death is inevitable. This age group should be told simple facts about the illness and its management, bearing in mind the likely limitation in abstract reasoning. Although adult minds shrink from approaching the topic of death because of its impact on them, talking to a young child about death is actually easier than approaching a teenager as its full implications are not feared so much as its possible discomfort and loneliness, and these can be assured of relief.

From 10 years onwards into adolescence the mind is slowly growing into adult stature, maturity again depending on intelligence and experience. At this age, the child may try to protect parents from the pain of discussion and should be given the opportunity to talk to someone else who is prepared to respond helpfully. The mother of a 12-year-old, dying at home, commented on long hours that he spent feigning sleep, following which he made oblique references to his coming death, comforting her with assurances that he would be in heaven and hopes that she would not then be losing weight and worrying about him. It needs to be remembered that the healthy brothers and sisters of a dying child are likely to have misconceptions and private fears which also need to be dealt with. Attention paid to the sick child may be seen entirely at face value and it is well for brothers and sisters to visit the hospital at treatment times as well as toy time! Parents may need prompting about when and how to share with their other children an impending death. These questions are easier to pose and to answer if the child is receiving terminal care at home (Cotton *et al.*, 1981). In his own way, a 15-year-old was able to tell his younger sisters, with a calmness which was itself reassuring, that he was going to leave them.

Listing symptoms and planning treatment

It is as well to remember at the onset that a child's symptoms can be due to physical or emotional discomfort, the latter sometimes provoked by spiritual searching or family and staff tension. In listing symptoms and planning appropriate treatment for each, the hidden areas of aetiology must always come up for consideration, particularly if symptoms persist after treatment (Fig. 14.3.).

Discomfort   Treatment
   vague symptoms
   pain   analgesics
   dyspnoea
   fever   antipyretics
   restlessness   anxiolytics

  ↑ ↓

Anxiety   communication
   general   diversion
   specific   watching
                    listening
                    talking

Fig. 14.3   Major problems and their treatment in terminal disease.

Common symptoms and their management

Symptoms

Discomfort of many kinds can make a child miserable, be it fever, headache, abdominal distension, dyspnoea or a vague general 'soreness'. Focal or referred pain is commonly from deposits in bone. We should first try to identify the causes of discomfort: thus treatment for constipation could relieve abdominal distension. If the cause is the incurable disease itself, analgesics should be given round the clock. *Nausea and vomiting* may be due to drugs, radiotherapy, disturbed biochemistry or diet as well as to the disease itself—and also to anxiety. The causes must all be considered before embarking on systematic antiemetics. *Anxiety* may present in various ways in childhood as with sleep or behaviour disturbances, abdominal pain or unaccountable tearfulness. It may be greatly relieved by bringing other symptoms under adequate control by round-the-clock medication. Anxiety can also be a reflection of other tensions, for which anxiolytics are but poor substitutes for diversion and discussion. In long drawn-out illnesses, *other symptoms*, such as muscle spasm, pressure sores and increasing isolation may also need attention.

Treatment

Drugs
There is a great need for the proper documentation of appropriate drugs and dosage for the control of symptoms in childhood disease. There are marked differences in the absorption, transportation and metabolism of drugs at different ages (possibly in different diseases), and young children may also react paradoxically both to standard sedatives and anxiolytics (Rylance, 1979). The suggestions here are therefore tentative: much more work is needed to substantiate them and we look hopefully to major centres for their findings (Rylance, 1980). Wherever possible, drugs are offered orally, intravenously into an existing infusion, or rectally, as intramuscular injections are themselves distressing to children.

1. *Analgesics* (Tables 14.2 and 14.3). Paracetamol and aspirin are both useful for mild and moderate discomfort or pain. Pethidine and methadone have little place except in the control of crisis pain: the first has a short action and the second accumulates. As it is important to demonstrate that discomfort can be controlled (for only so will anxiety be relieved), adequate round-the-clock dosage is a priority. Opiates may be needed to get symptoms under control but can often be replaced later (or a lower dose complemented) by paracetamol. The transforming effects of morphine can be dramatic, even when discomfort is due, for example, to intractable dyspnoea rather than to pain. We should not

Table 14.2 Analgesics for children

Symptoms	Drug	Presentation	Dosage
Mild or moderate pain	Paracetamol	Elixir: 120 mg per 5ml 500-mg tablets	Under 1 year: 25 mg per kg* 1 to 5 years: 240 mg 6 to 12 years: 250 or 500 mg
Mild or moderate pain	Acetylsalicylic acid	300 mg tablets (soluble)	1 to 6 years: 150 or 300 mg 7 to 12 years: 300 or 600 mg
Severe pain, 3- or 4-hourly	Papaveretum	10 or 20 mg per ml (by intramuscular, sueous or intravenous injection) 10-mg tablets (equivalent to 5 mg morphine by mouth)	2 weeks to 1 year: 0.2 mg per kg* 1 to 6 years: 2 to 5 mg 6 to 12 years: 5 or 10 mg Premedication: 0.6 mg per kg*
Severe pain, 4-hourly	Morphine	In syrup (not alcohol)	Over 2 years: 2, 4, 6 or 8 mg in 5 ml—older children may need 30 mg or more 4-hourly *NB*. Oral diamorphine is 1½ times as potent as oral morphine

* Per kg body weight.

Table 14.3 Dose adjustment when changing from oral morphine to injected diamorphine

Morphine (dosage in mg by mouth or per rectum)	Diamorphine (dosage in mg for intramuscular or subcutaneous injection)
5	2.5
10	5
20	7.5
30	10
45	15
60	20
90	30

be afraid to offer this drug to children, but bran or senna will be needed to counteract its constipating effect. Nausea from morphine rarely seems to be a paediatric problem and the euphoria produced may improve appetite.

2. *Antiemetics*. Vomiting is so common in normal children that its misery is not always taken seriously. As in adults (see page 104), phenothiazines, antihistamines or metoclopramide (Maxolon) may be useful. Unfortunately, chlorpromazine (Largactil), promazine hydrochloride (Stemetil) and metaclopramide can all cause oculogyric crises in childhood. Chlorpromazine seems to have the best record and its anxiolytic effect is also useful. Suggested starting dosages for chlorpromazine are:

orally: 0.5 mg/kg per dose 4–6-hourly,
rectally: 2 mg/kg per dose (up to an adult dose of 10–50 mg),
i.v.: up to 5 years not over 40 mg/day,
  5–12 years not over 75 mg/day.

If this causes drowsiness it may be be better to use domperidone as an antiemetic; appropriate dosage is still to be evaluated. The use of red towelling or tissues allays some of the anxiety provoked by haematemesis.

3. *Anxiolytics*. To relieve other symptoms is often to relieve anxiety. As some anxiolytic drugs have paradoxical effects on children, it is wise to give big doses of analgesics and small doses of anxiolytics as a first move. Chlorpromazine and morphine both have good effect on mood and may already be in use. Diazepam should be used cautiously, particularly for patients under 5 years of age, as it can cause agitation in susceptible children. If tolerated, the suggested dosage for children is:

all routes
up to 20 kg } 0.05–0.25 mg/kg per dose, 6–8-hourly,

over 7 years
all routes } 2–10 mg/dose 6–8-hourly.

4. *Other symptoms*. From the viewpoint of the bystander, some problems may seem small when considered against the enormity of the child's deterioration, but no distressing symptom is too minor to treat. The periodic review of symptoms with appropriate offers of treatment will do much to make the child's life as good as possible whilst it lasts (see Chapter 7, applying paediatric dosage; Insley and Wood, 1982; Kempe *et al.*, 1982). Muscle spasm may be helped by

diazepam or benztropine mesylate (Cogentin). When it is clear that the end is near, if the child is still in hospital, the need for intravenous therapy must be reviewed. Thirst is the main indicator for fluid, which can be given orally as iced lollies or jelly. The presence of an infusion may inhibit parents from holding a dying child and is so rarely needed that it should be removed.

5. *Relief of tension.* Diversion is important, both for preoccupation and as a means of communication. Play and painting are thus a serious part of treatment.

General diversion. A child in hospital can be included in the activities of the ward school or playroom, taking pleasure in watching other children, even if feeling too weak to participate personally. It is very demoralizing to be put on one side and left unstimulated, and all too often letters, gifts or messages slowly fade out as the child's state worsens (Herrmann, 1981). A side ward may give more privacy to the family if a child cannot go home, but given thought, any room can be kept colourful and interesting. Hints to the head teacher of the child's old school usually produce messages from old friends which are cheering.

Specific ideas for diversion will come from considering the five sensory pathways of touch, taste, smell, sound and sight: suggesting soft things to cuddle, fruit drops to suck, flowers to smell and tapes to listen to as well as collages, pictures and books to look at may all begin to fire the family's imagination for other ideas. A portable television is *not* enough.

Communication. A child may act out inner problems, either in play or through drawings, and it is important to make suitable provision for this. To give any insight or to be used as a lead into conversation, the child's messages must be received (Bluebond-Langner, 1980). Observers must watch, listen, interpret and be prepared to discuss. Pre-school children may be happier for such discussion to be mediated through parents, or at least relayed in their company. Older children may be offered private conversation with a nurse, doctor or clergyman and if this divulges something which parents ought to know, confidentiality must be honoured and the child's agreement obtained before sharing it with them. Children of all ages are usually responsive to offers of friendly help and relieved to have tension earthed. Adolescents may, however, be caught up in their own cycle of grief and need to feel that their counsellor is in no hurry and is also prepared to let them deny, denounce, despair—or develop—without preaching at them. To be given permission to express unpleasant feelings is in itself a relief. At this time, many teenagers begin to make spiritual searches: shyness on this topic may be relieved by a simple comment, 'Sometimes, being ill makes people wonder if there is a God'. If the topic is not taken up, it should not be forced, but, on the other hand, should not be ignored. To have seen a teenager's violent anger about his cancer transformed to serene Christian commitment is to be convinced of the need to attend to the health of the spirit despite the decline of the body—particularly as many families secretly go to faith-healers.

Functioning as a team

Those surrounding and supporting a child with malignancy may include family and friends, general practitioner, paediatrician, child psychiatrist, oncologist, radiotherapist, surgeon, ward sister and staff, social worker, teachers and workers for ecclesiastical, educational and paramedical services. Key people may be obvious to the professionals but the child and family can be utterly bemused. For the child, parents come first, probably followed by 'my nurse', or 'my doctor', both of whom are likely to be junior and so prone to an early disappearance. For the child's sake, therefore, parents must be seriously regarded as important members of the team and must be able to rely on communication being made with them regularly by other senior members: in hospital, usually the ward sister and consultant paediatrician, at home the general practitioner, community nurse and possibly also the consultant, or someone else skilled in terminal care. If parents relate better to a different team member, that person should be primed. In the hospital setting, information could get lost between so many people unless the team determines to meet regularly and discuss management. Parents will find it less intimidating to be given private sessions, but most other team members will find a voice over coffee together after the ward round. The less formal the meeting, the less muted the voices. Those working off the ward, such as child psychiatrist, chaplain or general practitioner may have vital contributions but will need due warning and may need to be contacted in some other way. Shared discussions can bring to light untreated symptoms, ineffective treatment, family problems requiring more exploration or support, as well as tensions amongst the staff themselves. The houseman who has for the first time experienced the anger of grief, either as the parents' target or in personal temper, may be relieved to find that this is normal. The student nurse may need permission to express sadness, even by tears. The concept that our support as a team is for each other, as well as for the child, is an important one to convey. As the child deteriorates, we need to help parents (and one another) to clarify the choices now open and whether or not the family would like to go home, even if initially 'for a trial run'.

Hospital, hospice or home?

To conduct a child's terminal care on a busy general ward is not easy, its only saving grace being when the child, family and staff are well known to each other and the team is genuinely prepared to change the direction of treatment. To transfer such a child to a strange hospice without maintaining contact with familiar people could be anxiety provoking. As many children with malignancy are likely to have been treated at regional centres away from their homes, to offer an undisturbed time at home before the end seems preferable, as long as treatment can satisfactorily be co-ordinated and the family supported (Martinson, 1978). If the regional centre has kept the local paediatric team involved during the period of active treatment, they, with the community team, could now take over. Even so, there is a real risk of families feeling abandoned and unsupported until the concept of proper terminal care has become generally practised. Until this happens, there may be a place for a hospice-trained team to be involved in a child's care at the regional centre and, on discharge from hospital, to offer a peripatetic domiciliary service, which then acts in integration with the peripheral services. Alternatively, a regional hospice could be a transit station (rather than becoming a terminus) for the establishment of symptom control after curative treatment has stopped. The first hospice for children in the UK, Helen House at Oxford, sees itself in this light, the expressed hope

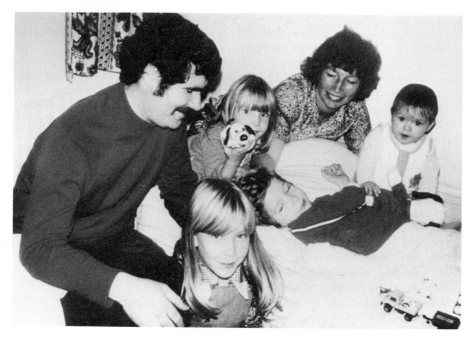

Fig. 14.4   'A brother dies at home.'

being that families will eventually feel supported enough to allow children to die at home (Fig. 14.4).

Ideally, the care provided by those attuned to terminal care in childhood should be available to all children who are dying, wherever they die. It is, after all, nothing more than the proper practice of paediatric medicine.

References

Beadle, M. (1970). *A Child's Mind*. Doubleday, New York.

Beard, R.M. (1969). *An outline of Piaget's Developmental Psychology*. Routledge & Kegan Paul, London.

Betjeman, J. (1980). A child ill. In *Collected Poems*, 4th edn, pp. 224–5. John Murray, London.

Bluebond-Langner, M. (1980). *The Private Worlds of Dying Children*. Princeton University Press, Princeton, NJ.

Bowlby, J. (1980). *Loss, Sadness and Depression*. Hogarth Press and Institute of Psychoanalysis, London.

Cotton, M., Cotton G. and Goodall J. (1981). A brother dies at home. *Journal of Maternal and Child Health* **6**, 288.

Court, S.D.M. (1976). *Fit for the Future*. HMSO, London.

Herrmann, N. (1981). *Go Out in Joy!* Kingsway, Eastbourne. (Reprinted 1981, Kingsway Publications, London.)

HMSO (1977). *Mortality Statistics in Childhood, England and Wales 1975*. HMSO, London.

Insley, J. and Wood, B. (Eds.) (1982). *A Paediatric Vade-Mecum*, 10th edn. Lloyd-Luke Medical, London.

Kempe, C.H., Silver, H.K. and O'Brien, D. (1982). *Current Paediatric Diagnosis and Treatment*, 7th edn. Lange, Los Altos.

Klaus, M.H. and Kennell, J. (1976). *Maternal–Infant Bonding*. C.V. Mosby, St Louis, Miss.

Martinson, I.M. (1978). Alternative environments for care of the dying child: hospice, hospital or home? In *The Child and Death*, pp. 83–91. Ed. by O.J.Z. Sahler. C.V. Mosby, St Louis, Miss.

Parkes, C.M. (1972). *Bereavement: Studies of Grief in Adult Life*. Tavistock and Pelican, London; International Universities Press, New York.

Pulaski, M.A.S. (1979). *Your Baby's Mind and How it Grows: Piaget's Theory for Parents*. Cassell, London.

Rylance, G. (1979). Prescribing in infancy and childhood. *British Journal of Hospital Medicine* **22**, 346.

Rylance, G. (1980). Drug level monitoring in paediatric practice. *Archives of Disease of Childhood* **55**, 89.

Ross, E.K. (1970). *On Death and Dying*. Tavistock, London.

Schiff, H.S.S. (1979). *The Bereaved Parent*. Souvenir Press, London.

15

Terminal care in the National Health Service

Gillian Ford CB*

'She saw that it was the whole world. . . .
Whatever she looked at, however far away it might be,
once she had fixed her eyes steadily on it, became quite
clear and close as if she were looking through a telescope.'
 (Lewis, 1956)

'Not only 1 per cent but one person is a relevant
statistic if it happens to be you or someone you love.'

Introduction

The terminal patient has been defined as one in whom, following accurate diagnosis, the advent of death is certain and not too far distant, and for whom treatment has changed from the curative to the palliative (Soukop and Calman, 1977). This chapter will cover the arrangements for looking after patients in the final stages of malignant disease, including the size of the problem, developments within the National Health Service, hospital services for cancer, hospice and other in-patient and community care for patients with terminal disease.

The size of the problem

The gradual elimination of early death from infectious diseases has thrown into prominence deaths from neoplastic disease. These now amount to about 120 000 each year in England and Wales—or one-fifth of all deaths. The age/sex breakdown of deaths from all causes and from cancer is shown in Table 15.1 and the rates in Table 15.2. Death rates from cancer, as from all causes, rise with age after 5 years. The tables show clearly that cancer deaths form a substantial proportion of early deaths (before 65 and this is most marked in women aged 25–64). The greater proportion of cancer deaths occur in hospital (Table 15.3). Deaths in NHS hospitals and at home account for almost 90 per cent of all cancer deaths—the remaining 10 per cent occurring in non-NHS hospitals or institutions or other accommodation, such as private residential homes. Over the last 15 years there has been a clear tendency for the proportion of deaths from cancer and from all causes occurring in hospital to increase, with a corresponding decrease in deaths at home.

*The views in this chapter are my own and do not necessarily commit the Department of Health and Social Security.

Table 15.1 Age/sex breakdown of deaths from all causes and from neoplastic disease in England and Wales, 1980

		All ages	0–4	5–14	15–24	25–44	45–64	65–74	75+
All deaths	M	29 869	5139	1063	3358	8913	65 746	91 188	113 462
	F	289 516	3946	722	1363	5632	38 614	64 087	175 202
Deaths from neoplastic disease (ICD nos. 140–239)	M	69 528	91	213	330	1799	19 637	26 462	20 996
	F	61 038	93	168	229	2444	17 346	18 109	22 649
Percentage deaths due to neoplastic disease	M	24	2	20	10	20	30	28	19
	F	21	2	23	17	43	45	28	13

Table 15.2 Death rates from all causes and from neoplastic disease per 100 000 population by age group and sex in England and Wales, 1980

		All ages	1–4*	5–14	15–24	25–44	45–64	65–74	75+
All causes	M	1 214	54	28	85	136	1 217	4 690	12 578
	F	1 146	47	20	36	88	683	2 462	9 201
Malignant neoplasm	M	289	6.0†	5.6	8.4	28	364	1 317	2 327
	F	242	4.2	4.6	6.1	38	307	696	1 189

* 1979 figures.
† 1979 figures for ICD 140–208.

Table 15.3 Total deaths and percentage of deaths occurring in non-psychiatric hospitals (NHS and other) and at home, in selected years between 1965 and 1979, England and Wales*

Year	All deaths (England and Wales)			All neoplastic disease		
	Total (1000s)	Non-psychiatric hospitals— NHS and other (%)	Home (%)	Total (1000s)	Non-psychiatric hospitals— NHS and other (%)	Home(%)
1965	549	50	38	107	60	37
1970	575	54	33	117	61.5	33
1974	585	56	31	123	64	31
1979	593	57	29	130	64	30

* For a fuller classification of place of death and breakdown by sex, see Table 14 of the Office of Population Censuses and Surveys' publication *Mortality Statistics, England and Wales, 1979*, Series DHI, No. 8.

This does not necessarily mean that cancer patients spend progressively less time being looked after in their own homes. Patients with malignant disease are spending shorter periods in hospital for episodes of treatment. Hospitals, whether private or public, clearly play a valuable part in the care of patients with terminal neoplastic disease, and in their deaths.

The development of the National Health Service

At its inception, the objectives of the NHS embodied the aims of the report (published in 1942) of the Planning Commission set up by the Royal Colleges, BMA and Scottish Medical Corporations in 1940. These were:

1. to provide a system of medical service directed towards the achievement of positive health, the prevention of disease and the relief of sickness;
2. to render available to every individual all necessary medical services, both general and specialist, and both domiciliary and institutional.

The ensuing debate and protracted negotiations in the 1940s centred on the methods of provision rather than the aims, and the latter have remained essentially unchanged for four decades.

The pattern of services provided in 1948 inevitably varied from place to place, not only because of the different level of capital investment in different parts of the country, but because perception of proper health functions varied between the local authorities who were then responsible for providing community and personal health and social services, some of which are now the responsibility of the District Health Authority. The 35 years which have passed since the original NHS Acts were put into effect have seen far-reaching changes in the distribution of facilities and their administration. Following the recommendations of Seebohm (1968), social work services were more sharply distinguished from health and became the responsibility of the local authority health department. The NHS Reorganisation Act of 1973 brought together hospital and community health services under one area health authority; these authorities were abolished in 1982 and their functions taken over by about 200 district health authorities in England and Wales. Bringing the health services under one authority had the important objective of reducing the gaps in care which could occur when one authority was responsible for hospitals and another for patient services in the community. Reorganization also made it easier to plan services for specific groups of patients who are extensive users of both hospital and community services, such as the elderly. The policy of providing services for the elderly in their own homes rather than admitting them to residential accommodation requires the efforts of both authorities. Providing services rather intensively for a period of weeks or perhaps months for the terminally ill patient at home also may need joint action by social and health personnel.

Regional health authorities (RHAs) plan and provide all the specialist hospital services and every region has at least one university hospital associated with a clinical medical school. These are foci for the development of the specialist work with a scientific and research basis and often act as centres of tertiary referral for patients whose treatment cannot be provided in the community or in the district general hospital.

Through the network of local services, including district general hospitals, the NHS provides, for most people during most of their lives, care and cure for illness 'events' either in hospital or at home. There are exceptions—for example, private medical treatment outside National Health Service hospitals is used by some patients and a number of charitably run homes supplement NHS or local authority accommodation for those who, because of age or disability, need a sheltered milieu.

Sometimes new developments in medical care are pioneered by university departments or other research institutes and these may bear a considerable treatment load before the NHS is able to take up the service commitments. Generally, such developments are absorbed as their value is recognized, but occasionally the 'non-NHS sector' makes a sustained contribution to care or treatment, or both. Terminal care is an important example. Of the 50 special units for those with terminal malignant disease open in 1980, 21 were administered by the NHS, and for a further 8 the NHS was the major provider of funds; smaller contributions were made to another 8 units (Lunt, 1980). A recent study (1983) of sources of revenue showed that 40-45 per cent of the 1700 beds available for terminal care in the UK are supported by the NHS. This total includes 104 beds in continuing care units in NHS hospitals but no beds in general wards are included. Apart from information furnished by the separate units which are devoted exclusively to care of the dying, there is little firm data on the nature and quantity of particular services for this group of patients. A Hospice Information Service based in St Christopher's aims to give help to individual enquirers and supplied the above information.

Hospital Services for cancer

A number of different medical specialists may be involved in the treatment of patients with cancer at some stage during the course of the disease—general physicians and surgeons, radiotherapists, oncologists and clinical pharmacologists. The central core of specialist medical services is the district general hospital, serving a population of the order of 100 000–250 000. Treatment for most types of cancer will begin within the district hospital where the general surgeon first sees and treats the patient, after referral from the general practitioner, and other specialists are brought in later if necessary. These specialties may or may not be present in the hospital to which the patient was first referred. Cancer services, such as radiotherapy, are provided at only a few specialist centres in each region. Concentration is economical of equipment and enables staff to sustain their skills, but one consequence is that patients may have to travel some distance if they are receiving regular radiotherapy as out-patients. This may be no more difficult than commuting to work in the Thames Regions but the patient who lives in Hereford and needs radiotherapy may have to go to Birmingham for it. The inconvenience of this has been partly eased in some places by building hostel-type accommodation so that patients can stay overnight without being admitted to a hospital bed. Treatment with cytotoxic drugs may be available in the same hospital as radiotherapy, but in only a few places are the cancer specialists grouped together in one department for the treatment of cancer. There is, however, an increasing trend towards co-ordination of the various specialties involved in cancer management.

In some hospitals, teams of specialists from different disciplines come together to plan the individual patient's management throughout the course of his or her illness. This approach is being developed in several NHS regions where some form of regional cancer organization (RCO) has been established. The provision of terminal care facilities, their integration with general cancer services, and the education of the profession in the particular problems of the patient with advanced cancer, are important elements in integrated cancer care. In Wessex Region, for example, a 25-bed continuing care unit has been built by the National Society for Cancer Relief in close association with the RHA and RCO, and two consultants who are responsible for the patient's continuity of care have been appointed; they are essential members of the cancer management team.

Some centres have been set up in the UK for the treatment of particular types of neoplasm, such as breast cancer (Guy's Hospital, London), choriocarcinoma (Charing Cross Hospital, London, and the Jessup Hospital for Women, Sheffield), and leukaemias (Hammersmith and Great Ormond Street hospitals, London). In the case of choriocarcinoma, as with most other rare types of malignant disease, it was clear that the results achieved by staff with experience were very much better than those achieved by staff who had little or no experience. The fact that only two units in England were necessary for the treatment of this rare condition will bring disruption to the family life of many of those needing treatment. The same problem may occur for others who suffer from rare conditions for which treatment facilities and expertise are concentrated in a few centres, but the chances of cure are better.

In-patient care for patients with terminal cancer

Diseases other than cancer may be responsible for distressing and disabling conditions prior to death, and by no means all patients dying from cancer require the prolonged pain relief and symptom control which are part of the specialist management of terminal disease. Nevertheless, it is commonly held by both the public and the professions that death from cancer is a prolonged affair, often painful and often accompanied by progressive physical deterioration. Many members of staff experience considerable difficulty in tackling the problems of pain, fear and grief common in these patients and their families. The special units for terminal care, which do not need to give preference to curative medicine, have cultivated the approach to death and dying which does not deny the fact of death, but sees that its attendant woes, whether of body, mind or spirit, receive attention.

General hospitals, including those which teach undergraduates, rarely have a section of the hospital set aside for patients who are terminally ill. This is generally deliberate policy to avoid part becoming known as a 'death ward'. What, then, are the arrangements for looking after such patients? In some hospitals the medical staff decide that each member remains responsible for his own patients from the time of initial treatment to the terminal stage, even if other disciplines are involved in clinical management during the intermediary stages. This often implies an undertaking to admit patients to the acute ward if symptoms or social conditions require it. Other hospitals may have the policy of admitting patients to the wards of the specialty providing treatment for that particular symptom or episode. Physical arrangements also differ. Side wards or single rooms, where they exist, may be used for very ill or dying cancer patients, but clinical practice and personal choice vary. Some patients do not like the additional physical isolation and the lack of distraction, and it places an additional burden both practical and emotional on the nurses. A small proportion of patients with cancer who are over 65 are treated in wards under the care of the geriatrician. Some GPs admit patients to small local hospitals near their homes. This may be necessary because constant nursing care or regular injections are needed, or because the family needs a break from caring for the patient, or simply because neither patient nor family wants death to occur at home.

The development of the hospice movement in the UK and the reasons behind it are discussed below. In 1983, 65 hospices in Great Britain provided 1560 beds, and numbers are still increasing. In addition to this total, there are also about another 120 beds in NHS hospitals.

Another development of recent years has been the institution of hospital symptom control teams. These consist generally of doctors and nurses and others who are expert in the control of pain and other symptoms which distress terminally ill patients and who are available for consultation. Much has also been achieved by nurses working on their own (see Chapter 12). The exact way of working varies from hospital to hospital: often advice and support only are given, but in some instances, if so requested, the team may take over clinical care of the patient. Such teams may be viewed with some suspicion in the early stages by colleagues who feel that some criticism of their own abilities is implied. Tact and a few successfully managed patients and some unexpectedly going home (Bates et al., 1981) soon dispel this, and they have become a well-accepted and highly valued part of the overall hospital services available for these patients. Their skills may sometimes be helpful in other, non-terminal patients. Also, in many hospitals an out-patient service is provided for patients who have been discharged from the hospital or who may be referred, directly, by their general practitioner.

Community services

In some instances, patients will reach hospitals because the community services have carried out screening services such as those of cervical cytology or chest x-rays, or because their general practitioners regard them as 'at risk' because of their age, family history or way of life, and are searching for early signs of malignant disease. Most commonly, however, patients are referred because of abnormal symptoms or signs. Later on, when the hospital treatment is complete, both the community services run by the health authority and those of the local authority may be involved in the continuing care of patients in their own homes with the object of sustaining both the patient and the family. Home helps are provided by the local authority to assist with the domestic care of patients. Volunteers from the Women's Voluntary Services (WVS), or perhaps the local church, may provide meals-on-wheels or just company, which is, in fact, often one of the most prized services. The social worker may have a difficult and 'ambiguous role' (Daniel, 1972), and while not providing direct health care may mobilize practical services, aids, money, and offer general support to the family. The NHS primary health care team consists of medical and district nursing staff, and health visitors and may be supplemented by Marie Curie Foundation nurses and other helpers and by home visits from occupational therapists and physiotherapists. This team is primarily responsible for dealing with all medical problems in the home.

There is increasing emphasis on community care for the dying and, if circumstances permit, this is often what the patient prefers. Some areas have special nurses to provide care for dying patients in their own homes, particularly in the evenings and at night when the ordinary district nurse is entitled to some leisure time. In other places similar services can be provided by charitable institutions such as the Marie Curie Memorial Foundation or the National Society for Cancer Relief. Many domiciliary care teams have also arisen from hospices which started as in-patient units. This is discussed in more detail below.

Changing patterns of care

The face of the NHS has changed as a result of the gradual development and improvement of services in the provinces, and through administrative changes. Many advances have changed medicine itself in a number of important respects: not only have the scope and range of therapy increased, but there has been consequential growth of team work in providing care and increasing fragmentation of medical specialities as the sum of knowledge is spread among many individuals.

Even the words 'medical care' now require definition. Provided by doctors? Not necessarily. Including curative and supportive elements? Probably, although care is sometimes used as the term for treatment which is not directed at cure. In recent years there has been general acceptance that 'care' provided by other health professions—nurses, physiotherapists, clinical psychologists— was complementary rather than subsidiary to that provided by doctors. The high standards of these professions, together with their own ethical codes and methods of enforcing them, place their members in the therapeutic team as a matter of right.

Most teams have a leader, and normally this will be the medical member, but increasingly the contribution to care of patients by the non-medical members has come to be recognized. Each member concentrates on what is naturally his or her sphere. Good nursing is not the appearance of order, but ensuring the well-being of the individual patient; this may mean the patient is out of bed learning to drive a wheelchair or walking, or anything else which retains independence, when the consultant comes to do his round. It also means that bedsores and constipation do not await the desultory attention which they might receive left to medical staff alone, but are tackled by nursing staff bent on their prevention. Even though medical treatment may at certain times not be appropriate, the skill of nursing staff and physiotherapist and attention from religious leaders and social workers will all help combat the multiple ills and sorrows that a cancer patient may experience.

Probably the growth of teamwork is even more important for patients ill with cancer who are still at home. Although the proportion of deaths occuring in hospitals is over 60 per cent of all cancer deaths, a substantial proportion of patients die in their own homes, while many more have spells at home before, or even during, the terminal stage. For them the services which can be provided at home are invaluable. Nurses, home helps, 'meals-on-wheels', general practitioner visits, may all be mobilized to provide care and support at home. Some other services are patchily available, such as a local authority laundry/incontinence service and night sitters.

The diversity of this community-based supporting team has its counterpart in the more purely medical skills concerned in treatment. Earlier, the different types of medical specialist concerned with cancer treatment and with terminal care were considered; any one of these may be the person responsible for the care of a particular patient at any one time—or possibly for the duration of his illness. The psychiatrist may also be involved, as may the anaesthetist, in providing special methods of pain relief.

The separation of different specialties within the main bodies of medicine and surgery has been an inevitable consequence of the development of medical knowledge and of different techniques, but effort is necessary to ensure that services a patient is receiving are not fragmented and unco-ordinated. Teamwork brings together people with necessary and complementary skills in the treatment of cancer, but it is possible that the patient feels that there is nobody in charge; this may become frightening if no more surgery is contemplated, a course of radiotherapy has just been completed, and the patient is at home with sundry unpleasant symptoms.

A common problem for hospital staffs, too, is that they do not know for certain who has been told what. Nursing and medical staff may be questioned and hope that their replies are appropriate for that particular question; the radiotherapist may be asked 'Did they take away all the ulcer?' The surgeon may be asked if plans can be made for a holiday. When the patient is at home, there is scope for the general practitioner to co-ordinate services, to explain again the rationale and side-effects of treatment, to prescribe for those symptoms with which the patient 'didn't like to bother the specialist'. Equally important, he can arrange for all the community services described earlier to be made available as required. It may be the GP who realizes that the patient is suffering from more pain than he is prepared to admit to during the course of a visit to out-patients: 'It wasn't my usual doctor and they were all so busy.' 'I know they've done their best and it seems ungrateful to complain that pain is still there even if it is in a different place.' Or, 'They told me at the hospital that they couldn't give me anything stronger.' Consultation on drug management between GP and hospital staff, or the exploration of the possibility of treatment by a nerve block, or referral to a hospital pain clinic, may then result.

In many ways, treatment provided for *any* patient is tailor-made for that individual, whatever his diagnosis. But the straightforward conditions are handled so easily by staff and patients alike that a real effort has to be made to sit down and think what to do for the patient whose problems will only be partly alleviated, if at all, by further treatment directed at the cause, who is likely to need underpinning by social and health workers, and whose family will need support and reassurance for an unpredictable length of time.

Home or hospital? Hospital or hospice?

The NHS combines community and specialist services in a unique way and it is likely that patients with cancer will get the best that these can offer. Bringing together the appropriate elements of both takes patience and perseverance, as a general practitioner well knows. Remaining as 'normal' as possible and staying at home are believed to be what most patients would prefer. Providing proper symptom control is achieved, and an intolerable burden is not put on relatives, domiciliary care is likely to be the 'best' solution, but if either of these breaks down, patients suffer and it may prove to be a 'worst' solution. Hospital specialist teams are not necessarily less good at providing care than the community team, but they do so within an institutional environment which is not home in spite of efforts to make it homely. Nevertheless, the rising proportion of deaths from cancer which now occur in hospitals and other institutions suggests that they are regarded as proper places in which to die, thus relieving families of some of the practical necessities associated with death.

Any precise policy laid down as to where terminal care should take place would be doomed to failure at the outset. It is not only a matter of the patient's medical condition, but the patient's own circumstances and preferences will also have a profound influence. Some staff feel that an acute general ward is not the ideal place to care for a dying patient because its pace and atmosphere are geared up to the acutely ill person. The regular drug round may be held up by an emergency admission so that a four-hour interval is stretched to six, and few people are prepared to discuss a patient's fears. Special arrangements, such as an evening at home, may seem trivial and burdensome to harrassed staff—and patients are often reluctant to bring their own needs to staff busy with other patients. Nevertheless, the patient may welcome returning to a ward with familiar faces and routine and, indeed, the majority of patients who die from cancer do so in ordinary wards in ordinary general hospitals, having spent varying amounts of time being actively treated in the same wards and without cause for any complaint.

It is obviously important that wherever a patient and his family decide is the right place for him to be, there are staff who are experienced in dealing with the problems and symptoms of terminal malignant disease. This was not often taught in British medical schools as a subject in its own right until latterly when the existence of special centres and public awareness and expectation have influenced traditional attitudes. It is being increasingly recognized that the surgical, radiotherapeutic or cytotoxic approaches are not the entire treatment, important though they are; nor is the patient the passive recipient—more an active partner. The difficulty lies in appreciating that handling the human approach to the patient, even after he has ceased to need the exercise of highly technical skills, is just as necessary as any other aspect of his treatment. This is not only to comply in a humanitarian way with patients' wishes to be treated as individuals, but also to lessen anxiety and tension (and perhaps, by so doing, diminish the need for, or the dose of, analgesics). Clearly, this art requires more than a theoretical exposition. The specialist units provide students with a short but valuable introduction. General practitioners have the opportunity through postgraduate medical education sessions to acquire the theory of terminal care, and some have studied the techniques at close range through courses organized in special units. Longer periods of study—the English National Board courses for nurses, residential or attachments schemes for doctors or students and other health workers—allow not only the principles of terminal care to be taught, but some chance of putting these principles into practice. Perhaps the most important part of such teaching is that a student should recognize that it does not require a purpose-built environment, or a profound knowledge of pharmacology, nor is it an art to which many cannot attain. With the acquisition of knowledge and experience comes confidence, and it is possible that general practitioners are now able to look after patients at home for longer periods and that this trend will continue. It would mean an extra load falling on the other domiciliary services—both health and social. The smaller families, more elderly population and working wives of today cannot manage death in the family without the help of others—be they trained personnel or neighbours. The medical and nursing professions recognize that the dying present problems which sometimes seem intractable. The future may perhaps see a build up of expertise at local level, a unit, a team, or perhaps a consultant with experience in the subject, whose skills could be drawn upon when the need arises.

Only comprehensive research on attitudes and expectation can reveal the extent to which the NHS meets the needs of cancer patients and their families during the terminal phase of their illness. Studies such as those of Cartwright *et al.* (1973), who looked at the lives and care of a random sample of adults who died, and Rees and Lutkins' (1967) comparisons of mortality and morbidity in bereavement after deaths at home and in hospital, and anecdotal evidence suggest that there are gaps which are most noticeable during the stages of illness when potentially curative therapy has ceased. Parkes and Parkes (1984) retrospective study of the relatives assessment of pain control indicates that patients suffered less distress and less pain in 1977-79 compared with 1967-69 and suggests that hospital staffs have learnt new skills. Hinton's encouraging comparative study of acute hospital wards, a Foundation Home and a hospice shows that good care is not confined to any one type of institution (Hinton, 1979).

The extent to which the special units have attracted local support suggests that they meet a perceived need, and the question must be asked, 'Is it right that hospices continue to develop through charitable and voluntary sources, and does this indicate that the NHS is not coping?' Trends in National Health

Table 15.4 Results of the survey into NHS funding of hospice beds in the UK—30 June 1983 (Hill and Oliver, 1984)

	Number of units in each category	Total number of beds per category	Number of beds funded by the NHS	Percentage NHS funding
Independent free standing units	37	775	268	34.5
NSCR units built on NHS grounds	11	265	265	100
Macmillan Mini Units	7	14	14	100
Continuing Care Wards in NHS hospitals	5	104	104	100
Sue Ryder Homes	6	108	17	15.7
Marie Curie Memorial Foundation	11	423	72	17
Total	77	1,689	740	43.8

Details of the numbers of independent free standing units receiving contributions from the NHS.

Contractual arrangements	14
Varying voluntary contributions	5
No contributions	18
Total	37

Service expenditure and in private and charitable expenditure suggest that this pattern of development will continue. In 1983 a study undertaken of sources of support (Hill and Oliver, 1984) showed that for the 37 free-standing units, 34.5 per cent of their expenditure was met from NHS sources, and that if the NSCR units within the NHS curtilage and continuing care wards in general hospitals were included, together with other hospices (Sue Ryder Homes and units supported by the Marie Curie Memorial Foundation), the total support from the NHS was 43.8 per cent. There is certainly an impression, despite many exceptions, that the NHS structure and the training and inclination of doctors and other health care professions favour systematic and technological aspects of patient care. This has left the initial development of some of those aspects of care relating to social, mental and spiritual well-being to people and agencies outside the NHS. But the essence of good care in terminal malignant illness, just as in other spheres of medicine, is in the attitude of the staff who provide it, and their readiness to search for and use better methods of practice wherever these have developed. The Royal Commission on the NHS concluded that, 'The most precious resource the NHS possesses is the people who work in it and for it, and the skill and application they bring to their work' (HMSO, 1976).

References

Bates, T., Hoy, A.M., Clarke, D.G. and Laird, P.P. (1981). The St Thomas' Hospital terminal care support team—a new concept of hospice care. *Lancet* **1**, 1201.

Cartwright, A., Hockey, L. and Anderson, J.L. (1973). *Life Before Death*. Routledge and Kegan Paul, London.

Daniel, M.P. (1972). *The Role of the Social Worker*. Paper presented at the National Symposium on Care of the Dying, held on 29 November, 1972. HMSO, London.

Hill, F. and Oliver, C. (1984). Hospice—the cost of inpatient care. *Health Trends* No 1, **16**, 11.

Hinton, J. (1979). Comparison of places and policies for terminal care. *Lancet* **1**, 29.

HMSO (1976). *The Task of the Commission*. HMSO, London.

Lewis, C.S. (1956). *The Last Battle*. Bodley Head, London.

Lunt, B.J. (1980). *Terminal Cancer Care: Specialist Services Available in Great Britain in 1980*. Wessex Regional Cancer Organisation, Southampton.

Parkes, C.M. and Parkes, J. (1984). 'Hospice' versus 'hospital' care: re-evaluation after ten years as seen by surviving spouses. *Postgraduate Medical Journal* **60**, 38.

Rees, D.W. and Lutkins, S.G. (1967). Mortality of bereavement. *British Medical Journal* **2**, 13.

Seebohm, F. (1968). *Report: Committee on Local Authority and Allied Personal Social Services*. HMSO, London.

Soukop, M. and Calman, K.C. (1977). Cancer patients: where do they die? An analysis. *Practitioner* **219**, 883.

Evolution in terminal care

Cicely Saunders

Modern 'hospice' or 'continuing' or 'terminal' care has long roots into the past. J. Englebert Dunphy, in a lecture on caring for the patient with cancer (1976), refers to his experience 30 years before in the wards of the Home of the Holy Ghost, Cambridge, Massachusetts (now Youville Hospital), and to the superb nursing care he found there. Worcester, in his lectures to medical students at Harvard in the 1930s, referred enthusiastically to the deaconess hospitals of Europe as well as to his own home care as a family practitioner (Worcester, 1935).

Those who are concerned with the management of terminal disease today (and not only with patients who are dying of cancer), can still learn from the experience of the past. Much of this experience has been in general or cancer hospitals, and many of the papers from which we have all been learning came from these sources, but since the end of the nineteenth century there have been special homes or hospices on both sides of the Atlantic, in Australia and elsewhere, deriving in their turn from the mediaeval resting places for travellers or pilgrims, the deaconess hospitals of Europe and from the work of the Irish Sisters of Charity in Ireland, Great Britain and Australia. Many of them are still active, continuing the work for which they were founded but gradually becoming involved with the new potentials in terminal care. (For example, The Hostel of God (now Trinity Hospice), St Luke's Hospital (now Hereford Lodge), St Joseph's Hospice and, from the 1950s, the Homes of the Marie Curie Memorial Foundation and others in the United Kingdom. In the United States of America, the Homes of the Hawthorne Dominicans, Youville Hospital, Boston (formerly Home of the Holy Ghost), Calvary Hospital and others.)

At the end of the 19th century, dying patients were often neglected or ostracized. It was seeing their desperation as they were banished to the almshouse on Welfare Island, New York, and to the Poor Law Institutions of London that impelled Rose Hawthorne and Dr Howard Barrett to begin their work at St Rose's Home and St Luke's Hospital. Hospices were needed because patients frequently had too *little* treatment, whereas today some of the 'hospice movement', especially in the United States, is stimulated by what is seen as too *much*, and often inappropriate, treatment. 'Medical headway has lengthened the average time which now elapses between the onset of a fatal illness and death. This is bringing in its wake exacerbated problems of chronic pain, fear, dependency loss of self-esteem, and progressive dehumanization for many persons' (Feifel, 1977). 'Physicians' failure to understand the nature of suffering can result in medical intervention that (though technically adequate) not only fails to relieve suffering but becomes a source of suffering itself' (Cassel, 1982). The hopes for success of some of the more recent treatments, even at a late stage of the disease, had made decisions concerning what is appropriate both more pressing and more difficult.

Surveys by the Marie Curie Memorial Foundation (1952) and Hinton (1963) revealed how much suffering was being endured by patients in their own homes and in general hospital wards. The trend for fewer deaths to take place at home isolated dying people from all that was familiar, often without offering them understanding or treatment appropriate to their special needs; many of those remaining at home also suffered intensely. Although the small number of special homes or hospices had much to offer, they were often prevented by lack of finance from having either adequate accommodation or staff (Glyn Hughes, 1960).

Work on the control of terminal pain in advanced cancer observed in St Luke's Hospital (founded 1893) from 1948 onwards was developed in St Joseph's Hospice (founded 1905) between 1958 and 1965 (Saunders, 1963). It was by then possible to exploit the therapeutic advances of the 1950s: new psychotropic drugs, synthetic steroids and the non-steroidal anti-inflammatory drugs, advances in cancer chemotherapy and palliative radiotherapy, the techniques of the new pain clinics and the greater knowledge of family responses to stress and bereavement.

When St Christopher's opened in 1967 as the first research and teaching hospice, it set out to begin laying the scientific foundations of terminal care (Symington and Carter, 1976) which could be interpreted in the home as well as in other settings and become a part of general medical, nursing and other teaching. It aimed to identify some of the common problems, to find some solutions and to spread this knowledge as widely as possible. Planned from the beginning, from 1969 onwards a domiciliary and out-patient service was based in St Christopher's with the support of the DHSS for a research and development project. By 1974, such a service had begun in New Haven, Connecticut, without any back-up beds of its own and with support from a Federal Research Grant, and showed how such a service could enable up to 70 per cent of patients to die in their own homes (Lack and Buckingham, 1978). In 1974, a separate ward on the lines of Horder Ward in the Royal Marsden Hospital (opened 1974) was established as a palliative care unit in the Royal Victoria Hospital, Montreal, with the addition of consulting and home-care teams and a full research and teaching programme. The unit had already completed a number of papers (Editorial, 1976; Melzack *et al*, 1976; Mount, 1976; Mount *et al.*, 1976) when, at a heavily over-subscribed conference on terminal care, Mount announced that the unit had ceased to be an experiment financed by the provincial government and would henceforth be an integral part of the hospital (Shephard, 1977). Since then, it has enlarged to a second unit and a home-care programme covering the whole city, and its leader is the first professor working exclusively in this field (Mount, 1980).

A small, multidisciplinary Hospice or 'symptom control team' began to operate in St Luke's Hospital, New York, in April 1975. This pioneer group had no beds of its own, but was called in by the physicians and their ward teams to see individual patients. The group was soon frequently consulted by the junior interns or housemen, with the encouragement of their seniors. The team's members worked alongside the ward staff, and their help in solving ward problems together led to their being accepted as a welcome resource. The team has been kept small and its case-load census has remained at about 40 patients (15 in-patients and 25 at home). One of the reasons for its speedy acceptance was the fact that several of its early patients benefited so much from the skilled control of their previous distress that, against all expectations, they were able to return home. A second reason was the ease with which the extra knowledge was incorporated into ward practice. This method of working has great potential for teaching and practice, and the first such team in the United Kingdom began operating on 1 January 1978 in St Thomas' Hospital in London. This team reported 225 referrals in 1982, with an average load of 12 patients in the hospital and 40 in the community. Both teams are led by consultant radio-therapists and/or oncologists and include part-time social workers and chaplains as well as their specialist nurses. St Luke's now has a full-time co-ordinator of volunteers. This is surely a most economical and direct way of tackling the problems of giving specialized care to a dying patient and his family in the wards of the general hospital and of sharing such experience day by day, and the present growth of such teams must be the most constructive way ahead for teaching and practice that will reach patients everywhere.

In the United Kingdom, the National Society for Cancer Relief frequently gave support to the independent homes and hospices. From 1975 onwards, this society then helped local groups to set up continuing care units of 25 beds built on National Health Service (NHS) land and then maintained as part of the NHS. Most of these are developed in close liaison with the local doctors and all have some form of domiciliary service. Some are much involved in graduate and undergraduate teaching. There is frequent interchange of staff and infor-mation between these units and those outside the NHS. There are other projects in the planning stage, developing both alongside and within the NHS, with a great escalation since the late 1970s (Hillier and Lunt, 1980). Some are staffed by part-time family doctors but the continuing care units and many others have appointed full-time medical directors. The society's present concentration has been on the provision of day centres (pioneered by St Luke's Nursing Home in Sheffield in 1976) and on teams and specialist nurses working mainly in the community. By June 1983, there were 70 such services with 177 nurses in post, some attached to units and others working independently.

Financial arrangements vary. Most of the units depend upon charitable sources for capital costs, but contractual arrangements with the district health authorities cover the cost of maintaining many of their beds, at a lower cost than most of the NHS beds these patients would otherwise have occupied. Each hospice has a number of 'free' beds and some have a very large financial gap to fill from gifts and donations. They normally have no private beds; money has never brought a patient into a hospice nor has the lack of it excluded those patients who need its care, but many families wish to give something towards the care that has been received. All these institutions owe a great debt to generous public support and could not exist without such local interest.

In spite of such voluntary enterprise and activity in setting up complementary local services, most patients who die of cancer will continue to do so in general wards, and much of our endeavour should be directed to developments which can be made there. Some of the essentials of good terminal management are more easily transferred than others—for example, the control of pain and of other symptoms can be practised anywhere. Other components may be more difficult to work for and must be included in whatever way is suited to local circumstances and available staff.

'A further advantage of the close involvement of hospices with the conven-tional services is that it has helped the hospice concept of care to become more widely known. The pioneers of the movement have never sought to retain a monopoly of their ideas. On the contrary, they have been keen to explain their philosophy and share their knowledge with those providing traditional forms of care. Like all good movements the impact of the hospice movement does not depend on bricks and mortar but on the interest its ideas generate and the changes in practical care which these have brought about.' (Young, 1981).

The DHSS Working Party (1980), many of whose recommendations were developed from hospice experience with patients and with their families, suggested that while there would be no advantage in promoting a large increase in hospices, yet they were needed to carry out research, educate and inform and as part of a local service for terminal care. It advised that their involvement should be integrated with the primary care sector and the hospital service.

Hedley Taylor (1983), in presenting a survey of the present situation, makes similar recommendations. Hospice units and teams are still needed, but today we must look beyond their special opportunities and experience to find their most important aim: that no dying patients, anywhere, should fail to find staff with sufficient awareness of their needs either to give help themselves or to call in others where they cannot do so.

References

Cassell, E. (1982). The nature of suffering and the goals of medicine. *New England Journal of Medicine* **306**, 639.

Dunphy, J.E. (1976). Annual discourse—on caring for the patient with cancer. *New England Journal of Medicine* **295**, 313.

Editorial (1976). Terminal care: towards an ideal. *Canadian Medical Association Journal* **115**, 97.

Feifel, H. (ed.) (1977). Death in contemporary America. In *New Meanings of Death*, p. 7. McGraw Hill, New York and Maidenhead.

Glyn Hughes, H.L. (1960). *Peace at the Last—A Survey of Terminal Care in the United Kingdom*. The Calouste Gulbenkian Foundation, London.

Hillier, R. and Lunt, B. (1981). Contemporary themes: terminal care: present services and future priorities. *British Medical Journal* **283**, 595.

Hinton, J. (1963). Mental and physical distress in the dying. *Quarterly Journal of Medicine* **32**, 1.

Lack, S. and Buckingham, R. (1978). *First American Hospice—Three Years of Home Care*. Connecticut Hospice, New Haven, Conn.

Marie Curie Memorial Foundation (1952). *Report on a National Survey Concerning Patients Nursed at Home*. Marie Curie Memorial Foundation. London.

Melzack, R., Ofiesh, J.G. and Mount, B.M. (1976). The Brompton Mixture: effects on pain in cancer patients. *Canadian Medical Association Journal* **115**, 125.

Mount, B.M. (1976). The problem of caring for the dying in a general hospital; the palliative care unit as a possible solution. *Canadian Medical Association Journal* **115**, 119.

Mount, B.M. (1980). Editorial. Hospice care. *Journal of the Royal Society of Medicine* **73**, 471.

Mount, B.M., Ajemian, I. and Scott, J.F. (1976). Use of the Brompton mixture in treating the chronic pain of malignant disease. *Canadian Medical Association Journal* **115**, 191.

Saunders, C.M. (1963). The treatment of intractable pain in terminal cancer. *Proceedings of the Royal Society of Medicine* **56**, 195.

Shephard, D. (1977). Principles and practice of palliative care. *Canadian Medical Association Journal* **116**, 522.

Symington, T. and Carter, R.L. (eds.) (1976). *Scientific Foundations of Oncology*, p. 673. Heinemann Medical, London.

Taylor, H. (1983). *The Hospice Movement in Britain: Its Role and Its Future*. Centre for Policy on Ageing, London.

Worcester, A. (1935). *The Care of the Aged, the Dying and the Dead*. Charles C Thomas; Springfield, Ill. (Reprinted 1977 under *The Literature of Death and Dying*. Arno Press, New York.)

Working Party Report on Terminal Care (1980). HMSO, London.

Young, G. (1981). Hospice and health care. In *Hospice, the Living Idea*, pp. 1–3. Ed. by C. Saunders, D. Summer and N. Teller. Edward Arnold, London.

16

Discerning the duties

G. R. Dunstan

Dying is a social activity, like being born. A report of someone being 'found dead' strikes a faint chill because (leaving aside occasions of foul play) it implies a being alone, unbefriended, neglected by the rest of us, in this last experience of life. Man is by nature social. As he is received, it is hoped, by welcoming hands at his coming into the world, so a hand—ministering, or friendly, or merely available—should attend his leaving of it. To discuss that attention in terms of duties detracts nothing from its humanity. 'Duty', like 'charity', has attracted the label 'cold'. The label is undeserved. To use the language of duty is but one means of knowing where we are, what we expect of one another, in a human relationship. Duty can be as warm as charity. It is useful to have it reasonably clear and understood as well.

Duty is mere debt: what we owe to one another. Some can give more, prompted by affection, human or divine—affection, that is, for the person or for God in Christ overflowing onto the person. But duty can stand without affection. Sometimes it is better so. Doctors and nurses are men and women; if every clinical relationship were compounded with affection, the strain would be more than most could bear. This is especially true in terminal care. Affection is proper to some human relationships; duty is proper to all. Duty is a formulation of apt responses to human claims.

The response is no less human for being dutiful. It is the more human as it is infused with the graces of an elevated, redeemed, humanity. Suppose that a patient is to be taken to hospital. In his sickness, in his helplessness perhaps and pain, he articulates a claim. The claim is met by an ambulance officer. His strict duty is to convey the patient to hospital with normal standards of care. If his personal response to the patient's claim is infused with courtesy, gentleness, a reassuring confidence and competence in knowing what to do and doing it, what to him is duty is to the patient more: it is a human relationship apt to his need, and he is comforted. They may never meet again. Yet something of eternal worth has passed between them, in terms of duty.

There are thus some elements in duty which can be prescribed; they can be stated as terms in a contract, explicit as between employer and employee, or implicit in an offer of professional service. These are duty's bare external features. Other elements cannot be prescribed; they can only be discerned. These lie at the heart of professional judgement. Where a discretion is allowed, where a choice is made or appropriate treatment decided, there the practitioner has to find or feel his way, within the terms of his general obligation.

He has general knowledge and experience to guide him—the accumulated wisdom of his profession, made his own by learning and by practice; he has a particular knowledge of his patient, his condition, circumstances, needs; he has colleagues to consult if he is in doubt; but his precise duty—what to do, advise or prescribe now—he can only discern, by a consideration of the empirical features in the light of his concept of the patient's interest or total good. As for the dispositions which grace the duty, those which the patient discerns and which, for the patient, lift the relationship above 'mere duty', these are hardly the practitioner's consciously to command; they become part of him as a result of a myriad choices and influences; they are his 'character', stamped upon him as by a seal upon cooling wax. They are beyond contract, beyond prescription; but they are real. Duty in its fullness is discerned.

The interests

The purpose of this chapter is to discuss the duties owed to the dying. First, however, we must expose the interests which the duties are to serve.

Dying matters to the patient. Rationally viewed, it will mean, when complete, an end to whatever suffering, pain, anxiety or undue dependency has troubled him in his illness. Considered, if at all, in terms of religion, dying may mean a passage to some new state: of waiting or expectancy it may be, or of purgatorial preparation or of enjoyment. What state is looked for depends upon the faith embraced. Few men with a religious conviction look upon death as the end. These are cerebral judgements, rational and religious. They possess some men in such a depth of their being as to create a great calm. Some, like Gerontius, they possess with awe, with a holy dread or with worse, before the calm (Newman, 1865):

'I am near to death ...
Pray for me, O my friends; a visitant
    Is knocking his dire summons at my door,
The like of whom, to scare me and to daunt,
    Has never, never, come to me before.

'Rouse thee, my fainting soul, and play the man;
    And through such waning span
Of life and thought as still has to be trod,
    Prepare to meet thy God.
And while the storm of that bewilderment
    Is for a season spent,
And, ere afresh the ruin on me fall,
    Use well the interval.'

Beneath are human feelings: in some, not far beneath; in many, dominating everything. At the level of feeling, dying means a severance with all that is familiar—relatives, friends, foes; a leaving of others with their mixture of griefs, regrets, freedoms, responsibilities.

Between life and death comes the process of dying. It holds many uncertainties. *Nihil certius morte, nihil incertius tempore mortis,** as men used to write when making their wills. Dying, viewed prospectively, is as uncertain in its manner

* Nothing is more certain than death, nothing less certain than the time of its coming.

as in its time. Rationally, men know that, given appropriate medical and nursing care, pain can be controlled. They know also that that quality of care is not yet available everywhere, and that death can still be painful. Judgement is further warped by talk of 'dying in agony', which used to attach to some illnesses inevitably, and which is still put about by the unthinking and by campaigners for euthanasia. It lingers in the mind. Men know, too, that if dying is protracted, there will be long dependency on others, whether at home or in hospital. Such knowledge, with its associations, brings emotion into play alongside reason. Reason and emotion may strive for the mastery; sometimes one may prevail, sometimes the other.

Instinctively man, as a biological organism, clings to life. Reason and emotion, locked in their own contention, may sometimes ally with instinct to preserve life; may sometimes, singly or together, go against instinct and prompt the ending of it.

Dying matters to the patient, therefore, principally because it puts him at the mercy of contending forces: between certainty and uncertainties; between human claims and obligations; between reason, emotion and instinct. The interest of the patient, therefore, is in the sort of terminal care which will enable him to reconcile and to override, so far as he may, that contention. This implies a wider care than one which concentrates only on the treatment of his medical condition or on the relief of its symptoms, important as both of these are. Duty begins with a recognition of the complex human interests, and with a gathering of resources to meet it.

Others beside the patient have interests. His immediate family and friends may be tied to him with the closest bonds of affection. They may need him, depend on him, emotionally, intellectually, physically, economically. His death may spell to them sheer loss. They may bear gladly the burden of his dependency, protracted though it may be; or they may grow weary under it, crave for relief, for freedom for other relationships and activities. His death, when it comes, may bring this freedom, and, perhaps, financial gain. Like the patient, therefore, they may be at the centre of a conflict. Their interest, then, is in such help and support as will enable them to come out of that conflict with integrity unimpaired and with human relationships undamaged or, if broken, reconciled.

Doctors and nurses have interests, involved with those of the patient and his kin. They have an interest in the advancement of their professional skills: their own personal fulfilment is involved in this in their awareness of work done as well as it can be done. They have an interest, not only in the integrity of their medical procedures and professional relationships, but also in an assured reputation for that integrity. When someone may benefit substantially from the patient's dying—or from his not dying at a particular time—his medical attendants must be free from all imputation of collusion. If public confidence in their integrity is weakened, the innocent will inevitably be suspected with the guilty, and vexatious litigation, and insurance against its cost, will grow.

Here are some of the interests to be served in terminal care. The related duties have to be discerned.

The duties

Of doctor and nurse

The terminal stage of an illness may be designated in terms of the patient's condition; it would describe the period when, with no prospect of remedy or remission, the only foreseeable course for the illness is towards the death of the patient. That designation would be matched in terms of the medical care offered; terminal care would be directed, not towards the cure of the fatal condition, but towards the care of the person dying. This would be to serve his interest in achieving a good death when it is no longer possible to serve his interest in living a healthy life.

This distinction is crucial for the appropriate management of the patient. Surgical intervention may be called for in terminal care for symptomatic control, for the alleviation of distress caused by the progress of the disease. But if such intervention went beyond this necessity and purpose, it would not serve the patient's interest in dying; it would be an imposition which might have been justified in the preterminal stage, when remedial action was a possibility, but it could be inappropriate now. Similarly, the decision whether to administer an antibiotic drug to combat infection would turn upon its purpose. If the purpose were to relieve a distress related to the malignancy, and if its action were specific to that end, then its administration would be appropriate. But if its purpose were to combat a supervening infection (of the lungs, for instance) which, if left untreated, might result in an earlier and easier release for the patient than that to be expected from his primary malignant condition, then its administration could frustrate the patient's interest in his dying. The duty is discretionary, dependent wholly upon the physician's clinical judgement of the patient's condition and upon his sense of timing.

It is sometimes argued that there is no moral difference between withholding a remedy which would prolong life and taking active steps to terminate it, between 'allowing to die' and killing—whether from a compassionate motive or not is beside the point (Glover, 1977). The argument does not carry conviction, certainly among practitioners actively caring for the dying, or among moral theologians (Mahoney, 1976). The critical questions concern the patient's interest and his corresponding right—that is, his claim upon professional duty. The interest of the terminal patient is in dying. The corresponding duty is to serve that interest, to assuage and support him in his dying. ('Allowing to die' is clearly an inadequate and pejorative mis-statement of this course of action.) The withholding of the remedy is not therefore a negligent act (and to that extent culpable) but a deliberate one, chosen because it is matched to the patient's condition and interest (and to that extent without fault). The patient's right to die (which would be infringed by inappropriate intervention to prolong life) may not properly be translated into a right to be killed, nor into a duty upon someone to kill him. Any act directly intended to terminate life would be culpable, in respect of the patient because it would infringe his interests both in life and in dying, and in respect of the practitioner—be he doctor or nurse— because it would infringe his basic professional principle as a servant of life. It would infringe also the right of the public to be able to trust him and his profession wholly as such. He is not authorized to kill.

Confusion surrounds the middle course also, between management without intervention on the one hand and an action intended to kill the patient on the other. This course arises when it becomes necessary to administer analgesic drugs in such quantity that they may predispose to a pulmonary infection from which the patient might die. Advocates of euthanasia claim a moral equivalence of this action with the deliberate administration of a lethal dose; they do so in order to advance the proposition that 'doctors kill already', that the public expects them to, and that it were both more honest and more safe to give them a statutory licence to kill in defined conditions.

This argument is fallacious. It is in the patient's interest to have his pain relieved, and it is the doctor's duty to relieve it by appropriate means—those effective for the purpose, with the minimum of harmful side-effect. If the side-effect can be remedied by means consistent with the patient's general interest in dying, then there is a duty to use those means. In the case under discussion, the analgesic drug is effective for its purpose. Control of pain may result in an improved general condition and spirits, and so prolong the patient's life. It may, however, predispose to a pneumonia which may shorten it. This would be a secondary effect, foreseeable as a possibility indeed, but not directly intended (and not avoidable) in the administration of the drug specific for the control of pain. Fault would not attend the giving of that drug, in law or in morals, no less drastic remedy being available. The intention is the control of pain, and this is the primary effect. A secondary effect, not intended, unavoidably accompanies the first. Moralists, on this account, are wont to cite the principle of 'double effect' in justification of the action; but the normal medical terms of 'appropriate management' are adequate to describe it (Percival, 1803; Duncan et al., 1981).

The withdrawal of intensive care may be considered in the same context. Switching off a respirator is not 'killing the patient', as it is sometimes said to be. 'Life-support systems' are more properly 'function- or organ-support systems'. They are used to support vital functions, either temporarily during surgical operations or temporarily after collapse in order to give time for spontaneous recovery of function, or for medical intervention to be organized, or to enable a clinical judgement to be made, whether spontaneous functioning will ever be resumed, or can be restarted, or not. To remove the support by switching off the apparatus is to give effect to a judgement that what is supported is not 'life' in the sense of an organic human activity controlled from the critical point of the central nervous system, the brain stem, but the functioning of organs, heart and lungs, already incapable of functioning by themselves because no longer in receipt of the appropriate stimuli from the brain. Their cessation, necessary (in the United Kingdom at least) for a clinical diagnosis of death to be made, is in truth the result of the cessation of internal stimuli, not of the withdrawal of external, artificial support.

The propriety of such action can stand on the basis of normally accepted medical ethics. If ecclesiastical warrant for it is required, it may be found in an address of Pope Pius XII to a congress of anaesthetists in 1957, in which he stated when it is permitted, and when it is a positive duty, to withdraw the apparatus of intensive care. He placed such procedures in the category of 'extraordinary means' which, in contrast to 'ordinary means' of care, a patient is under no obligation to request nor a doctor to administer (Pius XII, 1957;

C10, 1965; Duncan *et al.*, 1981). The argument, as before, can stand independently of the language in which it is expressed.

If, as has been said, the doctor's concern is with a person dying, and not only with a malignant disease, his duties will extend to the context of medical care as well as to the choice of care given. He may be faced with the question whether to tell a patient of his prognosis, his imminent death, or not. Clearly, he should not lie, if only for the pragmatic reason that lying erodes our common interest in truth and so undermines trust; and trust is too precious, too essential, in professional relationships to be so put in jeopardy. May he, then, by whatever prudent and diplomatic means, withhold the truth?

To answer this question we return to the basis of our argument: the doctor's duty is to serve the patient's interest in his dying. Within that interest are possibly conflicting considerations. The patient has an interest, certainly, in being spared unnecessary pain, shock and anxiety; this could be served by a prudent withholding of the truth about his condition. But he may have other interests which require him to know: his affairs to set in order, his worldly goods to dispose of or assign, his debts to pay; some obligations to fulfil; some persons from whom to seek forgiveness, some perhaps to forgive, some with whom to seek reconciliation; and himself to prepare, it may be, for a new awareness of the presence of God. On grounds such as these he has an interest in knowing the truth of his condition (Edmund Davies, 1973), of being helped into the truth (Mahoney, 1976). The conflicting interests in his nearest relatives may be similar. The doctor, therefore, has to discern his duty whether to communicate the truth or not to, and if so, how. Only personal and moral insight, gained from experience and matured in his own person, can help him to decide. He may well be spared the necessity of a decision if he can help the patient to face and articulate what the patient already knows.

With the doctor in terminal care are the nurses and other ancillary staff. They stand nearer the patient than does the doctor; they attend him for a longer time, more closely and more intimately. They may, therefore, from closer observation, contribute more knowledge of the patient (if not of the disease) than the doctor can attain. The doctor has a duty to respect that knowledge, to invite its communication, to be receptive to it; the knowledge ought to influence his decisions on apt or appropriate care. This same nearness to the patient can give rise to greater emotional attachment than the doctor has to experience; it should not be disregarded.

Of the patient's kin

If dying is the social event which we have envisaged it to be, the relatives and near kin are involved with the patient in his dying. The main points of their involvement have been touched on already; so has the ambivalence of feeling to which that involvement can give rise.

There is a sense in which those relatives attending the patient put themselves under medical tutelage, if not direction, in order that medical and family care can be concerted in the patient's interest. Yet there remains wide scope for initiative, for calm, imaginative energy, in the giving of appropriate support to the patient and his medical attendants. The quality of the interaction within the family group may affect profoundly the patient's well-being, and, therefore, the provision of medical care for him. The doctor may not subordinate his patient's interest to those of the relatives; but only a very shortsighted practitioner would act as though the relatives, with their own needs and feelings, were irrelevant to his patient's management. He has to take account of them for his patient's good. This mutual expectation, this reciprocity of duty, between the doctor on the one side and the patient-community on the other, needs more exploration than it is commonly given. Medical ethics are too often discussed in terms of the doctor's duties, what he may or may not do; that there are corresponding duties on the other side is generally forgotten.

Of the patient

The patient is in no condition to be lectured on ethics—his station and its duties. What he has not learned already, in the education of life, it is too late for him to learn formally in his dying. Yet there are other ways to discernment than instruction. In the long tradition of spiritual writing *de bono mortis*,* and of exhortation, *Disce mori*,† there is assumed a duty to make a good death, to be active in the management of it, not merely passive—a patient and nothing more.

The way to this he learns, discerns, in his interaction with the medical and nursing staff, his relatives and, if any, his priest. It would seem to lie in the right balance, if it can be found, of the active with the passive roles: knowing when to submit, certainly, and how to co-operate; but knowing also how to use the liberty given (when it is given) by relief from pain to attend to those inner recesses of being to which medical and nursing care may not penetrate.

An initiative is called for if personal obligations are to be met, affairs to be put in order, forgiveness to be sought and given, reconciliation to be effected. The initiative may cost effort, even pain. But the good relationship which is part of good terminal care may enable it. Death will come inevitably; a good death can only be achieved.

Of the priest

Every man is, in a sense, another man's priest, though the office is usually called that of the neighbour. It is to share the common human burden of mortality. It comes to one now; help him. It will come to you one day; you will welcome help.

There is also a special priesthood, derived from religion, from the common human faith in a relationship which transcends the human and is fulfilled in a divine being. This priest stands on the Godward side of man. He is a mediator of the things of God to man, and of the aspiration of man to God. He must act vicariously sometimes, saying and doing on behalf of men what he knows or must charitably suppose they would want to do and say for themselves. This office is called prayer, in its diverse forms. But, more than this, he is an enabler: he is to enable men to articulate themselves to God, to be themselves before God and so to offer themselves to God. This is his function, his profession, with

* On the good of death.
† Learn to die.

the living, from childhood to old age. The supreme test of his art is in his ministry to the dying, his contribution to terminal care (Hopkins, 1880).

He is one of a community of care—those whom in this chapter we have seen seeking to discern their duties. He must find his place, and hold it, in this community, this team. He must learn to respect the physical, with all its demands, restraints and limitations: 'first that which is natural, afterward that which is spiritual', St Paul wrote, in a related context (1 Corinthians 15:46). Yet he betrays his office if he forgets his primary commitment to the spiritual, if he sees for himself no role other than those discharged by the social worker, or psychotherapist, or voluntary hospital visitor. His unique place is 'on the Godward side', his unique care τὰ πρὸς τον Θεόν* the things pertaining to God (Hebrews 5:1).

This care extends beyond the patient to the whole attending community. Always his must be an available priesthood (Dominian, 1970); always on offer; never withdrawn; never grudged or brooded over because not always accepted. This is expected of him, even by those who ignore or reject his ministry. And as he is accessible to others, so he must have access to a counsellor of his own. He cannot care properly for the souls of others without care for his own; that care he is under duty to seek.

This is the office of priesthood. It has been written out of some understanding of Christian priesthood, just as the duties discerned, and the relationships, the forgivenesses and the reconciliations to be sought, derive from the Christian view of man and his calling. No apology is made for this; a man can write only of what he knows. If what has been written matches the need of men of other faiths, or of none, that is well. What is given is only what has been freely received. Were there no match, that would be sad. But the quest is open. Others may discern duties of their own.

Felix Randal

Felix Randal the farrier, O he is dead then? my duty all ended,
Who have watched his mould of man, big-boned and hardy-handsome
Pining, pining, till time when reason rambled in it and some
Fatal four disorders, fleshed there, all contended?

Sickness broke him. Impatient he cursed at first, but mended
Being anointed and all; though a heavenlier heart began some
Months earlier, since I had our sweet reprieve and ransom
Tendered to him. Ah well, God rest him all road ever he offended!

This seeing the sick endears them to us, us too it endears.
My tongue had taught thee comfort, touch had quenched thy tears,
Thy tears that touched my heart, child, Felix, poor Felix Randal;

---

* ta pros ton Theon.

How far from then forethought of, all thy more boisterous years,
When thou at the random grim forge, powerful amidst peers,
Didst fettle for the great grey drayhorse his bright and battering sandal!

Poems of Gerard Manley Hopkins

Third Edition, Geoffrey Cumberlege, Oxford University Press, London, New York, Toronto 1948.

References

CIO (1965). *Decisions about Life and Death.* Church Information Office, London.
Dominian, J. (1970). An available priesthood. In *The Sacred Ministry*, pp. 108–110. Ed. by G. R. Dunstan. SPCK, London.
Duncan, A.S., Dunstan, G.R. and Welbourn, R.B. (1981). *A Dictionary of Medical Ethics.* Darton, Longman & Todd, London, and Crossroad; New York.
Edmund-Davies, Lord E. (1973). The patient's right to know the truth. *Proceedings of the Royal Society of Medicine* **66**, 553.
Glover, J. (1977). *Causing Death and Saving Lives.* Pelican, London.
Hopkins, G.M. (1880). *Felix Randal.* See also *Times Literary Supplement* 19 March 1971, 331.
Mahoney, J. (1976). *The Way* (April) **16** (No. 2), 124.
Newman, J.H. (1865). *The Dream of Gerontius.* Set to music by Elgar in 1900.
Percival, T. (1803). *Medical Ethics*, IV, vi. Ed. by C.D. Leake. Williams & Wilkins, Baltimore.
Pius XII, Pope (1957). *Acta Apostolicae Sedis*, 1027. French translation in (1966) *Ethics in Medical Progress.* Ed. by G.E.W. Wolstenholme and M. O'Connor, J. & E. Churchill, London.

17

The law relating to the treatment of the terminally ill

Ian McC. Kennedy

That a book on the management of terminal disease should include a chapter written by a lawyer may seem odd. Surely, the argument goes, treating the terminally ill is a medical matter, properly and uniquely within the expertise of the doctor. The answer is that the law has something to say in this area just as in most other areas of activity. Doctors may resent what they see as the intrusion of law. Many have a stereotype of law as a body of irritating rules, insensitive and often irrelevant to their daily practice. This view is, however, ill-advised. In all areas of medical care, and the treatment of the terminally ill is a particularly obvious example, decisions are made and conduct engaged in which are based not on scientific but on normative principles. The very word 'management' in a medical context connotes a choice among alternatives—for example, whether to discontinue the administration of pain-killing drugs at the request of a determined but possibly confused patient. Such a decision is fundamentally a philosophical and moral one, for which the doctor, though he may have had greater exposure to it, has no greater training or expertise than the layman. Being so, the decision should be made in the light of principles deemed appropriate by society as a whole. Thus the doctor must observe not only the rules of his science and his profession but also those of society. Laws are one form of society's rules. They differ from, for example, morals or ethics in that they have the distinctive quality of being thought sufficiently important to be backed by sanctions for non-observance. They set standards for the regulation of conduct which purport to reflect a general popular consensus.

It is one thing to say that in the abstract the doctor must operate within the law; it is another to particularize that law. One of the greatest difficulties which confronts the medicolegal commentator in dealing with the treatment of the terminally ill is that techniques and technology have developed and changed with such rapidity in the past decade or so that it is only *vaguely* that the *problems* are perceived, let alone responded to, by developing a general consensus in the form of law. Some general legal rules do exist, but they assume a set of medical realities long overtaken by events. The sudden realization by the courts that respirators and cardiac pacemakers had made a legal definition of death based upon the absence of breathing and heart beat outmoded is a good example. Further, whatever legal rules do exist, deal largely with the conventional medicolegal issues of acute and emergency treatment and with malpractice. These rules are by and large irrelevant in dealing with the terminally ill patient who is, in a sense, in a special class. Such a patient is by definition going to die sooner rather than later, and the regimen of care adopted, overshadowed as it is by the mass of available technology, calls for distinct and very sensitive regulation. This regulation must take account of and seek to resolve one particularly intractable problem which bedevils all medicolegal discussions and is highlighted in the care of the terminally ill: the tension between the paternalism of the doctor and society and the right to self-determination of the patient. Traditionally, the law has been too ready to adopt as right whatever the doctor decides. Since the doctor's view can hardly be called objective and since the decision is philosophical rather than scientific in nature, legal rules must be developed which strike the appropriate balance between the two, according to the general popular consensus. Of course, doctors resent this attitude. It smacks of distrust. They would say they are good doctors who always act in the patient's best interests. But society and the patient need to provide for the eventuality that the doctor is not a good doctor (and these do exist) and what is in the patient's best interests is not always necessarily best answered by the doctor.

Moreover, not only have legal rules failed to develop, but the concepts which provide the stuff of legal rules are equally ill-equipped to respond adequately. For example, a legal system which sees the contact of a doctor with his patient as an assault or battery made lawful by consent, and rests so much on the notion of informed consent without showing any real understanding of the dynamics of the patient–doctor relationship, is in danger of losing respect.

In the light of the foregoing, I treat with some trepidation the invitation to spell out what exactly are the legal rules governing the treatment of the terminally ill. However, I will endeavour to do so in a series of propositions with explanatory additions where appropriate (Kennedy, 1976 and 1977).

1. A patient who is conscious and refuses further treatment of an aggressive or invasive nature must have his wish respected, whatever his condition, provided he is mature and lucid enough to make such a decision. This applies as much to the terminally ill as any other. The patient may not be abandoned, but the care given must change from treating for living to treating for dying. If the doctor thinks the patient is not sufficiently lucid or mature, then the decision should be ignored.

This stems from the proposition that any treatment which is administered without consent is unlawful. To abide by the refusal may be difficult for the doctor, but is required by law, the principle of self-determination overruling any notion that 'the doctor knows best'. In the unlikely event that a patient in a hospital refused even nursing care, for example bathing or changing sheets, different considerations would apply. The hospital's duty to maintain hygiene and protect the health of other patients would entitle the hospital to demand acceptance of such care as a condition for remaining in the hospital. Continued refusal would justify discharging those patients fit enough to be moved and with somewhere to go, and forcing the others to submit. This does not extend to feeding a patient against his will, which I regard as a form of aggressive treatment. Clearly, the crux of this proposition is whether the patient is lucid, that is, understands the nature and implications of the decision and is competent to make it. The final arbiter of this is, of course, the doctor. The decision is made harder by the knowledge that almost all terminally ill patients are receiving medication and may be suffering pain and distress, all of which could affect their mental competence, quite apart from some doctors' reluctance to 'give up'. Ultimately, the good faith of the doctor must guide his actions since complaints after the event by patients or relatives may founder for lack of proof. Putting the patient's request in writing may guarantee that his wishes are respected and protect doctors from later complaint.

2. When a patient is near death, a doctor is not obliged to embark upon or continue heroic treatment which has no prospect of benefiting the patient.

An alternative, more common, term than 'heroic' is extraordinary. It was Pope Pius XII (1957) who first advanced the view that doctors were not obliged to give, nor patients to accept, 'extraordinary medical measures'. The term has consistently been interpreted as meaning 'whatever here and now is very costly or very unusual or very painful or very difficult or very dangerous, or if the good effects that can be expected from its use are not proportionate to the difficulty and inconvenience that are entailed.' (Church Assembly Board, 1965). In the 1976 Stevens' Lecture, the Archbishop of Canterbury (1977) expressed his support for this as a moral principle. I take the view that it is also the legal principle. Indeed, I would go so far as to say that a doctor who continued treatment past this point would be behaving at least unethically if not unlawfully.

It is important to understand that it is never treatment in the abstract which can be described as extraordinary, but only treatment in the context of the particular patient being cared for (Dunstan, 1981). It is the particular patient's care which matters. The real question is whether, in the circumstances, it would be wrong to continue further intervention. This is often referred to as a consideration of the patient's future quality of life. Once this is understood, it is clear that terms such as extraordinary treatment, or quality of life, only state the problem. What still have to be worked out are the criteria which would justify not intervening aggressively, or (to put it another way) would amount to a quality of life which was not worth having. There is strong support for the idea that excessive pain, expense and hardship, together with no hope of benefit may serve as the starting points—though, obviously, words such as excessive need further careful explanation. Thus, the term extraordinary treatment is a conclusion rather than a starting point for analysis. As Dr Gillon argues, 'once the actual criteria of decision are specified, the misleading labels "ordinary means" and "extraordinary means" become superfluous.' (Gillon, 1981). I agree with Dr Gillon that it would be more helpful to use the terms 'ethically indicated' and 'ethically not indicated' instead of ordinary and extraordinary.

3. A doctor's obligation, in treating the terminally ill, is to make the patient comfortable, which includes easing his pain. If, to ease pain, the doctor must take measures which may hasten death, this is permissible, provided the doctor's principal and primary aim is only the relief of pain.

This reflects the so-called double effect theory and was incorporated into English law in one of the few decided cases in this area, R v Bodkin Adams (1957).

4. If the patient is competent, no one else may make decisions for him. Relatives should, of course, be involved but have no right to decide about treatment. If the patient is incompetent, only his parent(s) or legal guardian, but no one else, can speak for him. In so doing, they may only act in the best interest of the patient.

Incompetent patients are the unconscious, the mentally unfit, and immature minors. The test for what is in their best interests refers to general societal values rather than the views of the particular relatives. Thus, for example, the refusal by a parent or guardian, on the patient's behalf, of certain treatment need not necessarily be respected, if it may be in the patient's interests to treat him in this way. Equally, a doctor need not respect a parent's or legal guardian's demand that treatment be continued or altered if in his view it is pointless and the treatment would be categorized as ethically not indicated. This is because the law accepts that it may not always be in the best interests of the patient to receive further invasive or aggressive treatment.

Support for these propositions may be found in the judgment in the case of *In Re B* (a minor), (1981). The Court of Appeal had to decide whether to authorize surgery on a week-old child born with Down's syndrome and duodenal atresia. The child's parents took the view that surgery would be wrong and wanted the child to be allowed to die. Mr Justice Ewbank endorsed this view. But, on appeal the same day, Lord Justice Templeman, speaking for the Court, held that, 'the Judge erred because he was influenced by the views of the parents, instead of deciding what was in the best interests of the child.' Earlier in his decision, however, he had posed the question, 'was the child's life going to be so demonstrably awful that it should be condemned to die; or was the kind of life so imponderable that it would be wrong to condemn her to die?'. The implication would seem to be that some lives *could* be 'so demonstrably awful' that the doctor's legal duty was limited to making the child comfortable and allowing it to die. The Court does not offer any criteria of awfulness, but it may be that the law will reflect those factors involved in the analysis of the circumstances in which treatment is considered to be ethically not indicated. The significance of the decision, since the case concerned a child who was not terminally ill, is its recognition that it may not always be a doctor's duty in law to preserve life, provided certain conditions are met.

5. The doctor may not embark on any conduct with the primary intention of causing the patient's death.

This would be homicide. Put another way, euthanasia (whether or not at the request of the patient) is unlawful. The distinction between killing the patient and changing treatment so as to allow death to take place is sometimes a fine one and taxes philosophers and lawyers. Some see the distinction in terms of a commission which is unlawful and an omission which may not be. I do not adopt this distinction. Though it is part of the general law, I regard it as unhelpful here. The real argument is not how a doctor's conduct can be characterized, but whether in the circumstances he has fulfilled his duty to the patient to care for him in good faith. The principles of good faith reflect professional ethics and general social morality. Neither at present condones euthanasia, so that, to cause the patient's death, whether by omission or commission, would be a breach of the duty to care for the patient in good faith, and hence unlawful. Both, however, contemplate allowing the patient to die, if, in the circumstances, the illness is terminal and any other form of treatment, other than treatment for dying, would not be ethically indicated.

6. If a terminally ill patient expresses a desire to commit suicide, a doctor may not in law facilitate the suicide (Suicide Act, 1961). To do so would be a criminal offence, as the prosecution and conviction in November, 1981, of Nicholas Reed, the Secretary of the organization Exit, demonstrated.

For the majority of these propositions there is no authority in the sense of legislation or court decision. Though I am confident of their validity, it clearly is unsatisfactory for the law to remain a matter of conjecture. It follows that there is a need for some authoritative synthesis of the law. The form this should take is, in my view, a Code of Practice worked out by representatives of the medical profession together with lawyers, theologians, philosophers and other interested laymen. It would not be statute law in the first instance, since it takes so long to get proposed statutes passed into law. Also, there is a danger that in such a sensitive area a statute may well be a clumsy approach initially. A code could serve as a precursor. It would serve as the authoritative guideline while retaining flexibility and being easier to amend. Since, ultimately, the law has to be stated authoritatively, there is a case for passing a statute once experience of the working of the code had shown up any problems there may be. An example of the use of codes of practice is the Report (1979) of the Working Party on the transplantation of organs, produced under the aegis of the Department of Health, which itself incorporates an earlier code of practice on the diagnosis of death, contained in the Report (1976) of the Medical Royal Colleges and the Faculties in the United Kingdom.

References

Canterbury, Archbishop (1977). On dying and dying well: extracts from the Edwin Stevens Lecture. *Journal of Medical Ethics* **3**, 57.

Church Assembly Board for Social Responsibility (1965). *Decisions about Life and Death*, p. 52. CABSR, London.

Dunstan, G.R. (1981). Life, prolongation of ordinary and extraordinary means. In *Dictionary of Medical Ethics*, pp. 266–8. Ed. by A.S. Duncan, G.R. Dunstan and R.B. Welbourn. Darton, Longman & Todd, London.

Gillon, R. (1981). Editorial. *Journal of Medical Ethics* **7**, 55. *In Re B* (a minor) (1981), **1**, *W.L.R.*, 1421.

Kennedy, I. McC. (1976). The legal effects of requests by the terminally ill and aged not to receive further treatment. *Criminal Law Review*, p. 217.

Kennedy, I. McC. (1977). Doctors and the patient's right to die. *The Listener*, July 14, 42.

Pius XII, Pope (1957). *Acta Apostolicae Sedia* **49**, 1027.

R v. Bodkin Adams (1957). *Criminal Law Review*, p. 365.

Report of Working Party (1979). *The Removal of Cadaveric Organs for transplantation: A Code of Practice*. DHSS.

Report (1976). Conference of Medical Royal Colleges and their Faculties in the United Kingdom: Diagnosis of brain death. *British Medical Journal* **2**, 1187.

Suicide Act 1961, Section 2.

18

The philosophy of terminal care

Cicely Saunders

'The practice of medicine is an art, not a trade; a calling, not a business; a calling in which your heart will be exercised equally with your head.'
 (Osler, 1903)

The Shorter Oxford Dictionary includes among its definitions of philosophy: 'that department of knowledge or of study which deals with ultimate reality', and 'the study of the general principles of some particular knowledge, experience or activity'. Both definitions have been used to cover the substance of this book in the belief that, as in any field of care, we will only respond fully to the second if we give heed to the first. Here we are concerned with the nature of man, with living and dying, and with the whole man—body, mind and spirit—part of some family unit, with emotional and social as well as physical and practical needs for us to tackle with maximum competence.

The increasing knowledge of the underlying disease processes and the tested methods of relief which can and should always be given, form a large part of this book. Such knowledge has to be balanced with a detailed consideration of social and personal factors. 'Feelings are facts in this house, as one of the nuns of St Joseph's Hospice put it, and intuitive thinking has to be added to the discursive if we are to approach the full reality of another person. Much of what is written here is concerned with feelings, with emotional and family suffering. These have frequently been described as making up the complex 'total pain' (Fig. 18.1) which our patients have often endured before they come to us, though criticism has been made that this use of words carries the suggestion that such negative emotions should be avoided at all cost (Proudfoot, 1976). The automatic prescribing of antidepressant drugs or tranquillizers is to be deprecated; grief is appropriate, and the understanding of suffering and its creative handling may be as important as attempts at its alleviation. The use of

'Total Pain'

Physical

Mental

Social

Spiritual

Fig. 18.1 Total pain.

the word 'pain' was a deliberate attempt to stimulate students and others to look at the various facets of a dying person's distress, beyond the requirement for analgesics to the need for human understanding and practical social help. This does not preclude the use of such drugs but it puts them into perspective.

Some chapters may seem surprising for a medical textbook, but dying patients ask more than medical competence of their doctors. It is not only Mr A. 'Who happens to have terminal cancer' with whom we are concerned, it is also Dr B. 'Who happens to be looking after him'.

The use of words is always interesting. On more than one occasion, having given the title 'Dying, *they* live', I found the poster said, 'Dying *we* live'. And many years ago, I remember a patient reading the *Nursing Mirror* and finding my name under some such title as 'The Care of Terminal Patients'. She said, 'Doctor, I object! I'm not going to terminate, I'm going to die!' In one of those unpremeditated answers that are occasionally given to us, I found myself saying, 'But, Mrs T., it's your illness that is going to terminate, not you.' Since then I have not knowingly talked of 'terminal patients', only of 'patients with terminal illness'. Some believe that the end of the physical body with its burden of illness is the end of the person. Whether or not we believe this, we owe our patient our skill and our regard to the end.

'Wherever patients happen to be dying'

The preceding chapters have been written from individual and team experience and from widely differing backgrounds. Their suggestions can be put into effect wherever patients happen to be dying of cancer. Terminal care does not have to be carried out only in a geographically separate unit, though there are some patients and families who need the expertise and the space they should find there. Some separate hospices will be needed for patients with intractable problems and for research and teaching in terminal care, but most patients will continue to die in general hospitals, cancer or geriatric centres or in their own homes; the staff they will find there should be learning how to meet their needs.

The following list of the essential components of terminal care is the fruit of years of working in different units and of many discussions of the principles underlying standards for terminal care (Wald, 1979). Above all, it is the outcome of the good fortune which gave me the opportunity of listening to patients and their families during the 35 years since that first patient told me that he wanted 'What is in your mind and in your heart.'

Essential elements in the management of terminal malignant disease

Maximizing potential

A patient should be enabled to live until he dies, at his own maximum potential, performing to the limit of his physical activity and mental capacity, with control and independence wherever possible. He should be recognized as the unique person he is and helped to live as part of his family and in other relationships with some awareness from those around of his own hopes and expectations and of what has deepest meaning for him.

This demands full consideration both of the nature of his suffering and of the appropriateness of various possible treatments and settings in his particular circumstances. Alertness to any remission of his disease should accompany the effective control of all the manifestations of an inexorable advance; 'cure' and 'care' frequently overlap.

Even in the terminal stages of disease, it can be true that there is a 'potential for lives better than they had before cancer developed' (Fiore, 1979).

Place of choice

Patients should end their lives in the place most appropriate to them and their families, and, where possible, have choices in the matter. This does not necessarily mean total 'open awareness' on the part of the patient, but some insight into its serious nature will help towards making realistic decisions. Continuity of care can be maintained in the midst of change if there is effective communication and easy movement between different settings. For many this will be their own homes, for others the hospital and the staff who have carried out previous treatments, while some will need the smaller community of the separate hospice unit. These, increasingly used as 'tertiary referral centres', act as a *complementary* local service for particularly complex physical and social situations.

Alternatives need to be planned ahead and the patient and his family fully involved, visits arranged and flexibility maintained. A few days or even hours at home may intersperse with time in institutional settings, or the primary health care team may manage all needs alone or with the support of a team or a specialist nurse (see Chapter 13).

The patient and family as the unit of care

When a person is dying, the members of his family find themselves in a crisis situation with the joys and regrets of the past, the demands of the present and the fears of the future all brought into stark focus (Earnshaw-Smith, 1981). Help may be needed to deal with guilt, depression and family discord. Emotions are intensified and, although they may seem irrational, there is also the possibility of resolving old problems and finding reconciliations that greatly strengthen the family group.

If this time is to be fully used, there needs to be some degree of shared awareness of the true situation. Truth needs to be available (though not pressured) so that the family can travel together. Choices presuppose some degree of 'informed consent' and, in general, sharing is more creative than deception. The often-surprising potential for personal and family growth at this stage is one of the strongest objections most hospice workers feel for the legalisation of a deliberately hastened death.

Families should have every available option open to their choice and expect recognition of their cultural and individual needs. Once this has become part of the ethos of a ward, it appears to be largely self-perpetuating and emphasizes the importance of including the family in the care of any seriously ill person. Not everyone will have the time or the understanding to embark on long family discussions, but everyone can recognize the family by name, appreciate something of their distress and recognize when they should refer the family to others, such as the social worker or the chaplain. They must be accepted as an integral part of the team caring for the patient. We should aim to give the maximum of privacy to those who need it for peace and for the expressions of tenderness which are inhibited in a general ward. Separate units usually have more opportunity to give a special welcome to the solitary. Here, too, children can be welcomed, but wherever the patient may be, it is important that they are not excluded; this can leave serious problems in their bereavement.

Bereavement follow-up

Many hospitals make special arrangements for families who come to collect certificates and property, but our work should not end there. The family has to recover. A bereavement follow-up service will identify and support those in special need, working in co-operation with the family doctor and any local services which can be involved. Many doctors give such support as part of their service to the families thay have known over the years. Some of the bereaved are not so fortunate and a follow-up as described in Chapter 4 may fill this gap and ease the tragedy and long morbidity of some bereavements. Social workers and chaplains have initiated such work from general hospitals; some hospice groups work together with Cruse, while others have set up their own team to meet with those in need, with a leader to train and support the visitors themselves. There is no doubt that many families suffer from the sudden break from the people who have cared for the patient and have perhaps for a long time been a great part of their lives. In a small unit, families will be recognized as they enter the door and reception staff as well as ward nurses have a special role in this part of care for the bereaved. An informal welcome may be all that is needed, and many families will return spontaneously. Much still needs to be learned and tested in this area of terminal care.

Competent symptom control

The patient and his family will not use the time left to them to the full unless there is good control of pain and all the other symptoms that may arise. All doctors and nurses should be aware of the developments of these skills, and special units have a responsibility to initiate research and disseminate such knowledge. Terminal pain is so different in character and meaning from much of the pain met in a teaching hospital that the methods of giving relief and the standards of comfort and alertness which should be expected are sometimes difficult to establish in a general ward. Nevertheless, it is not impossible and this has been demonstrated through the initiative of both doctors and nurses. If patients are to have adequate treatment for the many symptoms that often accompany this usually generalized disease, it must be seen as relevant and possible everywhere. Once good symptom control is achieved it is then easier to become aware of the mental and social aspects of suffering. If pain and other distress are not controlled, neither the patient nor the family will be able to use the time remaining effectively.

Constantly reviewed analysis and assessment are aimed no longer at the diagnosis and treatment of the underlying diagnosis but at the details of the pathological processes of a now incurable disease. Once the 'Why' of a symptom is understood the 'How' of relieving it becomes more rational and effective and relates better to the approach and training of acute medicine.

This does not end until concern for the process of dying itself helps to ease such problems as the confusion or restlessness that may arise during the last 48 hours or so. *How* a patient finally dies remains in the memories of the families and of the other patients around who may be facing their own deaths.

An experienced clinical team

The team or unit for terminal care must carry out its practice in such a way as to earn the respect and co-operation of the doctors who refer their patients. Both there and where the patient remains under his usual clinicians, a multi-disciplinary medical approach is as important in the later stages of cancer management as in the earlier phases of the disease. Consultation will often be needed between physician, surgeon, radiotherapist, chemotherapist and some-times the psychiatrist or the clinician who runs the local pain clinic. It is no longer adequate medicine to try to cope alone with difficult decisions in terminal cancer management, even though the needs of many patients have been and still will be dealt with successfully by their own family doctors single handed.

A group of consultants in a unit or team may act merely as a resource while the patient remains in the care of his family doctor or of the clinicians who were involved with his initial treatment. A team may, however, take over his treat-ment completely, particularly if there is some special need such as intractable physical distress or complex family problems. There need be no feeling of rejec-tion if transfer to a special ward or hospice is carefully discussed and planned, but whenever the original doctor keeps in touch, his visits are likely to have a special place in maintaining a patient's morale.

Supportive team nursing

The definition by Henderson and Nite (1978) gives as the unique function of nurses:

> 'To help people, sick or well, in the performance of those activities contri-buting to health or its recovery (or to a peaceful death) that they would perform unaided if they had the necessary strength, will or knowledge. It is likewise the function of nurses to help people gain independence as rapidly as possible.'

The particular character of the nursing of dying patients illustrates this definition. It includes the time given to do things at the patient's pace, to listen to the fears that are often revealed first to the helper in an intimate situation, to offer tenderness, understanding and humour alongside practical deftness, and to greet and include the family both as cared-for and as carers.

A nursing plan or process helps to define appropriate goals and to give the patient a guiding voice and also to maintain excellence in symptom control to the end. Confident leadership by the ward sister or nursing officer in the com-munity helps to support and integrate a team approach, the best way to sustain this demanding branch of nursing and to emphasize its rewards.

An interprofessional team

This is not the field for total individual involvement, which can be most unhelpful for both patient and staff member. It takes time to build the way of working described in Chapter 11, but such interprofessional teams are to be found in other specialized units—for example, intensive care and renal dialysis. They are particularly needed by those who are grappling with emotional as well as with practical demands. Psychiatrists and social workers have frequently been involved as support. Volunteers may have an important role both within an institution and at home, but must receive sensitive selection, training and support.

Such a team, together with all its professional members, should be seen to include the ward orderlies, domestics and porters, often the people to whom hospital patients turn to most easily. Their support should not be underestimated or ignored. Students of all kinds may also assume this role, being themselves low in the pecking order, for the patient frequently feels that he himself is at the bottom. It is important that as many different members as possible meet for frequent discussion—referral notes are not enough. Though the clinician does not abrogate his clinical responsibility, each member should be ready to assume a degree of leadership concerning an individual patient or family.

A home-care programme

A home-care programme must be developed according to local circumstances and be integrated with the family practices of the area and any local beds that may be available. Patients can then be admitted at the moment of their choice and of accurately defined medical need, and they will also be able to move easily to and from the hospital or hospice wards for periods varying from days to weeks or months as short-term improvements are fully exploited in the place most suited to them. Skilled support and confidence in their potential may enable a family to keep a patient at home, often confounding all predictions. Where patients have access to adequate nursing, a 24-hour call service and other support, which may well include volunteers as well as good neighbours, home is likely to remain their choice. Even so, some people who have said they would like to die in their own homes need in-patient care, if only for the last few days. Some families find much greater relief and unity in a professional milieu in the last days, and others realize that they cannot face the thought of death at home after all. Both possibilities should be open to them.

Methodical recording and analysis

Recording such as is described on p. 13 makes possible the evaluation and monitoring of clinical experience and the establishment of soundly based practice. Research into the common clinical syndromes, into pharmacology and therapeutics and in psychosocial studies is needed to define and refine our practice and our attitudes.

Considerable progress has been made, both in direct hospice approach (Walsh, 1984) and in related fields (Wall, 1984) but the scientific foundations of this field are only now being recognized. Conferences of those who are active in the work further the exchange of views on practical problems at local, national and international levels and give encouragement to those who feel that they are battling against much inertia or opposition and who need to keep alert their spirit of enquiry. This is a challenge to those who feel that 'tender, loving care' is all that is needed. Nothing can take its place, but terminal care of the 1980s developed from and should not now be the same as that of the 1900s or even the 1960s. 'Efficient loving care' is our aim and—as this book shows—every resource of clinical and social medicine has to be exploited.

Teaching in all aspects of terminal care

Teaching in this field is much in demand by students and graduates of all the disciplines concerned as it has only a meagre place—if any—in general curricula. The subject is tackled in conferences and seminars, in workshops, lectures and ward rounds and as in-service experience, both within the units and in outside visits by members of the staff. We find that any lectures and ward rounds of this kind are likely to be overcrowded. However (in spite of encouraging comeback, often years later, from those who have attended only one session), there should be reinforcement of such teaching for medical, nursing and other students in their own hospital wards. One of many groups of medical students who visited St Christopher's Hospice at their own request wrote afterwards: 'It was a relief to be able to discuss freely a subject which is usually actively avoided in a large teaching hospital'. Though much of the future development must be more closely integrated with general teaching centres, the special units are likely to maintain their role of stimulating initial interest and organizing courses for those who will in their turn be concentrating in this field. This is no longer a discipline in which no past special experience need be required.

Imaginative use of the architecture available

Dying patients may be nursed in a separate unit or in a ward or a section of a ward in a general hospital, but most patients will and should return to their own hospitals, to a general ward. Wherever it may be, there should be space for families and opportunities for patients to move around; room for staff to work easily and to relax; and 'transition spaces' for the anxious to take time off or to brace themselves for a meeing. Emphasis should be given to the need for spaces for private talk; these must be found, whatever the area offered. Above all, a feeling of openness to the world outside and good public transport are chief among the needs of any unit for terminal and long-term care. Some of us have been fortunate enough to plan for the purpose, others have learned to adapt whatever they could find, and successful practice has often arisen from the imaginative use of structural peculiarities.

The proportion of single rooms to bays or wards dictates the way a ward team handles the patient's last hours and the needs of his family at that time. Some feel strongly that no patient should be expected to witness the death of another person dying in the same room or bay. Others, mainly those with fairly generous space and windows, find that this can usually be managed so that the reaction of most patients and their families is almost entirely positive. The peaceful death of a patient who shows no distress in breathing or in any other way, who is not left alone and, above all, one who is not hidden behind screens and curtains, frequently enables other patients to feel more confident about their own end. A distressing death would indeed have the opposite effect, but those who are expert in such care should not let this occur. Patients and families admitted within a very short time of death will usually require single rooms. Longer-stay patients play a special role in the life of a ward as part of its hospitality and support although, like the staff, they will need a holiday from it at times.

Families in the bays talk with each other and with other patients, and most hospices find it is rare for them to return for the practical business of the next day without going to see those they have known to give thanks for the friendship that has comforted them both.

A mixed group of patients

Although the homes or hospices which welcome only dying patients have given superb care for many years, and by doing so have frequently outweighed any fear locally of a 'death house', yet we do not believe that this should now be the ideal. A good community is usually a mixed one.

St Luke's Day Centre was a pioneer in the field and adds a welcome dimension to hospice work, and some of the new continuing care units are adding such centres, including a proportion of patients with non-malignant diseases of a longer-term nature. St Christopher's Hospice has welcomed 10–20 per cent of its patients from this group, and has always had a wing for a group of elderly people who live in their own bed sitting rooms. Transfers to and from the wards are fairly common and most of the newer residents are former volunteers or members of staff. It will be well if we all look more widely; the person with the prognosis of some two years often has more difficult problems to handle than the one with only some two months to live, and there are other disadvantaged groups whose need for competent and compassionate terminal care is not yet adequately met (Klagsbrun, 1981).

Hospice care should not be limited to those who are dying but may be offered to all those who need more personal and less technological care than is usually easy to give in an acute general ward. It takes place in many of the special centres mentioned, while cottage and community hospitals have long concerned themselves with such work.

Supportive administration

Efficiency is very comforting and competence in administrative detail gives security to patients, families and staff. It eases the liaison with outside contacts that is so essential for the small, specialized unit and supports those who are managing such work among other pressures.

All members of staff will at times become drained by the work of the wards and in other contacts with the families of patients. Informal safety valves should arise spontaneously according to local personalities and surroundings, but care must be taken to see that not only regular off-duty but study leaves and extra time off are arranged before a crisis is reached. Staff members must be prevented from investing all their emotional commitment in their work and be given a chance to talk with those who are are more detached from it, who can emphasize realistic goals and appropriate successes.

The search for meaning

The work will at times cause pain and bewilderment to all members of the staff. If they do not have the opportunity of sharing their strain and questions, they are likely to leave this field or find a method of hiding behind a professional mask. Those who commit themselves to remaining near the suffering of dependence and parting find they are impelled to develop a basic philosophy, part individual and part corporate. This grows out of the work undertaken together as members find that they each have to search, often painfully, for some meaning in the most adverse circumstances and gain enough freedom from their own anxieties to listen to another's questions of distress.

Most of the early homes and hospices were Christian foundations, their members believing that if they continued faithfully with the work to which they felt called, help would reach their patients from God. Some of the traditional ways of expressing this faith are being interpreted afresh today and there are also many people entering this field who have still to consider their own religious or philosophical commitment. This is not an optional extra; it has a fundamental bearing on the way the work is done, and everyone meeting these patients and their families needs to have some awareness of this dimension.

In considering these essential components of terminal care it is important to distinguish between the general principles being interpreted at St Christopher's Hospice and its own peculiar characteristics, stemming from the personalities of its staff and, above all, from its Christian foundation. The seed from which the hospice grew was a gift of £500 left by a man from the Warsaw ghetto who died of cancer in a London hospital in 1948. His promise, 'I'll be a window in your home', was fulfilled 19 years later when the first patients were admitted. That phrase and his other request, 'I want what is in your mind and in your heart', summed up the need of all patients for the skill combined with friendship that make up terminal care. The original gift of £500 had grown to £500 000 when the hospice was opened in 1967. Now, 17 years later, the need to extend its research further into the control of suffering in all its aspects and the ever-increasing demands for teaching have grown far beyond its original ideas, but they must still be balanced to the daily needs of each patient, family and staff member.

Many are convinced that the time and manner of this beginning and growth were the work of the God who said, 'My grace is sufficient for thee: for my strength is made perfect in weakness' (2 Corinthians, 12:9). Our confidence in this grace has grown as we have seen that the patients have always been the central members of the community. Every day they bring their pain and their feelings of anger, bitterness and grief into the hospice as they are admitted. Yet the overwhelming majority find the atmosphere is peaceful, welcoming and often joyful, and their pain and many of these feelings are continually being transformed. We believe this is the work of the spirit of God in all men, however they may seek for truth and interpret the meaning of their lives in response to 'the true Light, which lighteth every man that cometh into the world' (St John's Gospel, 1:9). St Christopher's Hospice, whose founding patient and present Chairman both belong to the Jewish faith, which has turned as a whole to find help in a recent Jewish contribution on the problem of suffering (Kushner, 1982), is yet fully committed to the belief that, in Jesus of Nazareth, God knew a human life and the ultimate weakness of death as we know them, and on behalf of all men, whether or not they yet believe. 'In all their affliction he was afflicted, and the angel of his presence saved them' (Isaiah, 63:9). Only a God whose love fully shares all pain from within can still our doubts and questions, not because we can understand, but because we can trust. There is a sense in which we say, 'This is His Body' of each dying person and in which the small transformations that we witness continually speak of new meaning and a Resurrection which will finally redeem and encompass all creation. This is the edge of that unsearchable abyss of deity which we meet in our daily experience, the beyond in our midst.

It seems to us that only the belief that all men belong to the family of a God who shared and still shares their suffering and death can bring an answer, not only to those whom we try to help but also to the millions of the deprived and wronged; not only to those who face their end with peace and fulfilment but also those who have never had any chance of finding either a worthwhile life *or* death. That all wrongs will be righted and all the comfortless comforted should be the perspective of the individual, personal care that is offered in a hospice.

This is also the perspective in which the St Christopher's Hospice staff say to those of different beliefs or none, together with the atheist doctor and the priest in Camus' novel, *The Plague*, 'we're working side by side for something that unites us—beyond blasphemy and prayers' (Camus, 1948).

> 'Finally, the physician should bear in mind that he himself is not exempt from the common lot, but subject to the same laws of mortality and disease as others, and he will care for the sick with more diligence and tenderness if he remembers that he himself is their fellow sufferer.'
> (Sydenham, 1666)

References

Camus, A. (1948). *The Plague*. Hamish Hamilton, London.

Earnshaw-Smith, E. (1981). Dealing with the disadvantaged: dealing with dying patients and their relatives. *British Medical Journal* **282**, 1779.

Fiore, N. (1979). Fighting cancer—one patient's perspective. *New England Journal of Medicine* **300**, 284.

Henderson, V. and Nite, G. (1978). *Principles and Practice of Nursing*. Macmillan, New York and London.

Klagsbrun, S. (1981). Hospice—a developing role. In *Hospice: the Living Idea*, pp. 5–8. Ed. by C. Saunders, D. Summers and N. Teller. Edward Arnold, London.

Kushner, H.S. (1982). *When Bad Things Happen to Good People*. Pan, London and Sydney.

Osler, W. (1903). *The Master Word in Medicine*.

Proudfoot, W. (1976). Commenting on 'Living with dying', Saunders, C.M. *Man and Medicine* **1**, 246.

Sydenham, T. (1666). *Methodus Curandi Febres*. London.

Wald, F. (1979). Report of international work groups in death, dying and bereavement: proposed standards for terminal care' *Nursing Times* **75**, 69.

Wall, P. and Melzack, R. (1984). *Textbook of Pain*. Churchill Livingstone, Edinburgh. (In press)

Walsh, T.D. (1984). Opiates and respiratory function in advanced cancer: a preliminary report. *Recent Advances in Cancer Research* **89**, 115.

Walsh, T.D. (1984). Oral morphine for chronic cancer pain. *Pain* **18**,1.

Index